IBS For Dummies®

Cheat Sheet

Finding the Right Doctor for You

If you suspect that you have IBS, you want to find a caring doctor with a history of working with IBS patients. How do you do that? When you meet a new doctor for the first time, take this list of questions along with you. And be sure to check out Chapter 6, where we offer more suggestions.

- **Do you have patients with IBS?** This may be the only question you need to ask. Keep in mind that up to 11 per cent of the population suffers from IBS. If a doctor says that she doesn't have patients with IBS, she may have selective vision.

- **What do you think causes IBS?** Lots of theories exist about what causes IBS. Ideally, you want a doctor to admit that the medical community hasn't identified a single cause, but many triggers (such as diet and stress) play a role. If she claims to know what causes IBS 100 per cent of the time, ask for clarification, and be prepared to walk away.

- **How do you diagnose IBS?** If your doctor mentions something called the Rome III criteria (which we explain in Chapter 2), that's a great sign. You also want to hear that she runs tests to rule out other bowel conditions, as well as to rule out conditions with similar symptoms.

- **What role does diet play in IBS?** Most people with IBS are very aware that what they eat can trigger symptoms. You want your doctor to know that connection exists as well and to be aware that food allergies and intolerances can masquerade as IBS.

- **How do you treat IBS?** You want to hear a doctor say that a variety of treatment options exist, and the right treatment plan is one that you and she create together. She should mention the importance of improving your diet, getting regular exercise, and reducing stress. She may also mention medications or dietary supplements. An answer focused solely on medications should raise a flag: While drugs help some people with IBS, they don't cure the condition, and they don't work for everyone.

Eliminating Common Triggers

An IBS trigger is something that sets off a chain reaction in the body leading to symptoms of diarrhoea or constipation (or both). We talk a lot about triggers in Chapters 4 and 17. Here's a short list of things you want to avoid while you're getting your IBS symptoms under control:

- Alcohol
- Antibiotics
- Aspartame
- Carbonated drinks
- Dairy
- Monosodium glutamate
- Processed foods
- Spicy foods
- Stress
- Sugar

For Dummies: Bestselling Book Series for Beginners

IBS For Dummies®

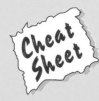

Charting Your Symptoms

In Chapter 7, we suggest various pieces of information to take to your doctor in order to have a fruitful discussion about your condition. For example, you want to know if anyone in your family has a history of bowel trouble and be able to explain when your symptoms began. You want to tell your doctor what treatment options you've tried and how successful they've been.

It's also useful to fill out a questionnaire about your symptoms, such as the one below.

Describe your symptoms. Check all that apply.

❑ Abdominal cramping

❑ Abdominal pain on the left side

❑ Diarrhoea

❑ Bloating

❑ Constipation

❑ Straining with a bowel movement

❑ Wind

❑ Other _____

How long have you had these symptoms?

❑ A few weeks

❑ About 12 weeks

❑ About 6 months

❑ Less than 1 year

❑ Less than 5 years

❑ 5 to 10 years

How often do you have these symptoms?

❑ Once per month

❑ Once per week

❑ Every day

❑ Several times per day

❑ Constantly

For Dummies: Bestselling Book Series for Beginners

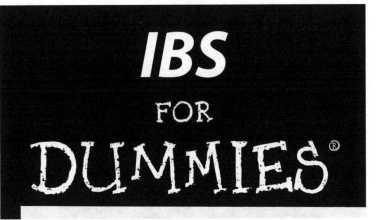

IBS
FOR
DUMMIES®

**This book is to be returned on or before
the last date stamped below.**

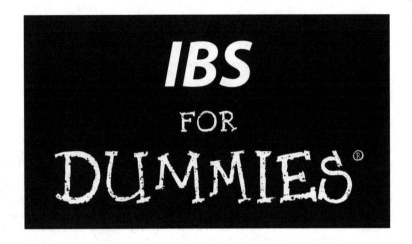

IBS FOR DUMMIES®

by Dr Patricia Macnair, Dr Carolyn Dean, and Christine Wheeler

WILEY

John Wiley & Sons, Ltd

IBS For Dummies®

Published by
John Wiley & Sons, Ltd
The Atrium
Southern Gate
Chichester
West Sussex
PO19 8SQ
England

E-mail (for orders and customer service enquires): cs-books@wiley.co.uk

Visit our Home Page on www.wiley.com

For general information on our other products and services, please contact our Customer Care Department within the U.S. at 800-762-2974, outside the U.S. at 317-572-3993, or fax 317-572-4002.

For technical support, please visit www.wiley.com/techsupport.

Wiley also publishes its books in a variety of electronic formats. Some content that appears in print may not be available in electronic books.

British Library Cataloguing in Publication Data: A catalogue record for this book is available from the British Library

ISBN: 978-0-470-51737-6

Printed and bound in Great Britain by Bell & Bain Ltd., Glasgow

10 9 8 7 6 5 4 3 2 1

WILEY

About the Authors

Dr Patricia Macnair is a physician working part-time in Medicine for the Elderly at Milford Hospital in Surrey, UK. Ever since she was a teenager reporting for her college magazine, she has had an interest in journalism and this continued with work for BBC Radio while she studied Medicine at the University of Bristol. After qualifying in 1982, Trisha worked for several years in a variety of specialities within hospital medicine, before rekindling her early interest in writing and radio.

For the past 17 years she has worked as a freelance medical journalist and broadcaster, writing, reporting and presenting on health for BBC Radio, BBCi Health (the BBC Health website), and a number of TV programmes. Trisha has written many articles for national newspapers and magazines, and in recent years has had a number of books published. These include a series of children's books on the human body, a workbook for health professionals, and a fun guide to living longer.

In 2001 Trisha completed an MA in Medical Ethics and Medical Law at King's College, University of London, and in 2005, after a long spell out of clinical work, she returned to the hospital wards. There her patients present a myriad of different medical problems during their rehabilitation after major illness.

In those rare moments between working and looking after a busy family, she relaxes by playing guitar in a rock band, and forlornly striving to improve her tennis.

Dr Carolyn Dean is a rare breed of medical doctor. She is one of a handful of doctors who has received dual degrees in medicine and naturopathic medicine and bridges the gap between the two. Dr Dean graduated from Dalhousie Medical School in Nova Scotia in 1978. She is also a graduate of the Ontario Naturopathic College and is presently on the board of the Canadian College of Naturopathic Medicine in Toronto, Canada.

Dr Dean is licensed to practice medicine in California, but her base is in New York, where she publishes, writes, consults, and travels frequently to present rousing lectures to eager listeners on health and wellness issues.

In her private practice, which she ran for 12 years in Toronto (from 1979 to 1992), Dr Dean treated thousands of patients who came to her with symptoms of IBS. Having seen similar symptoms in her own family and she, herself being sensitive to wheat and dairy, Dr Dean understands the impact of diet, exercise, and stress on the bowel.

Dr Dean has written many books, including *Natural Prescriptions for Common Ailments, Menopause Naturally, Homeopathic Remedies for Children's Common Ailments, The Miracle of Magnesium, Death by Modern Medicine,* and *Hormone Balance.* She has also co-authored *Women's Book of Natural Health* and *The Yeast Connection and Women's Health.* She is an advisor to *Natural Health* magazine and the medical advisor for www.yeastconnection.com. Dr Dean is a regular guest on TV and radio, appearing many times on *The View* as well as Fox, CBS, and NBC, and she has her own radio show.

Christine Wheeler has been a freelance researcher and writer for 15 years. For the past seven years, she has focused mainly on health and medical topics, including extensive research on the health benefits of nutritional products. She has especially enjoyed providing writing and editorial support to Dr Dean on various book projects.

In 1999, Christine discovered Emotional Freedom Techniques (EFT). After extensive training and preparation, she opened her private practice in 2002. She has worked with hundreds of people to help them alleviate stress, anxiety, emotional traumas, and the accompanying physical manifestations, including IBS symptoms.

Having had a brush with IBS herself, and using EFT to alleviate the condition, co-writing this book seemed to be a perfect fit and a unique opportunity to help others suffering with this condition.

Dedication

Carolyn would like to dedicate this book to the memory of her parents, Rena and Harold Wheeler. To Mum for her wry sense of humour and amazing spirit, and to Dad for his way with words. And to both of them for giving us early insight into the world of IBS.

Christine would like to dedicate this book to her sweetie, husband, partner, and spouse, Ken Lawson, a constant support and source of fun and inspiration while she worked on what was affectionately known as 'the poo book.'

Trisha would like to dedicate this book to her family, who burst through the closed study door at frequent intervals to offer sustenance and light relief, her son Rory for his big hugs, her daughter Lottie for her hilarious anecdotes from *The Simpsons*, her husband Duncan for much needed gin and tonics, and Esmie the cat for providing welcome excuses to get out into the fresh air and hunt for a mouse.

Authors' Acknowledgements

From Carolyn and Christine: We would like to acknowledge each other — this sisterly collaboration made for a sometimes riotous voyage through the research and writing on this serious yet scatological topic.

We thank our agent, Jacky Sach of Book Ends, for offering the opportunity to do this project and helping to get it underway. We have great appreciation for Stacy Kennedy, our acquisitions editor at Wiley, who felt we had what it took to get to the bottom of IBS. We thoroughly enjoyed working with Joan Friedman, our editor at Wiley. She took great care of our words while patiently guiding us through the Dummies process.

We would also like to thank Dr Irene Grant, our professional reader, for her input and kind words about the book. And thanks to Pam Floener for her insights on the topic of mercury poisoning and mercury detoxification.

We especially appreciate our past and current patients and clients with IBS who, in their efforts to find relief from their condition, have given us the gift of learning. We hope that this book is helpful and that we can continue the dialogue as they delve into this material.

Christine would like to thank Therese Dorer for her limitless friendship, crystal clear insights, and the great rounds of laughter. And to her in-laws, Doug and Sherry Lawson, thank you for understanding when she couldn't come out to play.

From Trisha: My greatest thanks have to go to the editorial team at Wiley – in nearly two decades of writing I have never come across such sharp eyes and focused minds, especially developer Colette Holden, copy-editor Charlie Wilson, and development editor Simon Bell. I have no doubt that without them this book would be a flabby shadow of what it is, and I would like to borrow them for every future project I work on! Many thanks too to Samantha Clapp, who first commissioned me to write this book.

I'd also like to acknowledge the efforts of the Medicine for the Elderly consultants at the Royal Surrey County Hospital in Guildford for helping me back into clinical medicine after nearly 20 years out of the world of patients and ward rounds. With their encouragement, and confidence in my abilities, I have been able to rediscover the satisfaction of working with people to manage their diseases, rather than just talking or writing about doing so. This has helped me to gain fresh insight into the art of practising medicine, which I hope is reflected within this book. Finally I would like to thank my sister, Dr Gill Jenkins, a GP in Bristol who has kept me firmly in touch with a primary care perspective on managing both my patients and IBS, and calmed my tendency as a hospital physician to get overexcited and keen to intervene.

Publisher's Acknowledgements

We're proud of this book; please send us your comments through our Dummies online registration form located at www.dummies.com/register/.

Some of the people who helped bring this book to market include the following:

Acquisitions, Editorial, and Media Development

Development Editor: Simon Bell

Content Editor: Nicole Burnett

Commissioning Editor: Samantha Clapp

Copy Editor: Charlie Wilson

Technical Editor: Irene H. Grant, MD, CAC

Publisher: Jason Dunne

Executive Project Editor: Daniel Mersey

Cartoons: Ed McLachlan

Composition Services

Project Coordinator: Erin Smith

Layout and Graphics: Stacie Brooks, Reuben W. Davis, Alissa D. Ellet, Barbara Moore, Ronald Terry, Christine Williams

Proofreaders: Laura Albert, Robert Springer

Indexer: Cheryl Duksta

Contents at a Glance

Introduction *1*

Part 1: Just the Facts about 1BS.....................................*7*
Chapter 1: What Is IBS? Classifying the Condition 9
Chapter 2: Your Gut: Working Well 21
Chapter 3: Your Sensitive Gut: Working Not So Well....................................41
Chapter 4: Considering Causes and Targeting Triggers 65
Chapter 5: Who Gets IBS and Why 93

Part 11: Getting Medical Help *105*
Chapter 6: Working With Your Doctor 107
Chapter 7: Looking into the Problem 129
Chapter 8: Treating IBS Symptoms with Drugs 145

Part 111: Healing and Dealing with 1BS......................*169*
Chapter 9: Controlling Your IBS 171
Chapter 10: Eating an IBS-Friendly Diet 183
Chapter 11: Alleviating IBS with Exercise...205
Chapter 12: Managing Emotions and Stress..217
Chapter 13: Evaluating Complementary Therapies 231

Part 1V: Living and Working with 1BS *253*
Chapter 14: Taking Responsibility: Reclaiming Your Life............................255
Chapter 15: Working with IBS 275
Chapter 16: Helping Your Child Cope with IBS..285
Chapter 17: Keeping Up-to-Date with IBS 299

Part V: The Part of Tens *311*
Chapter 18: Ten IBS Triggers to Avoid...313
Chapter 19: Ten Things to Do for Your IBS 321
Chapter 20: Ten Ways to Get Help for Your IBS 329

Part V1: Appendixes *339*
Appendix A: Soluble and Insoluble Fibre Chart...341
Appendix B: Glossary 343

Index *353*

Table of Contents

Introduction 1

About This Book..2

Conventions Used in This Book 2

What You're Not to Read 2

Foolish Assumptions 3

How This Book Is Organised..3

　　Part I: Just the Facts about IBS 3

　　Part II: Getting Medical Help 4

　　Part III: Healing and Dealing with IBS.................................4

　　Part IV: Living and Working with IBS....................................5

　　Part V: The Part of Tens...5

　　Part VI: Appendixes..5

Icons Used in This Book 5

Where to Go From Here...6

Part 1: Just the Facts about 1BS 7

Chapter 1: What Is IBS? Classifying the Condition 9

Tackling IBS head-on..9

Considering a Condition That You Can't Put Your Finger On...............10

Searching for Evidence..11

Meeting the Rome Criteria 12

Spotting Primary Symptoms...13

Recognising Other Common Symptoms 14

Looking at Less Frequent Symptoms...15

Dealing With Mild Cases..16

　　Morning movements 16

　　Three a day...17

Linking Other Problems to IBS 17

Separating IBS from IBD 18

Knowing That IBS Isn't Just Imaginary.......................................19

Chapter 2: Your Gut: Working Well 21

Getting to Know (and Love) Your Gut 22

Getting to Know the Food You Eat...23

　　Understanding why fresh food matters..............................23

　　Gathering info on what's good to eat..................................23

Thinking of Your Gut as a Food Processor 24
    Chewing and swallowing 24
    Sloshing in the stomach 26
    Slipping through the small intestine....................................28
    Transforming food into you 29
    Looking at your liver 29
    Pleasing your pancreas..30
    Heading deep into the large intestine................................30
Good Bacteria v. Bad Bacteria...32
All You Ever Wanted to Know About Gas 35
Finding Out About Faeces 35
Understanding What Controls Your Gut 37
Timing Is Everything...39
Protecting Your Gut 40

Chapter 3: Your Sensitive Gut: Working Not So Well 41

Sussing Out Your Sensitive Gut 41
    Homing in on hypersensitivity 42
    Evaluating visceral hypersensitivity.................................42
    Reviewing the roles of anxiety and other factors 43
Finding Out about Faulty Functioning.......................................44
    Gut reactions: Dealing with dodgy digestion...................45
    Getting food moving through the gut 46
    Talking about trapped wind 46
    Looking at the leaky gut 48
Understanding What Happens When Your Gut Goes Wrong.....50
    Reflux and heartburn...50
    Nausea and vomiting 50
    Belching and Flatulence...53
    Indigestion...54
    Abdominal distension and bloating 54
    Tummy ache...56
    Diarrhoea...57
    Constipation..59
    Urgency and faecal incontinence 61
    Incomplete evacuation 62
    Pain in the bum...63

Chapter 4: Considering Causes and Targeting Triggers 65

Defining Our Terms...65
Looking at What Makes the Gut Sensitive..................................66
    Investigating infection and inflammation.........................67
    Sussing out your souped-up immune system.....................69
    Meeting the new neighbours: Changes in the bacteria
        that keep you company 70
    Controlling Candida 72

Finding Out Whether Food's a Factor...72
    Getting the terms straight 72
    Watching what and how you eat 74
    Looking at lactose 74
    Surveying sorbitol 76
    Figuring out fat..76
    Wondering whether wheat can make you wobble 77
    Focusing on fantastic fibre 78
    Being coy about soy..79
    Keeping blood sugar on an even keel 79
    Seeing the sense and sensitivity of allergy testing..........80
Stamping Out Stress...82
    Letting your head rule your gut 82
    Linking your emotions and your gut...............................82
    Counting on stress 84
Weighing Up Nature and Nurture 84
Making the Chemical Connection 85
    Avoiding antibiotics 86
    Analysing other medications 86
    Focusing on food additives 87
    Moving away from mercury 87
    Sounding out smoking 88
    Finding out about fluoride toxicity 89
    Managing magnesium levels 89
Homing in on a Holistic Theory of IBS 90
Leaving No Trigger Unturned 90

Chapter 5: Who Gets IBS and Why **93**
Stating the Statistics 93
Singling Out Women...94
    Grappling with the gender gap 95
    Realising that the gender gap starts early 96
    Putting up with pain..97
    Homing in on hormones 97
    Planning for your period 99
    Avoiding misdiagnosis 99
Linking IBS and Your Upbringing 101
Taking Action 103

Part II: Getting Medical Help..*105*

Chapter 6: Working with Your Doctor **107**
Knowing When to Get Medical Help 108
    Sussing out your symptoms before you see a doctor ...108
    Sounding the alarm 109
    Reviewing red flag symptoms..110

Finding the Right Doctor for You 111
Believing in IBS 111
Building a Partnership with Your GP 112
    Getting over the embarrassment 113
    Stating your symptoms 114
    Ready, steady, flow! Noting when symptoms started 115
    Asking questions 116
    Having a physical examination 118
    Seeking specialist help 120
Preparing for Your First Appointment 123
    Filling out a questionnaire 123
    Charting your symptoms and diet 125
    Perusing previous test results and family history 126
    Packing for your appointment 127

Chapter 7: Looking into the Problem **129**

Considering Key Investigations 130
    Physical and rectal examination 130
    Faecal occult blood test 131
    Blood tests 132
    Pelvic examination 133
    Sigmoidoscopy and colonoscopy 134
    Barium enema 136
    Upper gastrointestinal series 137
    CT and MR scans 137
    Tests for lactose intolerance 138
    Tests for gluten intolerance 139
    Food allergy tests 140
    Comprehensive digestive stool analysis (CDSA) 141
Differentiating Your Diagnosis 141

Chapter 8: Treating IBS Symptoms with Drugs **145**

Trying Not to Expect Too Much from Drug Therapies 146
    Waiting for better drugs 146
    Reviewing clinical trials 147
Dealing with Diarrhoea 148
    Co-phenotrope 148
    Loperamide 149
    Colestyramine 150
    Bulk-forming agents 151
    Serotonin blockers (5-HT antagonists) 152
    Probiotics 153
    Codeine 154

Controlling Constipation 154
    Focusing on triggers first 155
    Knowing your options 156
    Bulk-forming laxatives 156
    Osmotic laxatives 158
    Saline purgatives 158
    Prokinetic agents 159
    Stimulant (irritant) laxatives.......................................160
    Lubricant and softening laxatives 160
    Laxative mixtures 161
    Suppositories and enemas 162
Dealing with Pain...163
    Treating spasms 163
    Using antidepressants 165
Working with Wind..167

Part III: Healing and Dealing with IBS 169

Chapter 9: Controlling Your IBS 171

Self-Managing Your Symptoms 171
Relying on the Doctor Within 172
    Assuming power 172
    Dealing with your IBS...173
    Developing a healthy scepticism 173
Keeping a Diary of Symptoms and Life Events....................174
    Recording each day...175
    Paying attention to your body......................................176
    Reducing the stress in your life 176
Eating for Health...177
Encouraging Good Bowel Habits..178
Taking Regular Exercise 179
Relaxing – Your Way...179
    Making time for you 180
    Sleeping for health 180
Talking to Others..181

Chapter 10: Eating an IBS-Friendly Diet 183

Keeping a Diet Diary 184
    Watching what you eat 185
Dodging disastrous diets..186

Making Smart Food Choices 187
    Combining food wisely 187
    Reducing fats 188
    Knowing what's healthy for you 189
Eliminating Possible Food Triggers 190
    Taking two weeks towards better health 190
    Doing the detox 192
    Challenging individual foods 193
Translating Your Results into Better Habits 194
    Substituting good foods 195
    Planning and shopping for health 196
    Choosing healthier ways of cooking 197
Treating Symptoms with Supplements 198
    Healing with herbs 199
    Dosing on digestive enzymes..201
    Probing probiotics..202
Seeing How Diet and Stress Interact.......................................203

Chapter 11: Alleviating IBS with Exercise 205

Defining Exercise..206
    Allowing air in...206
    Building strength 207
    Finding flexibility 207
Benefiting from Exercise 207
    Reducing health risks 209
    Maintaining your muscles 209
    Focusing on psychological fitness 210
    Relieving pain...210
Taking the First Steps 210
    Checking your attitude 211
    Getting – and staying – motivated......................................211
Exercising Choices 212
Loving Yoga...213
    Happy baby 213
    Ankles crossed, knees to chest 214
    One-legged forward bend 214
    Supine twist..215

Chapter 12: Managing Emotions and Stress 217

Keeping on Top of Life..218
    Considering catastrophising and panic.............................218
    Assuaging your anger 220
    Being assertive...220
    Dealing with despair 221

Unravelling the Meaning of IBS 222
Sounding Out Psychotherapy.................................223
    Choosing the therapy for you.........................224
    Brooding over behavioural therapy................225
    Assessing psychoanalytical psychotherapy....227
    Sussing Out psychodynamic interpersonal therapy 228
    Concentrating on counselling.........................228
    Finding a therapist 229

Chapter 13: Evaluating Complementary Therapies 231
Getting Started with Complementary Therapies.............232
Pondering the Placebo Effect 233
Helping with Homeopathy 234
    Trying homeopathy for IBS 234
    Finding a homeopathic therapist 236
Pinning Down IBS with Acupuncture.......................237
    Achieving balance 237
    Healing with heat...238
    Finding an acupuncturist 238
Ruminating on Reflexology 239
Relaxing Your Way to Health 239
Homing In on Hypnotherapy 241
    Directing the gut..241
    Hypnotising yourself......................................242
    Finding a hypnotherapist 242
Appraising Aromatherapy.....................................243
Feeling Fine with Therapeutic Massage 244
Opting for Osteopathy and Chiropractic 245
Cracking Down on Colonic Irrigation 246
Taking Control with Biofeedback...........................247
Nailing IBS with Naturopathic Medicine 248
Integrating Complementary and Conventional Medicine....249

Part IV: Living and Working with IBS..........................253

Chapter 14: Taking Responsibility: Reclaiming Your Life 255
Asserting Yourself...256
Enjoying the Life You Deserve..............................257
Dealing with Family and Friends 258
Coping with Journeys 259
Taking Steps Towards Better Health......................260
    Surveying the effects of IBS...........................260
    Focusing on the financial costs of IBS 261
    Emphasising the emotional costs of IBS 262

Tackling Social Situations..264
Experiencing faecal incontinence 264
Covering up odours 269
Connecting with Others 270
Supporting someone with IBS......................................270
Communicating with your partner..............................271
Having sex 271
Telling your friends 272
Making Web connections..272
Taking Baby Steps 273

Chapter 15: Working with IBS 275
Facing Facts about IBS on the Job 276
Producing less work..276
Passing up promotions 276
Suffering from stress 277
Making Your Work Day Bearable..277
Starting your day in the right way 277
Enjoying an accident-free commute............................278
Dealing with an attack at work 279
Talking to Your Boss and Colleagues..................................280
Deciding when to tell 280
Deciding what to say...281
Working from Home 282

Chapter 16: Helping Your Child Cope with IBS 285
Realising That a Tummy Ache Is Something More 286
Finding out what's wrong 286
Ruling out other conditions 287
Struggling with the pain...288
Overcoming the Stress of IBS 289
Maintaining Balance at Home...293
Working Through Your Child's Emotions.............................294
Being there for your child 295
Listening to your child..295
Helping your child take action.....................................296
Nailing negative emotions 296

Chapter 17: Keeping Up-to-Date with IBS .299
Raising Awareness of IBS...299
Marketing medications 300
Sharing your knowledge with a self-help group 300

Surfing the Net..303
    Impinging on your doctor's turf?................................304
    Knowing your source 305
    Seeking alternatives 305
    Reaping the benefits 305
Seeing Possibilities in Serotonin Research 306
    Finding abnormal serotonin levels in the IBS gut 306
    Realising that your gut has a nervous system...............307
    Supplementing your serotonin 308
    Expecting more research..309

Part V: The Part of Tens 311

Chapter 18: Ten IBS Triggers to Avoid 313
Apprehending Your Alcohol Intake....................................313
Avoiding Antibiotics 314
Ending Erratic Meal Times..315
Fathoming the Facts about Fibre 316
Ferreting Out Fatty Meals 317
Finding the Foods that Faze You 317
Handling Hormone Horrors...318
Losing the Late Nights..319
Stamping Out Stressful Situations....................................319
Trying Not to Do Too Much 320

Chapter 19: Ten Things to Do for Your IBS 321
Cutting Back on Medications..321
Developing Regular Habits..322
Eating a Healthy Diet 323
Exercising Every Day 323
Joining or Starting a Support Group.................................324
Listening to Your Body and Taking Charge........................324
Planning Your Next Move..325
Releasing Your Anger..326
Weeding Out Worry...326
Working with a Doctor You Can Talk To.............................328

Chapter 20: Ten Ways to Get Help for Your IBS 329
Joining an IBS Organisation 329
Looking for Local Groups..330

Making Web Connections...331
    Signing up to a Mailing List Server..332
Informing Your Family 333
Growing Your Own Support Network 334
Unearthing Exercise Resources..334
Stamping Out Stress Relief..335
Discovering Diet Data 336
Taking Note from Other Diseases..337

Part VI: Appendixes...*339*

Appendix A: Soluble and Insoluble Fibre Chart 341

Appendix B: Glossary 343

Index..*353*

Introduction

・・

*I*rritable bowel syndrome (IBS) is a functional medical problem that's something of a well-kept secret, even though perhaps 11 per cent of the population suffers from it. We use the word *functional* to describe IBS because the condition doesn't cause structural changes in the body and no laboratory tests exist that can diagnose it. We call it a well-kept secret because even though up to 6 million people in the UK may have IBS, you don't hear much about it in the media. These days, most medical conditions and diseases have networks of fundraisers and public events to help raise money for research. But not many celebrities want to be identified with a bowel disease.

Having IBS can be a very isolating experience, so we want you to know up front that you aren't alone. Most people with IBS don't talk about their problems – not even to their families or doctors.

The Internet has really opened up the dialogue on IBS. More people seek information and help on IBS Web sites than ever before. And you can even order books like this online, which may prevent some embarrassment.

Chances are you know all too well what having IBS is like. IBS is a condition of bowel disruption. Constipation, diarrhoea, or alternating constipation and diarrhoea are the hallmarks. Abdominal pain, gas, and bloating make people miserable and unable to function normally. If you're reading this book to better understand what a loved one is going through, think back to a time when you had food poisoning or stomach flu and you couldn't stop running to the toilet. Or think about the worst constipation you've ever experienced. Now, imagine those sensations going on for weeks and months, and you have some idea what having IBS is like.

Some people have a hard time accepting IBS as a valid diagnosis and seem to think it's just a state of mind. Some people dispute the degree of disability and suffering it creates. But we're here to tell you that IBS is real, and it causes real pain and misery.

Despite what you may have read or heard, stress does not cause IBS. Stress is very often a part of the problem and can certainly aggravate your symptoms, so you want to keep it to a minimum. But we don't yet know the cause of IBS – it's probably a combination of several factors and you certainly aren't in any way to blame for bringing IBS upon yourself.

No single cure, no simple drug or treatment, works for everyone. However, many helpful remedies exist, which we discuss in detail in this book. Knowledge is the first remedy, because if you can identify what triggers your IBS, you have the means to halt your symptoms. (And you may even discover that your symptoms aren't the result of IBS at all but a condition that's been hiding from you for years.)

About This Book

Our goals in writing this book are to confirm that IBS is real and to show you the many ways you can successfully deal with your symptoms. Because no wonder drug exists that cures IBS, people desperate for help try all sorts of therapies to find relief. We sort through the good, the bad, and the ugly and present you with the best of the best remedies and therapies for IBS.

Although reading this book from beginning to end would make you an IBS genius, you don't really have to do that. You can read Chapter 1 and get a great overview of the book. You can check out the Part of Tens chapters at the end of the book for some great food for thought. Or you can use the table of contents or index to locate chapters and sections that interest you most.

Conventions Used in This Book

The following conventions are used throughout the text to make things consistent and easy to understand:

- New terms appear in *italics* and are closely followed by an easy-to-understand definition.
- **Bold** is used to highlight key words in bulleted lists.
- All Web addresses appear in `monofont`.

What You're Not to Read

Although we're really fond of this book and have obsessed over every word, we recognise that you don't need to read every word in order to benefit from the book. If you're looking for just the facts you need to start managing your IBS effectively, you can skip two types of text without missing crucial information:

✔ Sidebars, which appear in shaded gray boxes, include information that may interest you but isn't critical to your understanding of IBS.

✔ Paragraphs that appear next to the icon called 'Technical Stuff' may contain a bit more detail than you want, depending on how intense you want to get in your study of IBS.

Foolish Assumptions

In writing this book, we made some basic assumptions about you. We assume that:

✔ You have IBS, think that you may have it, or have a friend or family member with IBS.

✔ You want information that can help you or a loved one manage IBS more effectively.

✔ You want to understand how your bowel works.

✔ You want to know whether your symptoms may be caused by something other than IBS.

✔ You want information on the latest treatments for IBS.

✔ You want to work with your doctor to obtain optimal care.

✔ You want to take charge of your body.

How This Book Is Organised

We have divided this book into six parts so that you can skip directly to the bits that draw your interest. Following is a brief overview of each part.

Part 1: Just the Facts about IBS

IBS is not something you'd wish on your worst enemy, but the more you know about it, the better your quality of life can be. In this part, we first explain what IBS is, what it isn't, and how it differs from bowel conditions that have similar symptoms. Next, we give you the rundown of how your gastrointestinal tract is supposed to work and what can go awry.

Identifying what triggers your IBS symptoms is crucial to improving your health, and in this part we offer a comprehensive discussion of known IBS triggers. Finally, we explain who is most at risk for having IBS and why. (Here's a hint: We're guessing that a large proportion of the people reading this page are women.)

Part II: Getting Medical Help

We all want doctors who are knowledgeable and up-to-date on the current research, have great bedside manners, and work with us to provide the best care possible. That's doubly important for someone with IBS. Because this is a functional condition, your doctor first has to understand that IBS is real and know how to diagnose it. Then your doctor needs to be willing to help you sort through various treatment options to find those that make the most sense for your situation.

In this part, we offer suggestions on when to seek medical help and how to find a doctor that's right for you. We also explain the steps you can take to work with your doctor and make his job easier. Then we discuss how doctors diagnose IBS so that you can talk knowledgeably with your doctor about the tests you may need.

Finally, we devote a chapter to current medicines for IBS that you and your doctor may consider. No wonder drug exists that alleviates IBS symptoms in everyone, so you need to think long and hard about whether medication is the right avenue for you. We provide the pros and cons so that you can make the decision more easily.

Part III: Healing and Dealing with IBS

'Healing' is a powerful word, and in this part we aim to give you power over your IBS symptoms.

We start by discussing how you can take charge and become self-reliant in managing your own condition. Next, we move to the all-important topic of diet; an IBS-friendly diet is the cornerstone of any IBS treatment plan. Exercise is also key to good health, especially if you have IBS-constipation, gas, and/or bloating.

Stress and difficult emotions are the next subject for our attention, with a raft of information on eliminating some of the most important triggers of your IBS symptoms. We cover helpful therapies such as acupuncture, biofeedback, and hypnotherapy. Lastly, we turn the spotlight on complementary therapies and look at how a long list of different treatments may have something to offer you.

Part IV: Living and Working with IBS

Having IBS can make you feel isolated, embarrassed, and afraid. The condition can greatly affect how you interact with your family, your work colleagues, your friends, and the world at large. In this part, we offer specific suggestions on how to tackle your worst fears about public embarrassment so that you don't feel trapped in the house. We also discuss how to minimise the impact of IBS on your work life.

Children with IBS require special care. The emotional trauma from having such a debilitating condition has the potential to cause lifelong strain. In this part, we offer tips for parents so that they can help a child with IBS to cope.

Finally, we show you how to keep up to date with current knowledge about IBS, and look at some of the most promising new research that may translate into improved quality of life in the near future.

Part V: The Part of Tens

This part is a standard in the For Dummies series. The chapters are short and chock-full of crucial information. We present ten common IBS triggers to avoid, ten things you can do when you're diagnosed with IBS, and ten ways to get help and more info on IBS.

Part VI: Appendixes

The first appendix is a chart that shows you common sources of two types of fibre: soluble (which you want to eat lots of) and insoluble (which you may want to limit or avoid). The second appendix is a handy glossary of IBS-related terms.

Icons Used in This Book

We use icons in the margins of this book to help you find specific types of information. Here's what each icon means:

We use this icon when we tell a story about a patient.

This string around the finger highlights information you may want to tuck into your mental filing cabinet for future reference.

The paragraphs next to this icon contain material that's a little more detailed than the rest. You don't need to read these paragraphs to effectively manage your IBS, so you can skip them if you prefer.

This icon points out practical information that you can put into use immediately.

When you see this icon, be on alert: The text next to it warns of potential problems or threats to your health.

Where to Go From Here

This book is designed to be so user-friendly that you can dive in anywhere that interests you and get valuable information. It's a reference book, so you don't have to worry about keeping up with the plot. You can even read the last chapter first if you like.

Part I
Just the Facts about IBS

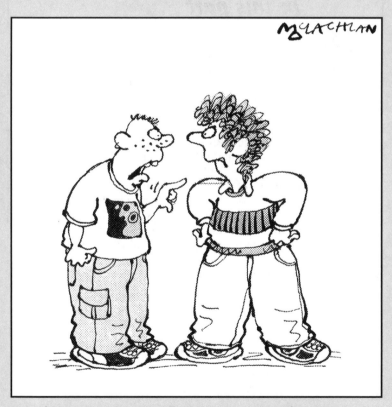

'oh yeah? — Well, I bet _my_ dad's bowel syndrome is more irritable than _your_ dad's bowel syndrome.'

In this part . . .

We wish it were easy to give you a list of facts about IBS and move on. But it's not an easy topic. IBS is a *functional* condition, which means it doesn't create structural symptoms in your body to help with diagnosis. Neither does it have a specific medical treatment. And IBS is sometimes mistaken for other conditions.

In this part, we classify IBS and distinguish it from inflammatory bowel disease and other bowel conditions. We give you a peek at your gastrointestinal system, show you how digestion is supposed to work, and tell you why it can go wrong. Triggers for IBS, which we discuss in detail in this part, are especially important to know about because you can avoid many of them and decrease your IBS symptoms. Finally, we let you in on who gets IBS and why.

Chapter 1

What Is IBS? Classifying the Condition

In This Chapter

▶ Getting some basic facts

▶ Recognising your symptoms

▶ Linking mind and body

*I*BS is a reality for many people. Up to 11 per cent of the British population have IBS symptoms, and no single definitive cure is in sight. That's quite a double whammy.

But we have some good news: We know a whole lot more about IBS today than we did even five or ten years ago. And although no miracle drug exists that can cure IBS, we do have a lot of treatment options that can provide relief if you're willing to take some time to figure out what works for you.

In this chapter, we paint a picture of IBS with a broad brush. We give an overview of what having IBS is like, look at the typical symptoms, and find out how doctors define IBS. We also talk briefly about other medical problems that frequently occur alongside IBS. We explain which diseases can sometimes be mistaken for IBS, and we strip away the confusion surrounding the role that psychology plays in the condition by asking whether IBS is 'all in the mind'. Many of the issues we touch on in this chapter we cover in depth in later chapters.

Tackling IBS head-on

Even though around 6 million people in the UK have IBS, many won't even mention it to their doctors. The reason is partly embarrassment and partly a perception that nobody can help. But a lot of confusion also exists about what is normal and when you need medical help. People with IBS often remark (at least at first) that they just assumed their gut was having an off day or two and that things would settle down. That may sound odd when you are running to the toilet dozens of times a day or rolling about in agony, but it's surprising what we tell ourselves about ways our bodies behave. Perhaps you have a desperate optimism that things will get better and you won't need to have any nasty tests or treatments, or get a diagnosis that you don't want.

If you have mentioned your symptoms to your GP, she may told you not to worry – but that's easier said than done when you have pain and your bowels are acting like they're inhabited by alien beings. Perhaps your doctor told you to increase the fibre in your diet, which made you feel even worse. Or maybe your doctor prescribed some medications that didn't work. These experiences can affect your attitude towards your condition, perhaps making you feel that you don't really have a medical condition that can be treated or that your situation is hopeless and nobody can help.

The end result of these influences – embarrassment, helplessness, and denial – is that a majority of people with IBS suffer in silence. But IBS is a real condition, with very real symptoms – as you know all too well – and many treatments and therapies can make a difference. To get on top of your condition you need to believe that it exists and know that you are able to do something about it.

As we discuss later in this book, doctors (especially GPs) are often limited in the medications that they can prescribe, and even more limited in the time they can spend with each patient. This means that your doctor may not be able to give you the best tools available to manage your condition and counsel you in depth about diet, exercise, stress reduction, and how to handle the emotional impact of IBS. Throughout this book, however, we give you those tools and offer a wealth of information about IBS that may just change your life.

Considering a Condition That You Can't Put Your Finger On

IBS is a *functional* condition. That means IBS doesn't cause structural damage to your body the way that a disease does, but it changes the way your body operates or functions. Your doctor can't see the results of IBS on a scan or order a lab test to get a quick diagnosis. To diagnose IBS, your doctor rules out a whole list of other possible bowel conditions and diseases first, such as food allergies and intolerances, or bowel cancer. All this uncertainty makes IBS seem unreal to some people, who may wonder whether the condition is 'all in your head'.

But although IBS may be invisible to others, its symptoms certainly make their presence felt. You know IBS couldn't be more real when your symptoms impinge on your daily life. Having to urgently go to the bathroom may wake you up in the morning. Or you may get up feeling fine but be gripped by painful gas and bloating as soon as you eat your first bite of breakfast. If you have constipation, you may have incredible discomfort, and even though you always feel a certain pressure that makes you think your bowels are about to move, nothing much seems to happen to alleviate your discomfort.

You can't put your finger on a lump or bump that is IBS, or show your friends and colleagues a picture of it (although they may get a feel for the condition if they look at the images at `www.aboutibs.org/site/about-ibs/art-of-ibs/gallery` that people with IBS have sent to the International Foundation for Functional Gastrointestinal Disorders to express their condition). However, you can certainly pinpoint the disruption that IBS causes to your life, and the misery of your symptoms.

Searching for Evidence

The medical world these days looks for evidence about every aspect of disease. Rather than the old-fashioned 'doctor knows best' approach to treating conditions, people want solid statistics and scientific principles – *evidence-based medicine.* What proof is there, doctors now constantly ask, that diseases first described hundreds of years ago actually exist and that treatments long recommended really work?

Asking questions, debunking myths, and setting the facts straight is healthy and often worthwhile. Take stomach ulcers, for example: For many years, doctors thought ulcers were the result of excessive acid eating away at the lining of the stomach. But in new, more powerful tests scientists discovered that a bacterial infection causes ulcers. Ulcer treatments changed overnight: Instead of giving powerful drugs to suppress the production of stomach acid, doctors swapped to offering a short course of antibiotics. In this way science can provide new evidence which makes doctors completely rethink a disease. This is beginning to happen in IBS, as researchers are demonstrating changes in the levels of serotonin (a neurotransmitter or chemical signal) in the gut (Chapter 17 has more on the latest avenues of research). These new findings may one day provide some insight into the cause.

But if, so far, doctors haven't been able to put a finger on the cause of IBS, where's the evidence that the condition is real? Unfortunately, evidence-based medicine is fairly thin on the ground in the realms of IBS. The most powerful evidence for the existence of the condition used to be the sheer numbers of people describing a similar group of symptoms – one in ten of the population have trouble with abdominal pain, bloating, changes in bowel habits, and flatulence. Laboratory tests were normal and researchers couldn't find any strange pathological specimens, but arguing that 6 million people imagine their problems is difficult.

But now 21st-century medicine is providing harder evidence that something is amiss in IBS. One group of researchers suggest that in at least some people with IBS, an inflammation exists that hasn't been detected before. Meanwhile, other researchers have evidence of excessive numbers of bacteria in the small intestine in people with IBS; these bacteria may ferment food to generate methane gas, which in turn can alter the *motility,* or movement, of the bowel. Yet more scientists report disruptions in the interaction between the gut and the brain in people with IBS.

Meeting the Rome Criteria

As we explain in Chapter 7, your doctor only *officially* diagnoses IBS after she rules out all other conditions such infections, cancer or food allergy. Therefore, most doctors depend on looking at the pattern of symptoms to define the disease.

Rome seems to have a special place in its heart for IBS. In 1988, the 13th International Congress of Gastroenterology was held in Rome. The congress developed the Rome Diagnostic Criteria for IBS, published in 1990. In 1999, the Rome Foundation revised this list of symptoms and signs that guide a doctor to the diagnosis of IBS to form the Rome II criteria, which provide a more detailed and accurate definition of IBS. Yet further revisions, based on new evidence, led to the Rome III criteria, which are even more precise about symptoms, especially of pain.

 If you think figuring out whether or not you have IBS is hard, you're in good company. It took ten multinational working teams collaborating for more than four years to arrive at a consensus for the following symptom-based diagnostic standards.

The Rome III Diagnostic Criteria presume 'the absence of a structural or biochemical explanation for the symptoms', and describe IBS as consisting of recurrent abdominal pain or discomfort on at least three days per month in the past three months associated with two or more of the following:

- ✓ Improvement with defecation
- ✓ Onset associated with a change in frequency of stool
- ✓ Onset associated with a change in form (appearance) of stool

These criteria must have been fulfilled for the past three months with symptom onset at least six months before diagnosis.

In the definition, 'discomfort' means an uncomfortable sensation not described as pain. The Rome III committee also advised that 'in order for subjects to be eligible to take part in pathophysiology research and clinical trials in IBS, they should have a pain/discomfort frequency of at least two days a week'.

Some doctors try to sub-classify IBS according to what sort of bowel habit is predominant. Researchers use a guide known as the *Bristol Stool Form Scale*. Devised by gastroenterologists in Bristol, this guide (which comes with handy pictures!) classifies stools into seven types, according to their appearance as seen in the watery depths of the toilet. Type 1 consists of separate hard lumps ('like nuts', the guide says) – this sort of stool has spent a long time in the colon and is hard to pass. At the other end of the scale, type 6 stools are 'fluffy pieces with ragged edges, a mushy stool' and type 7 stool is 'watery, with no solid pieces'.

About a third of people with IBS have mostly diarrhoea (type 5, 6, or 7 stools). They have *diarrhoea-predominant IBS,* (sometimes called IBS-D). Another third have *constipation-predominant IBS,* (IBS-C) (type 1 or 2 stools). The remainder have a *mixed bowel habit,* with both loose and hard stools (IBS-M). Some people, called *alternators,* can't seem to make their minds up and switch subtype frequently.

Most of the published data on the incidence, prevalence, and natural history of IBS do not distinguish between different subtypes of IBS. This may be especially important when it comes to trials of different drugs, because some drugs work better for diarrhoea-predominant IBS and others for constipation-predominant IBS.

Spotting Primary Symptoms

IBS has a way of interfering with your quality of life – your home life, work, sleep, social life, travel, diet, and sex. IBS also creates a financial burden, costing you directly for medical expenses and indirectly for time off work or school and lost productivity. The costs of decreased quality of life are immeasurable. We discuss these various issues in detail in Part IV of this book.

In the following sections, we describe the various symptoms of IBS and talk about the spectrum of severity that people with IBS can experience. IBS has several major symptoms, and not everyone with IBS has all these symptoms. Some people have a predominant symptom, such as diarrhoea, constipation, or pain 30 minutes to two hours after eating.

The symptoms of IBS that most people experience are:

- **Abdominal cramps:** These cramps can be achy or colicky and tend to occur in the lower abdomen. They are sometimes relieved by a bowel movement or passing gas. If they start up in a public place, you probably automatically try to put a clamp on them for fear of passing gas or having a messy accident. That reaction only adds to the pain.

  Many women with IBS, both with constipation-predominant IBS and diarrhoea-predominant IBS, report abdominal cramping and pain which they say is comparable to child birth. Although seemingly unbearable pain is rare, it's very frightening and can result in trips to the accident and emergency department at the hospital.

- **Bloating:** Seventy-five per cent of people with IBS regularly undo their belt to accommodate bloat. Bloating comes and goes so fast that you may know you can't wear anything tight around your waist – low-rider jeans were just made for people with IBS.

- **Constipation:** Chronic constipation is often characterised by straining and pain and a feeling of not fully evacuating the bowel. Although you may have a bowel movement only three or fewer times per week, we know you probably spend much of your time contemplating the relief it brings. When the evasive bowel movement comes, the stool is often hard and lumpy, and your relief is rarely absolute.

- **Diarrhoea:** Diarrhoea may be the most distressing symptom of IBS. Running to the bathroom, especially at work or in public, can be embarrassing. The anxiety of worrying about finding a toilet and getting there in time only adds to the problem. Everyone has the odd anxious moment when the trigger from the brain makes the bowels churn. For people with IBS, that moment may occur many times a day.

- **Alternating constipation and diarrhoea:** Having alternating diarrhoea and constipation may not seem so bad in theory. But when your days of running to the bathroom constantly are replaced by broken promises of a bowel movement, you end up with another kind of misery. Whereas a bowel movement can relieve the pain and cramping of gas build-up, constipation makes you feel like an uncomfortable beached whale.

Recognising Other Common Symptoms

As well as the main symptoms of IBS, some people with IBS also experience the following:

- **Diarrhoea after eating or after waking in the morning:** IBS is particularly harsh when the mere act of eating causes your symptoms. For many people with IBS, the stomach, intestinal juices, sphincters, and muscles go into overdrive when you chew and swallow. For other people, the very act of opening your eyes first thing in the morning stimulates your metabolism and triggers the urge to go. Standing up adds to the process as gravity drops your intestinal contents to their inevitable end.

✔ **Excessive gas:** Having gas and burping or passing gas is not life-threatening. Most gas is odourless, consisting of oxygen (from swallowing air), nitrogen, hydrogen, and sometimes methane (which is what students light at parties). The noxious odour we associate with flatulence is produced by sulphur-based compounds, such as hydrogen sulphide and methyl mercaptan.

✔ **Incomplete bowel movements:** When you have an incomplete bowel movement, you have the sensation that there's more to come. When you experience that sensation, you may or may not actually have more stool to pass. The feeling is strange and makes you *too* aware of your bowels. It's difficult to know what causes the sensation, but it may be due to mucus in the intestines.

A severe form of the sensation of an incomplete bowel movement is called *tenesmus,* where the constant feeling of the need to go is painful and involves cramping and involuntary straining efforts. Tenesmus is not associated with IBS but is a symptom of inflammatory bowel disease.

Another cause of incomplete evacuation is a *faecolith,* a hard intestinal mass formed from faeces. If a faecolith partially blocks the rectum, it can cause symptoms of alternating constipation, diarrhoea, pain, and an obvious feeling of incomplete evacuation.

✔ **Mucus in the stool:** Don't be alarmed if you see mucus in the toilet. Mucus that coats the stool comes from an irritated intestinal lining from all the cramping, gas, and bloating. The mucus is actually trying to coat the intestines and protect them from the irritation.

✔ **Nausea:** Feeling queasy is pretty easy when your stomach and intestines are bloated and pressing up into your diaphragm. The gut–brain axis (which we describe in Chapter 2) is highly tuned – nerves that detect distension of the intestines send signals into areas of the brain, including those that specialise in nausea, so fullness in your digestive system can make you want to gag.

Looking at Less Frequent Symptoms

In this section we mention some other IBS symptoms, some of which occur in the colon and others in the stomach and oesophagus. These symptoms are rarer than the others we discuss in this chapter.

The following symptoms may occur in the large intestine:

- ✔ Pain under the left ribs that is not relieved by a bowel movement
- ✔ Bloating that subsides at night but comes back the next day
- ✔ Stabbing pains in the rectum, called *proctalgia fugax*

The following symptoms may occur in the stomach:

- ✔ Stomach pain that can be confused with ulcers
- ✔ Inability to eat a large meal due to pressure from bloating

The following symptoms occur in the oesophagus:

- ✔ A sensation like having a golf ball in your throat, which does not interfere with swallowing (called *globus hystericus*)
- ✔ Heartburn, which is burning pain often felt behind the breastbone
- ✔ Painful swallowing, which is called *odynophagia*

IBS does not cause food to become lodged in the oesophagus. This problem is called *dysphagia*. If you experience dysphagia, get checked out by your doctor because it can be a symptom of narrowing of the oesophagus due to cancer, or due to scarring from the inflammatory bowel disease, Crohn's disease.

Dealing With Mild Cases

IBS symptoms come in various shades of mild, moderate, and severe. Some fortunate people with IBS have only mild symptoms and just an occasional flare-up when the triggers turn into explosions (see Chapter 4 to find out what your triggers may be). The majority of people with IBS are lucky enough to be in this group, and if you are, you may never see a doctor about your symptoms. Perhaps you picked up this book just to see whether having three bowel movements a day was abnormal. Rather than make you read the whole book to find out, we can tell you right now – you're probably just fine.

Morning movements

Many people have two or three bowel movements in the morning, which is perfectly normal. The excitement of getting up, the pressures of gravity, having breakfast, and maybe drinking one too many cups of coffee may be enough to give you an extra bowel movement or two.

But, as we mention in the previous section 'Recognising Other Common Symptoms', the rise and shine time can trigger IBS in some people. The stress of getting ready for your work day can increase your urgency to visit the bathroom. And a few extra trips to the bathroom in the morning can make you run late and further increase your stress, thus increasing your symptoms.

 If we've just described your morning, here's a simple solution: Set the alarm 30 minutes earlier, and allow your bowels to get moving. You have a more relaxed preparation time and perhaps reduce bowel stress. If you have more time before running out the door, you may spend less time running to the bathroom.

Three a day

Having three bowel movements a day, especially if they come shortly after meals, is not a symptom of IBS. In fact, it's just what the doctor ordered. Some doctors believe that a single bowel movement a day is normal, but others – especially those who practise medicine that deals with dietary supplements and natural remedies – think otherwise.

Think of your body this way: When something goes in, something else must come out to make room for it. So when you push a meal down at one end of the gut, it makes perfect sense that your body goes into action to move things out at the other end. Perhaps you're wondering why we don't just absorb more of our food to avoid the need to excrete the waste. But, as we discuss in Chapter 2, the waste we produce isn't just left-over food particles. Instead, as nutrients are removed from the gut contents, so their place is taken by millions of friendly bacteria which live in the intestines. Along with dead cells which are constantly shed from the lining of the gut, these bacteria account for a large proportion of the stool that you pass.

 Even though having more than three bowel movements a day is one criterion for IBS, it's only *part* of the whole picture. If you don't have pain and bloating as well, you probably don't have IBS – your symptoms may be due entirely to what you eat.

Linking Other Problems to IBS

A whole host of problems may relate to your IBS. In other words, if you have IBS, you have a greater chance of having these other conditions. We talk more about these problems in Chapter 5, but here is a list of possibilities:

✔ Back and groin pain

✔ Depression

✔ Fatigue

✔ Frequent urination

✔ Insomnia

✔ Painful periods

✔ Pain during intercourse

If you're experiencing one or more of these problems, your doctor may treat each as if it does not relate to IBS. We encourage you to ask your doctor about the possible connection so that you won't be treated for symptoms instead of addressing IBS.

Separating IBS from IBD

As we explain in Chapter 7, IBS is a diagnosis of exclusion. That means your doctor has to rule out the really bad guys before settling on a diagnosis of IBS. Some of the worst bad guys in this story are Crohn's disease and ulcerative colitis. Together, these are called *inflammatory bowel disease* (IBD) and they affect about 1 in 1,000 people. IBD causes damage to the gastrointestinal tract that shows up on an X-ray, through a endoscope (a flexible tube that doctors pass into the bowel to examine it internally) or even on blood tests.

The symptoms of IBS can mirror a mild case of an IBD. For that reason, diagnosing abdominal pain and diarrhoea based on symptoms alone can be difficult. However, moderate to severe IBD has many associated symptoms such as fever and a bloody discharge or actual bleeding from the bowels, which quickly set it apart from IBS (where fever and bleeding don't occur).

In general, Crohn's disease and ulcerative colitis affect two different areas of the bowel. Crohn's mostly attacks the small intestine (although it can cause problems at any point from mouth to anus) while ulcerative colitis attacks the large intestine.

Bleeding from the bowel always need proper investigation, so make an urgent appointment to see your GP if you notice small amounts of bright red blood on the toilet paper after opening your bowels. But if you are losing anything greater than a smear of blood, put down this book and call your doctor immediately, or go to your nearest Hospital Emergency Department. You don't have IBS but may have a more dangerous condition such as a cancer or stomach ulcer, and you could lose a lot of blood.

Knowing That IBS Isn't Just Imaginary

It's hard to think of any condition known to medicine where mind and body remain coldly and cleanly separated and where the illness can be said to be either all in the body or all in the mind. Mind-related conditions such as anxiety and depression cause real physical signs such as a fast pulse, sluggish bowels, or weigh loss, and body-related conditions such as an arthritic joint or an in-growing toenail can cause mind symptoms, including low mood, irritability, and tiredness. The mind and body are inextricably linked and the more we find out about ourselves the more intricate these links appear to be.

The latest research on IBS focuses heavily on the relationship between the brain and the gut, known as the *brain–gut axis,* and the influence the brain has on the function of the intestines via the special nervous system of the intestine (we explain this in Chapter 2). IBS is no more 'all in the mind' than it's 'all in the gut'.

We suspect that people who worry that they are somehow imagining their IBS – perhaps thinking that they may be fussing unnecessarily over something that is really quite normal – aren't looking for an analysis of the anatomy of the nervous system. Instead, they need warm reassurance that their condition is both real and can be treated, that their symptoms are valid and not trivial, and that their despair is not a madness. They are asking for help – not dismissal. Most doctors are aware that their patients fear being branded time-wasters, whingers, or lunatics, and try hard to show their concern and belief in the problem. If your GP seems to think that your IBS is all in your mind, then maybe it's time to find a new one. This book is full of information and therapeutic ideas that should convince even the most hardened sceptic to take IBS seriously.

Science is helping to dismiss the 'all in the mind' myth as it churns out research that is slowly pin-pointing abnormalities in the gut. Meanwhile, several important international research groups are working hard to tell anyone who'll listen that IBS is not a psychological or psychiatric disorder. Even though test results may be normal, stress is an important factor, and no obvious damage to the tissues can be found, IBS is a very real bodily affliction.

Chapter 2

Your Gut: Working Well

In This Chapter

▶ Looking at the different parts of your gastrointestinal tract

▶ Discovering how your digestive system works

▶ Finding out what friendly bacteria do for you

*Y*our gut, or *gastrointestinal track* (GIT), can act just like a *git* sometimes – annoying, troublesome, unpleasant, and thoughtless. But problems with your gut usually happen when you eat or drink something that upsets it.

Your gut is an independent system that consists of a long tube that passes through your body from mouth to anus. Some researchers say that the gut is a *complete* system within the body. However, your gut needs help from two major organs – your pancreas and your liver – so many doctors consider these organs to be part of your gut. The main function of your gut is to process foods and liquids. Everything we eat or drink goes through that long hollow tube and is worked upon by dozens of different chemicals.

Don't take your digestive system for granted. Your gut is constantly working, digesting, and processing your food without you having to think about anything. However, considering what your gut does for you is a good idea, especially if you have a gastrointestinal disorder such as IBS.

When you eat or drink something that your gut doesn't like or can't process, your whole body can suffer. To understand how true that statement is, have a look at Chapter 3, where we list many symptoms that are attributable to IBS.

Unfortunately, your mouth does not have a guard making you stay away from things that are bad for you. Instead, you have to be the guard for your gut, because you want to avoid your gut reacting harshly to the things you eat.

In this chapter, we take you on a journey through your gut. Reading this chapter gives you an idea of what goes on in a healthy gut. Then, in Chapter 3, we explain what happens if your gut has gone awry.

Getting to Know (and Love) Your Gut

We go into much more detail later in this chapter, but for now here are some basic facts about the structure of your gut. Your gut is an enclosed system that travels from mouth to anus with about 6 metres of small intestine and 1.8 metres of large intestine in between. The main part of your large intestine is called the *colon,* which you can see in Figure 2-1.

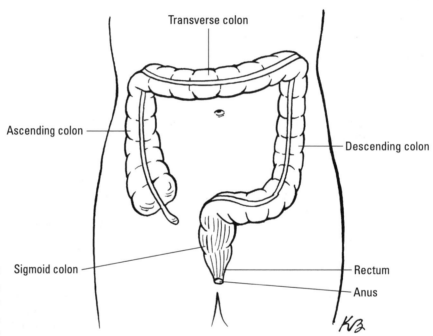

Transverse colon

Ascending colon

Descending colon

Sigmoid colon

Rectum

Anus

Figure 2-1:
A healthy colon.

If you've ever eaten a lot of corn on the cob, you may have witnessed how things can go in one end and come out the other undisturbed. The point of your gut, however, is to transform those corn niblets into something that helps build or repair your body – which is what digestion is all about.

Don't be confused if, during a meal, you have to run to the bathroom. You aren't eliminating your present meal but the one you ate a few hours earlier. We give you some clues on how to determine the transit time of food entering and leaving your body in the section 'Timing is Everything', later in this chapter.

Getting to Know the Food You Eat

You can make a big difference to your IBS symptoms by changing your lifestyle, and one of the most obvious areas you can change is the food you eat, and how you cook it.

Modern society places a premium on speed and convenience in food preparation, but it doesn't have to be a chore to choose and prepare food which is good for you.

Understanding why fresh food matters

Let's talk for a minute about how food gets to your table. Our days of hunting and gathering – of living off the land and enjoying its bounty – are far behind us. Our new hunting and gathering skills consist of finding the time to walk or drive to the nearest supermarket and stock up for a few days or a week with fresh, frozen, canned, and packaged food items.

Many of these food items come from thousands of miles away. Fruits are mostly picked before they ripen, and they go through the important ripening process deep inside storage vans. Many other foods are processed beyond recognition and mixed with dozens of ingredients.

Because we are so removed from our food supply, you may not realise that the processing, the chemical additives, and the multiple combinations of ingredients in a food product may not be good for your body and can easily throw your digestion out of whack. Your gut may not look kindly upon chemical additives, powerful spices, or ingredients it has never come across before. Instead, your gut wants mainly fresh foods from natural sources, especially if you have IBS.

Your digestive system has a lot of work deciding what is natural, safe, and digestible versus what is foreign, unsafe, and indigestible. Sometimes your gut rebels and rejects foods that are too complex or too spicy or contain too many chemicals: This is part of your gut's way of protecting your body. Your gut appears to have a wisdom of its own and may reject a food or drink today that was acceptable yesterday.

Gathering info on what's good to eat

Knowing what you are eating and knowing what to eat may be the most important way to protect your digestive system. For example, you may find it useful to know whether a food contains MSG or aspartame, two of hundreds of chemicals that can irritate your intestines. Be your own scientist: Reading the label is your first clue to what's in a food. Most labels are complete, but some problem chemicals may not be immediately apparent – MSG, for example, may be covered by the term 'hydrolysed protein' on the label. We talk about MSG, aspartame, and other additives in Chapter 4.

Buying basic food ingredients and making meals from scratch may not be what you had in mind when you picked up this book, but these activities may help heal your bowels. We talk more about diet in Chapter 10, with a focus on finding safe foods that probably won't bother you.

In the next section, we discuss the impact of your senses on the digestive process. Perhaps the most important sense for proper digestion is common sense. Everyone agrees that IBS can be triggered by what you eat and how you eat, so getting a handle on what goes in your mouth is very important. See Chapters 4 and 10 for much more information about how food can affect your IBS.

Thinking of Your Gut as a Food Processor

Have you ever looked at some food and noticed that your mouth started watering? Have you ever been overcome with the memory of a delicious meal and felt saliva burst into your mouth?

Smell is often the first sense that triggers the digestive process. The aroma of a home-cooked meal filling the kitchen can certainly get the digestive juices flowing. (People who don't have a sense of smell don't enjoy their food nearly as much as those who do.)

Digestive juices consist of digestive enzymes in your saliva and in your stomach that start pouring out to help break down a meal. If the smell or sight of delicious food triggers these juices and you don't start eating soon, you begin to drool.

But if you're like us, you probably don't wait too long before diving into that delicious food. In the following sections we explain the whole chain of events that begins when you start eating.

Chewing and swallowing

Your teeth are designed for ripping, grinding, and chewing. Your gnashers chop up food into smaller pieces that are more manageable in the mouth. While your teeth are doing their work, your salivary glands pump out saliva, which is loaded with chemicals called enzymes that work to break down or digest your food.

Triggering the production of saliva is the start of the digestive process, and any of your senses may be involved in that work. Right now, if you think about the taste of fresh raspberries bursting into your mouth, you may start salivating on the spot.

We produce about a litre of saliva every day and barely even notice. Only when you get a sore throat do you become aware of how many times a day you swallow.

Saliva is sticky with mucus. Mucus is important because it helps coat your food so that digestive enzymes don't simply wash away down your throat but remain glued onto the food particles where they can do their work. The enzymes are mainly *amylase* enzymes, which digest carbohydrates, especially grains.

Kick-starting good digestion

Why are we talking about something as mundane as chewing? What does chewing have to do with IBS? Well, here's some food for thought: If you chew your food properly, which means at least 30 times per bite, you can accomplish almost one-third of your digestion in your mouth. This means that great lumps of completely undigested food don't pass down into the stomach, and makes it easier for the digestive process to run efficiently further down the gut

Your teeth are so important in eating that dental problems, badly fitting dentures, and problems with the joint where the lower jaw attaches to the skull either side of your face (known as temporomandibular joint (TMJ) dysfunction) can adversely affect your whole digestive system because of increased pressure and inflammation in your jaw. If you have trouble chewing because of one of these problems, you may gravitate towards a less healthy soft and sweet diet instead of a healthier diet consisting of hard vegetables and tough whole grains.

Make sure your mouth is in tip-top condition by brushing your teeth in the morning, at night and after meals. Flossing is important too, as are regular checkups at your dental surgery. Don't leave dental problems lurking: Take action as soon as possible to keep the top end of your gut working well.

Sidestepping proper chewing

Okay, we agree: Almost nobody chews food 50 times per bite – some people don't even chew their food 10 times. The downside to not chewing properly is that your stomach has to work overtime to break down food that falls into your stomach in lumps. Each step of the digestive process makes the food ready for the next. If the stomach doesn't do its job properly, valuable nutrients locked inside the food lumps may not be absorbed into your bloodstream.

To make matters worse, food that is not digested properly by the time it hits your large intestine becomes a feast for bacteria, resulting in gas and bloating. We talk about the billions of bacteria that live in your gut later in this chapter and in Chapter 4.

Flushing down food with water or any other drink dilutes the enzymes in your mouth and the digestive juices in your stomach. Too much fluid can also push food out of your stomach before it has a chance to be broken down fully. Drink plenty of water between meals, but take small sips instead when you eat.

If food feels stuck when you swallow during a meal, get up and move around before trying to flush it down with a beverage. Try standing on the balls of your feet and gently bouncing a few times: You may feel the food move along. However, if you repeatedly feel food getting stuck during swallowing, make an appointment to see your doctor.

Poor eating habits and lack of nutrients can cause a deficiency in stomach acid and in the enzymes required for digestion. You are what you eat, and if you eat junk, you are going to look and feel like junk.

Sloshing in the stomach

Your *oesophagus* is a hollow tube through which food moves from the space at the back of your mouth (the pharynx) to the stomach (see Figure 3–2). But that statement doesn't capture the whole picture: Your oesophagus is more than just a hollow tube, because you can still swallow food when you are upside down. How? A team of muscles in your oesophagus propels the food down your throat, through the chest area, and into your stomach for the next part of the digestive journey. Once in the stomach, food is trapped behind a special valve called the *oesophageal sphincter,* which stops it from travelling back up towards the mouth.

Food in your stomach is broken down by gastric acid, which is released by special glands in the stomach when they know that they have a job to do. The same sensors that perceive food and pump acid also close the oesophageal sphincter and open the *ileocecal sphincter* (the opening between the small intestine and the large intestine). Making room for the food coming in by opening the door to move the waste out is good sense. We discuss the ileocecal sphincter in the section 'Heading deep into the large intestine', later in this chapter.

Gastric juice breaks down protein very effectively because it contains hydrochloric acid. Certain stomach cells produce this acid, which is so concentrated that a drop of it eats through a piece of wood. Fortunately, other stomach cells produce a thick layer of mucous gel, which coats your stomach lining and protects it from harm, and your very own supply of bicarbonate of soda, which neutralises the acid.

Powerful muscles in the wall of your stomach contract rhythmically to knead and churn the food inside. This activity helps to mix the food with the acid and physically break the solid food down to particles less than 1 millimetre in diameter.

How big is your stomach? Here's an easy way to estimate: Hold out both hands, fingers together and little fingers touching, and make a basket of them – that's about the size of your stomach. This measurement gives you an idea of the maximum amount of food you can eat at any one time and still feel comfortable. Too much food in your stomach doesn't leave enough room for the mixing and churning that has to occur for stomach acids to do their work.

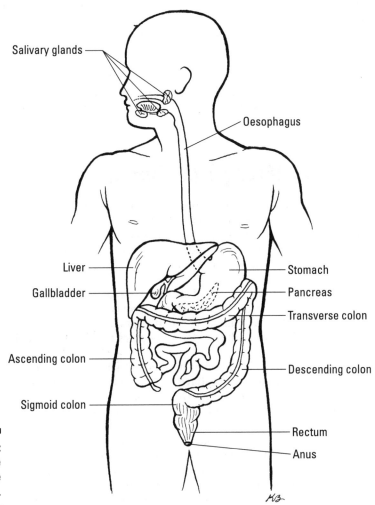

Figure 3–2:
The digestive system.

Different foods digest at different rates:

- ✔ Liquids pass through your stomach within minutes.
- ✔ Fruit takes about half an hour.
- ✔ Vegetables take about 45 minutes.
- ✔ Whole grains take two hours.
- ✔ Protein takes three to four hours.
- ✔ Fats take the longest time – at least six hours.

Tea and coffee speed up the whole digestive process and can push foods out of your stomach before they are completely broken down. They can also irritate the stomach lining. Having a relaxing cup of tea or coffee after a big meal can relax your digestive system so much that you don't actually digest your meal.

When the stomach phase of your digestive process goes amok, a whole host of symptoms can make your life miserable. Many of these symptoms are associated with IBS, such as acid reflux and heartburn. In Chapter 3 we talk more about these problems.

Slipping through the small intestine

When your stomach has finished its work, a mass of acidic sludge (which was your last meal) is squirted out into your small intestine. This thick creamy fluid is called *chyme,* and its arrival immediately triggers special mucous cells in the lining of the small intestine to spray copious amounts of mucus onto the walls to protect them from the acid.

Another mixture, this time full of alkaline bicarbonate and containing a different batch of digestive enzymes that digest all types of food, moves in from the pancreas. Bile that is made in the liver and stored in the gall bladder is squeezed out from the gall bladder and enters the mixture to help digest fats.

We haven't yet talked about what happens to sugar. Sugar molecules, such as lactose, sucrose, and maltose, have to be broken down just like any other food. Specific enzymes that come from cells in the intestinal wall break down sugars, which end up as simple sugars: glucose, fructose, and galactose.

All the different parts of your gut work like an orchestra to put together the complex piece of music that is digestion, with contributions at different times and from different parts. A combination of nerve signals and hormonal messages act as the conductors to tell each section of your gut what to do and at what pace to work. For example, as your stomach empties, your small intestine sends signals that slow down your stomach and give your intestines time to neutralise their acidic contents and absorb incoming nutrients.

Transforming food into you

Next, food is transformed into you. All the mixing and churning in your small intestine finally breaks food down into molecules that are building blocks or energy for tissues throughout your body. Your bloodstream or lymphatic circulation can now absorb these molecules through the wall of your small intestine and disseminate them throughout your body. Vitamins and minerals are also worked on and absorbed, mostly in your small intestine.

You are probably familiar with your lymphatic tissues, but you likely know them as 'swollen glands' – those painful lumps and bumps that swell up under your chin when you have a sore throat. These clumps of tissue exist all over your body and are connected by tiny passages much like blood vessels. But your lymphatic circulation doesn't have a heart pumping it and depends entirely on body movement to do its job right. This is one reason why exercise, such as a gentle stroll after a meal, can help digestion – the movement of the body helps increase lymphatic circulation, so helping to carry nutrients away from the gut to the rest of the body.

Your body tissues and organs are in a constant cycle of growth and repair. For example, your body replaces your stomach lining every two to three weeks by breaking down old cells and replacing them with new ones. In the time it takes for you to read this sentence, 50,000 cells have died and been replaced. So if you can remove the causes of an intestinal condition and give your body the right building blocks, you can have a whole new colon in a matter of a couple of weeks!

Looking at your liver

Although not directly inside the gut, your liver has many vital functions that impact the workings of your gut. The liver is a miracle organ that carries out more than 500 different chemical processes necessary for your body to function normally. Your liver is like a huge factory inside your abdomen that makes, processes, and disposes of all sorts of different molecules. One of your liver's most important digestive functions is to produce bile from cholesterol – bile is necessary for breaking down fatty foods.

Your liver is a necessary stop on the journey food takes through your body. It processes protein, carbohydrates, and fats and then sends them to various body tissues to take part in energy production, growth, and repair. Some of these nutrients may be stored for future use. A large part of your liver's function is to neutralise toxins and dispose of them through the kidneys in the urine; the intestines by way of the stool; or the skin through sweat.

The key to a healthy liver is moderation. You can overwork your liver if you ask it to process too much alcohol, too many drugs (legal or otherwise), or too much food. If your liver does not immediately deactivate drugs and toxins in your body, they can end up circulating in your bloodstream and may damage your organs before they are eliminated from your body.

Pleasing your pancreas

Your pancreas is responsible for two main functions concerned with digestion:

- ✔ Producing bicarbonate to neutralise the partially digested acidic food mixture that is dumped into the small intestine from your stomach
- ✔ Producing and releasing enzymes that break down protein, fats, and carbohydrates

If your pancreas does not produce enough bicarbonate to neutralise stomach acid, you can develop ulcers where the stomach meets the small intestine. Lack of sufficient pancreatic enzymes results in severe malnutrition even if you eat well.

Beyond digestion, the pancreas has a whole other life dealing with the end products of digestion and the transformation of sugar in the blood (called glucose) into energy. The pancreas produces *insulin,* a hormone with the unique ability to open up doorways in cell membranes and allow glucose to enter. Glucose then acts as the fuel for metabolic systems that create energy for running all the activities in the whole body.

Heading deep into the large intestine

Your large intestine – a deep, dark continent in your gut – is mainly a waste-recycling depot. If your small intestine does its job properly, it removes most of the nutrients and about 90 per cent of the water from the food you eat, and the remaining fibre and other non-digestible waste passes through the ileocecal sphincter (the point at which small and large intestine meet) into the large intestine.

Your large intestine has three main functions:

- ✔ Reabsorbing remaining water and salts.
- ✔ Breaking down indigestible particles through microbial fermentation.
- ✔ Forming, storing, and ejecting faeces.

We discuss each of these in the following sections.

Recycling and reabsorbing water and salts

The litres of saliva, gastric juices, and pancreatic liquids that travel to the large intestine would make every bowel movement very loose and also cause dehydration if your large intestine didn't vacuum up those liquids and recycle them. Salts such as sodium and chloride are also reabsorbed in the large bowel.

Microbial fermentation

Many indigestible molecules reach your large intestine. One of the main examples is cellulose, a giant sugary molecule that is the main component of the cell walls of plants. The more fruit and veg you eat, the more cellulose arrives in your gut. Because your body can't break down cellulose, you rely on a bit of help from some friendly bacteria that live in your large intestine. These bacteria (which are discussed in the following section, 'Good Bacteria v. Bad Bacteria') produce enzymes that can break down cellulose and other indigestible elements.

Forming and transporting faeces

When the large intestine works well, it creates faeces or stool (or poo, to use its more common name) by pulling out as much water as possible but still leaving the stool soft and well-formed so that you can pass it easily. Although juicer manufacturers won't appreciate the comparison, think of the waste that you create when you put fruits and vegetables through a juicer. The juicer pulverises the fruit, we drink the juice (which contains the nutrients) for energy, and we dump the waste.

Just like the oesophageal sphincter, the ileocecal sphincter is a one-way trip into the large intestine with no way back. And that's a good thing, because it would be a disaster if sugar-loving bacteria and yeasts got into the small intestine, where they could feast on sugar, and cause gas, bloating, and diarrhoea.

The cells that make up the lining of the large intestine secrete large amounts of mucus to protect the lining from being irritated by faecal waste, which usually contains a large amount of potentially irritating undigested fibre and bile salts. In healthy people, the bulk of stool is composed of *friendly* bacteria, which has many functions, including the breakdown of hormones and indigestible molecules.

After generating stool, the large intestine gently moves the stool up the right side of your colon, across the top of your abdomen, and down the left side into your rectum. Stool gathers in your rectum and builds up pressure until you feel that you want to empty your bowels.

Food and waste are transported through both the small and large intestines by automatic waves of movement through the gut that are caused by muscles not under our conscious control. These muscles, in the walls of the intestines, are called *involuntary* muscles. They react to fullness in the intestine and begin a rhythmic contraction that ripples along the intestine, squeezing the waste matter along towards its final end. The intestinal muscles push a meal through the small intestine and finally empty the leftovers into the large intestine.

There may be different types of activity in the muscles within the walls of the large bowel. For example, frequent small irregular contractions help to mix the contents of the colon while 4 to 6 times a day a large wave of muscular contraction passes all along the colon, carrying large amounts of faeces towards their final destination. Although you won't feel these large waves of muscular contraction, they may trigger an overwhelming urge to open your bowels.

Exercise seems to be important in helping these waves of muscular activity to be strong and regular. Working your limb muscles, whether you take a stroll through the countryside or race around a squash court, gives your intestinal muscles a workout too, moving food through the gut and reducing the likelihood of constipation.

When a full load reaches the rectum, a certain amount of voluntary muscle action can help push it out, but that's about the extent of our control. Conversely, if you are trying to hold back a rush of diarrhoea when you are in the middle of an airport queue, the only muscles on your side are the voluntary muscles around your anus, which keep the end of your gut shut.

Voluntary muscles are muscles that move at your command, for example leg and arm muscles. Involuntary muscles just keep working on their own. Heart muscle, intestinal muscle, uterine muscle, and muscle in blood vessels are involuntary muscles. We talk more about the two different kinds of nervous systems that control voluntary and involuntary functions in your body in Chapter 4.

Good Bacteria v. Bad Bacteria

Ten per cent of our body weight is made up of microorganisms. If that makes you squirm, keep reading to find out why that fact isn't all bad.

About 400 species make up the trillions of microbes that live in the warm, protected environment of your large intestine, where no harmful acid (which you find in the stomach) and no harsh alkaline bile (which you find in your upper small intestine) exist. The acid in your stomach and the bile in your small intestine are designed to eliminate infectious organisms as far as possible. But those nasties that survive the journey – and many do – live off undigested foods, especially sugar, and can cause gas, bloating, abnormal bowel movements, and cramping pain.

The microbes in your large intestine consist mostly of bacteria and make up the bulk of the stool – at least for people who live in Western countries. (In some cultures, indigestible plant fibre makes up the bulk of the stool. We talk more about fibre and its benefits for both diarrhoea and constipation in Chapter 10.)

There can also be worms, parasites, and yeast in the stool. Some people believe that an overgrowth of yeast in the large intestine can play a significant part in causing symptoms of IBS, but this is controversial. You can read more in Chapter 4 about theories on the yeast *Candida* running amok in the gut.

Scientists who devote their lives to studying stool know that a diet low in fibre and high in protein is less likely to encourage friendly bacteria to thrive in the gut. Meanwhile, the types of bacteria that do like this sort of food break down the proteins and amino acids into chemicals called putrescine and cadaverine. These chemicals have a particular smell. In contrast, a diet high in complex carbohydrates (vegetables and whole grains) promotes the growth of beneficial bacteria, which have a much less offensive odour. Many people with IBS talk about an unpleasant odour that accompanies their bowel movements – perhaps they are picking up the signal that they need to increase the amount of fibre in their diet.

Here are some of the reasons why having bacteria in your gut is a good thing:

- ✔ **Keeping your mucosa healthy:** The cells that form the *mucosa,* or lining, of the large intestine can't get all the nourishment they need from your blood supply. Instead, they rely on beneficial bacteria that break down complex carbohydrates within the cavity, or *lumen,* of the intestines to provide a local source of nutrients and energy directly to the cells. The beneficial bacteria are known as *probiotic bacteria,* and the fibrous foods and complex proteins that they break down are called *prebiotics* or *colonic foods.*

- ✔ **Increasing immune protection:** About 70 per cent of your body's immune tissues are in your gut, poised ready and waiting to scrutinise everything that floats past and prepare the defences against anything that looks foreign. Just by being there, the microbes in your intestine provide a constant workout for the immune system. Your body continually makes antibodies against all bacteria because your immune system is always on guard for a life-threatening invasion.

- ✔ **Controlling yeasts and parasites:** Teams of bacteria that are lords and masters of the gut prevent the yeast and parasite populations from overproducing.

✔ **Producing antibiotics:** A number of bacteria actually produce their own antibiotics to keep invaders in check in your gut.

✔ **Producing vitamins:** Bacteria in the large intestine (especially the bacteria that don't like oxygen) produce tiny amounts of usable vitamin B, vitamin B_{12}, pantothenic acid, pyridoxine, biotin, and vitamin K.

If you take antibiotics for an infection, be sure to also take *Lactobacillus acidophilus* (abbreviated to *L. acidophilus*) or *L. plantarum* to replace the good bacteria that the antibiotics kill indiscriminately. Just take Lactobacilli two hours apart from your antibiotics. Lactobacilli (and other beneficial bacteria) come in capsule, liquid, or powder forms – ask at your pharmacy or health food store. "Live" yoghurt containing probiotic bacteria such as Lactobacilli, or plain kefir (a fermented milk drink available from most health food outlets) can also provide a source of beneficial bacteria. However, some experts argue that the levels of bacteria in these foods are not high enough to be effective, and that you would need to swallow several pots of probiotic yoghurt every day to counter the effects of antibiotics.

You may want to ask your GP about Lactobacilli supplements at the time that they prescribe antibiotics for you. The topic of probiotics (foods which provide a source of good or friendly bacteria such as Lactobacilli) is causing a big stir in the medical world and increasing numbers of doctors and nurses are becoming convinced of their importance. However some doctors are not yet persuaded that there is enough clear scientific evidence about exactly how and when probiotics should be used. Your GP may recommend Lactobacilli and explain where you can purchase supplements locally (they are not yet available on prescription on the NHS).

However, some GPs are uncertain about the value of probiotics and don't recommend them. If your GP is one of these 'non-believers' there is still nothing to stop you from trying them yourself. You also don't need to worry about probiotics interfering with other medicines that you might be taking – there is no evidence yet that supplements of friendly bacteria can cause any problems.

You may also hear about a strange-sounding organism called *Saccharomyces bourlardii*. Numerous experiments showed that this type of yeast helps to repopulate the gut with good bacteria while pushing out the bad bacteria. Scientists aren't sure yet exactly how *Saccharomyces bourlardii* has its positive effect but some studies have suggested that harmful bacteria may stick to the surface of the yeast and be carried out of the intestines on it when the bowels empty. *Saccharomyces bourlardii* may also rev up the immune response by increasing the production of immunoglobulins (chemicals which protect against harmful microbes). This probiotic, like *L. acidophilus* and *L.plantarum,* is available in capsule form at health food stores.

All You Ever Wanted to Know About Gas

Finding gas within the gut is perfectly normal, and we expel between 200 and 2,500 millilitres of it every day through the anus. But although gas may be a source of great mirth for young boys, it can cause a lot of unhappiness and discomfort for others, and bloating and excessive gas production are common symptoms in IBS.

The gas that bubbles though your gut has three main sources:

✔ **Air swallowing:** This is the major source of gas in your stomach. Every time you gulp down food or saliva, several millilitres of gas go down with it. Most of this gas comes back out the way it went down, as burps and belches. Very little gets through into the small intestine.

✔ **Gas production in the small intestine:** The acidic stomach contents mixing with the alkaline bicarbonate produced by the pancreas create carbon dioxide. Most of this gas is absorbed into the blood.

✔ **Fermentation in the large intestine:** Fermentation of undigested food by the bacteria in the large intestine produces much more gas. Some foodstuffs, such as starchy vegetables, beans and pulses, are more likely to reach the large intestine not fully digested, and are therefore more likely to produce gas. The main gases produced by fermentation include methane, hydrogen, carbon dioxide, lactic acid, and volatile fatty acids, including acetic, propionic, and butyric acids. These volatile fatty acids can be absorbed back into your body, but the other gases are mostly passed through the anus as *flatus,* or farts.

The five gases – nitrogen, oxygen, carbon dioxide, hydrogen and methane – that account for more than 99 per cent of flatus are all odourless. The unpleasant smell is due to very small amounts of other gases, particularly hydrogen sulphide.

 Keep a food diary to help battle bloating. By looking carefully at what you are eating, and how well the food is digested in your stomach and small intestine, you can cut back on the amount of undigested foodstuff you feed to your colon and so reduce gas production.

Finding Out About Faeces

Faecal waste contains undigested food – mostly indigestible plant cell walls from vegetables – as well as bacteria, yeast, intestinal secretions, and debris from dead cells flaking off the gut lining.

In a recent European survey, nearly one in ten of the UK population said they had suffered from constipation in the last 12 months. We think that, if asked carefully, many more may admit to the problem. Women seem to suffer more than men, and older people more than younger people. Research shows that about five in ten women strain to open their bowels at least a quarter of the time, compared with about four in ten men. In 2001, doctors in England wrote about 12 million prescriptions for *laxatives* (drugs to help the bowels move), and many more people buy these laxatives over the counter without ever talking to their doctor. We talk about the dangers of overuse of laxatives in Chapters 4 and 8.

Here are some stool facts to keep in mind:

- Stool is normally yellow-brown, coloured by bile salts from the gall bladder. The colour may vary, however, from pale brown to quite dark brown or greeny brown.

- Red stool is often due to eating beetroot.

- Fresh blood in the stool (either mixed in or on the surface) is what doctors often refer to as an "alarm" or "red flag" sign – this means a warning sign of a problem (usually at the lower end of the gut) which needs urgent investigation. If you see blood in the stool, you should talk to your doctor as soon as possible. Most often, fresh blood in the stool is caused by haemorrhoids (piles) or a small tear in the surface of the anus. Rarer but more serious causes include bleeding from an ulcer or damaged blood vessel, or a cancer of the rectum. Read more about blood in the stool in Chapter 7.

- Black tarry stool is another alarm or red flag sign, because it may be the result of bleeding high up in your gut, for example from a stomach ulcer. .Initially bright red, the blood passes through the intestines and is broken down into much darker compounds so that by the time it exits your body it is no longer red but black and thick. Because the blood has to pass through the intestines before it appears, there may be considerable bleeding before the problem is recognised. Just as with bright red blood in the stool, you should get urgent medical advice if you notice that your motions are unusually dark and like tar. You'll find information about tests to help you detect blood in the stool, in Chapter 7.

- Very pale stool ('chalky' stool) may be an alarm sign indicating a blockage in the bile duct or hepatitis, both of which keep bile from entering the intestines and lending its normal yellow-brown colour. Talk to your doctor if you notice that your stools are very pale – they will probably want to check a sample and take some blood to test how well your liver is working.

- Stool that is loose and frothy (as opposed to watery) is an alarm sign that often indicates a problem known as malabsorption, where nutrients from food aren't able to pass from the intestines into the body as they normally should be. As a result, such stool may contain fats, shreds of mucus, or recognisable bits of undigested food. When malabsorption occurs, your body fails to get some of the essential nutrients it needs from food, leading to weight loss or disease. Some conditions that cause malabsorption, especially Gluten Intolerance, can easily be mistaken for IBS. In Chapter 4 we explain the tests used to check for Gluten Intolerance.

- Stool that floats on the surface of the water in the toilet is full of fat – this indicates that fat is not being taken into the body from food as it should but remains in the intestines mixed with the stool. So floating stools are another alarm sign for malabsorption, which you need to discuss with your doctor.

- Watery stool of any type is usually called diarrhoea. There are many causes for diarrhoea, from infection to IBS – you'll find a lot of information on diarrhoea in this book because it is one of the main symptoms of IBS. Chapter 3 has a whole section on diarrhoea, while Chapter 8 looks at treatments for this often-persistent symptom.

- Mucous stool indicates that excessive mucus is being produced in the intestines and can be an alarm sign warning that an underling bowel irritation or inflammation exists. Let your doctor know if you are passing a lot of mucus – they may want to look at stool samples or arrange a endoscopy test to look inside the bowel. Chapter 7 provides the low-down on endoscopy.

- Constipation involves stool that is hard and dry and comes out painfully in pebbles. Bowel movements are usually fewer than three per week. Constipation is another common symptom in IBS but it may be an alarm sign of a blockage in the intestines, so it should be discussed with your doctor, who may decide to investigate it further. We discuss constipation in depth in Chapter 3 and offer suggestions for treatment in Chapter 8.

- The colour and consistency of normal stool can vary greatly for any individual, often reflecting variation in the foods we eat and the amount of fluids we drink.

Understanding What Controls Your Gut

The gut isn't just a long tube through which food falls. Your gut's a sophisticated processing machine that extracts a myriad of ingredients essential for your body's needs. And like any complex machine, your gut is under careful control.

Imagine you've been drawn into your local bakery by the delicious smell of fresh warm bread. Even before you rip open the paper bag and start shovelling that bun into your mouth, your gut turns on switches and gets its machinery rolling, increasing the flow of saliva in your mouth ready to start digestion. Within minutes of swallowing your first bite of bread, signals fly from your stomach to your large intestine, ramping up the action to move contents on through your gut in order to make way for fresh supplies at the top end.

All this activity is synchronised by the nervous system and hormonal (endocrine) system, which work closely together to control the gut. These two systems influence every process, including motility (the activity of the bowel that moves food through it), the secretion of chemicals such as digestive enzymes, the absorption of nutrients and fluid, the opening and closing of sphincters, and the speed at which blood flows through the gut. The gut has its own private nervous supply – the *enteric* or *intrinsic* nervous supply – which works alongside the central nervous system and the autonomic nervous system.

In addition to the nervous system, the endocrine organs release a number of hormones into the blood stream in order to regulate the working of your gut. The trigger for the release of these hormones is usually a change in the internal environment of the body. These chemical messengers travel to their targets elsewhere in your gut, where they may activate or inhibit different actions. Hormones actually made in your gut have the most profound effect. Three of the main ones hormones made in your gut are:

- **Gastrin:** This hormone is released by the stomach and controls the release of acid.
- **Cholecystokinin:** Produced by the small intestine, this hormone gets the pancreas and gall bladder going, with the release of pancreatic enzymes and bile.
- **Secretin:** This hormone from the small intestine stimulates release of fluids rich in bicarbonate from the pancreas and liver.

For example, imagine that by now that warm bun from the bakery is nicely mixed with stomach acid. Signals in your nervous system are relaxing the pyloric sphincter (which normally holds the entrance to the stomach shut tight) and contracting the muscular stomach walls to squeeze the mixture out into the small intestine. The arrival of this acidic glop triggers the secretion of the hormone secretin from endocrine cells in the lining of the small intestines. Secretin whizzes through the blood stream to the pancreas, telling it to release bicarbonate-rich fluids that neutralise the acid. Once the acid is neutralised, the trigger for secretin production is lost.

Timing Is Everything

Transit time is the time it takes for food to travel from your mouth to your anus. The extremes can be several hours to several weeks, but the normal transit time is about 24 hours.

A transit time much shorter than 24 hours means the small intestine doesn't have enough time to extract the nutrients from your foods. Although the more easily digested carbohydrates may be broken down, protein and fats may not. Your stool may reflect this fact by floating on the surface (because it's filled with fat) or containing undigested strands of meat. Remember: If you are not digesting a food, you are not gaining nutrients from the food – and gaining nutrient is what digestion is all about.

Now that we have seen the incredible orchestration necessary to digest a meal, we can recognise some of the many causes of digestion gone awry:

✔ Eating too quickly (so that the teeth, for example, don't have time to break down food adequately in the mouth).

✔ Drinking too much fluid with a meal (so that food is washed through the mouth or stomach very quickly).

✔ Eating large meals (so that too much food enters your system in too short a time).

✔ Not eating enough fibre (fibre can help increase transit time. With low fibre levels, transit time may be slow and constipation becomes a problem).

✔ Not getting enough exercise to help stimulate movement in your intestines (and lymphatic system).

✔ Lacking proper nutrition to make necessary enzymes, bile, and immune factors.

✔ Eating when stressed – stomach tension can shut down blood flow and diminish production of gastric juices, which means that the back flow of caustic juices from the small intestine can cause stress ulcers.

Curious about your own transit time? The *beetroot test* is the time it takes for the natural red dye in beetroot to go from one end of your digestive system to the other. If your stool is red within 24 hours, you have a good transit time. If your stool is much faster, you have fast digestion and may not be getting the best out of your food before it's flushed out the other end. Taking two days or longer to come through is not good either, because you are absorbing toxins from waste that's lying around in your intestines for too long. You can do the same test with corn on the cob: Just look out for bits of corn rather than red stool.

Protecting Your Gut

From the eyes, nose, and mouth to the anus, each of us has many resources that protect the gut from harm. Your senses – sight, smell, and taste – warn you away from foods that are rancid, mouldy, and poisonous. However, parasites, viruses (cold, flu, and hepatitis), and harmful bacteria can be mixed up in foods without you knowing it. These organisms don't wave flags as they stealthily slip into our bodies.

Most of the time, we are not affected by the many microbes swimming in our environment because of all the defense mechanisms built into our bodies. For example:

- ✔ In the mouth, saliva contains immunoglobulin A (IgA), an immune substance that can bind bacteria and deactivate certain parasites.

- ✔ In the stomach, strong hydrochloric acid kills off foreign microbes and helps break down protein that can produce allergy reactions if it remains undigested.

- ✔ Enzymes from the pancreas that squirt into the small intestine continue working on the protein and can also attack parasites.

- ✔ Any invader that has made it as far as the small intestine is attacked by more IgA made in your gut's lymphatic tissue and lurking in the intestinal mucus.

- ✔ Bile from the gall bladder is also on the offensive. One of its chemicals is strong enough to kill microbes.

Chapter 3

Your Sensitive Gut: Working Not So Well

In This Chapter
▶ Finding out about functional problems
▶ Getting to grips with gas
▶ Understanding and dealing with your gut symptoms

*W*hen your gastrointestinal tract or gut works well, it's a fantastic factory, taking in raw ingredients at one end and processing them into energy and waste in a series of co-ordinated steps. But often your gut doesn't work quite so well. Like any complicated production line, many different things can throw a spanner into the works, resulting in symptoms ranging from heartburn at the top end to unpleasant rumblings at the bottom end. You can look closely at many of these symptoms later in this chapter.

But when you have IBS, what is happening in your gut to upset your system? Whatever the cause (you can read about many of them in Chapter 4), one of the most important underlying features of IBS appears to be an increased sensitivity, or *hypersensitivity,* to all the nerve signals or chemical messages that constantly whiz to and fro between your brain and your gut.

Sussing Out Your Sensitive Gut

To understand the idea of a 'sensitive' gut, picture the nerve pathways that link your gut and brain. Nerve pathways send sensory information from your gut to your brain. Your brain then fires back control messages to your gut, a bit like a conversation. The whole set-up is known as the *gut–brain axis.* When you have a sensitive gut, the conversation in your gut–brain axis may be confused, as one of the 'participants' misunderstands what the other says.

Homing in on hypersensitivity

Doctors use the term 'hypersensitivity' to describe the gut overreacting to incoming information. That information may be signals coming from your brain through your gut's own nervous system (the *visceral nervous system*) or chemical signals coming from ingredients in the food you eat. An overreaction may, for example, cause your intestines to contract far more frequently or strongly than is necessary, leading to painful *spasms,* or muscle over-activity, and a rush of diarrhoea.

You may be starting to worry that perhaps IBS is therefore all in the mind rather than real. But this is not what hypersensitivity means. It's not just a matter of the brain overreacting to what is happening in the gut, but your gut physically overreacting to the signals it receives. For example, when your gut detects fats arriving within food, it normally switches on production of moderate amounts of fat-digesting enzymes. But in IBS it seems as though all the dials are turned up much higher and those fat-digesting enzymes come pouring out.

Evaluating visceral hypersensitivity

So your sensitive gut may be the result of hypersensitivity in the nerves that control it – your visceral nervous system. Although we've emphasised that IBS is not all in the mind, experts feel that when you have IBS, the whole gut–brain axis (that is the nerves of the brain, the gut and all the connections in between) is turned up to full volume. Therefore your brain may also be more sensitive to the signals coming from your gut. Most of the time, most people have little perception of every alteration in the way the gut is working, unless the gut needs a response from the rest of the body – for example, when your rectum fills and you need to open your bowels.

Despite the fact that the sensory nerves constantly buzz with information such as the composition of food just eaten, or the amount of acid in the stomach, only a small fraction of sensory information ever reaches your consciousness. You don't normally feel anything when your stomach starts emptying your lunch into the small intestine or when the arrival of unfamiliar food into the colon activates the cells of your immune system. Powerful mechanisms keep events in the gut – whether contractions, the production of gas, or low-grade inflammation – out of your mind.

But in IBS, your brain may be listening in almost too intensely to every little squeak of the bowel. Many symptoms relate to an increased awareness of sensations originating in the gut, such as distension of the intestines by gas (which leads to a sensation of bloating), or muscular contraction of the intestinal walls (causing cramping, churning pains). People with IBS become abnormally sensitive to what are normal gut activities.

When researchers measure pressures inside the bowel, people with IBS tend to report discomfort at lower levels of pressure or distension than people without IBS. This increased perception of activity within the gut is known as *visceral hypersensitivity*. People with IBS also seem to have altered perception from other systems in the body too, such as the urinary system or the muscles and joints, which means that they're more likely to report symptoms not directly related to the gut such as discomfort passing urine or aching limbs.

Two possible mechanisms are at work in visceral hypersensitivity: Your nervous system may detect more signals from your gut and send more information to your brain; alternatively, there may be alterations in the way the nervous system suppresses signals, so that you become aware of activities in the gut that the brain normally ignores. People with IBS, for example, often describe a sensation of excessive gas and bloating. However, researchers consistently fail to demonstrate any alterations in gas production within the bowel that matches these symptoms. So why do people get this sensation? It may be that normal levels of gas trigger many more signals in the nervous system than usual, so the brain misreads the signals as high levels of gas.

Reviewing the roles of anxiety and other factors

Most people have a sensitive gut at times. If you eat a really hot curry, for example, you may well have symptoms resulting from powerful GIT sensations – symptoms that people with IBS are all too familiar with. But normally those symptoms settle quickly and don't disable you.

In IBS, symptoms persist because of how you react to the sensations you feel. Anxiety is a common reaction in IBS. Unfortunately, however, your GIT is particularly sensitive to anxiety. So, your initial symptoms of IBS lead to anxiety, which increases your GIT symptoms, causing more anxiety, and so on. Spiralling out of control in this way is why managing stress (which further increases anxiety) is so important in relieving IBS.

The idea of a sensitive gut still doesn't make clear the exact cause of IBS or why your gut becomes sensitive in the first place. But the concept does link up earlier theories about IBS, such as it being a disorder of gastrointestinal contractions. Current research includes exploring the factors that may be to blame for making your gut more sensitive, such as food allergies, inflammation, viral infections, wonky genetic signals, stress, and a chemical called serotonin. We look at all these factors in more depth in Chapter 4.

Scientists cannot be sure what goes wrong with serotonin in people with IBS, but theories include inadequate production of serotonin in the body, damage to the receptors on the nerves that detect serotonin, and problems with the system that supports serotonin. Wherever the fault lies, the result may be abdominal pain, altered bowel habit, and bloating. Drug treatments that increase the amount of serotonin or its receptors in the body may offer effective treatment for IBS in the future.

Finding Out about Faulty Functioning

IBS is defined as a 'functional condition', a term we consider in Chapter 1. This definition is important because it helps both doctors and patients to move on from wondering what causes IBS and instead focus on ideas about managing the condition. We tackle the definition of 'functional' here.

We recognise that the symptoms of IBS are real. Certain people with IBS diarrhoea have 10–15 bowel movements a day and all the associated painful cramps, gas, bloating, and social discomfort. But IBS does not damage the colon: No bleeding, ulcers, or tumours occur, and visceral hypersensitivity does not show up on any test currently used. Therefore, IBS is not a diagnosable disease where changes to the tissues or structure of the organs can be pinpointed. In the future, a blood test, a tissue sample of the colon, or a brain scan showing sensory signals from the gut may help to identify the ailment, but until then doctors describe IBS as a *functional bowel disorder* (FBD).

Functional is another way of saying, 'Sorry, pal, we really don't know what's happening, but we do admit that something is wrong, mainly because you keep bugging us about it and running to the bathroom and using up all the toilet paper'. Don't quote us on this definition, but many people with IBS spend years trying to get a proper diagnosis as their doctors rule out all sorts of possibilities. If that's been your experience, the definition probably rings true.

Science is based on observation, X-rays, laboratory blood tests, and evidence of disease. But the sum total of your intestines' daily output is not what doctors and researchers are looking for. Because doctors find no structural damage in your colon and no biochemical changes in your blood, the only explanation for your symptoms is that your colon isn't functioning properly. Such a functional impairment results in very real twisting, spasming, gripping, and swelling of the colon, but the colon does not become inflamed as it does in other colon diseases, such as ulcerative colitis and Crohn's disease. (We discuss inflammatory bowel diseases in Chapter 7.)

Because of the lack of structural evidence of disease, a diagnostic cloud hangs over IBS. Even though the words 'Irritable Bowel Syndrome' do quite neatly conjure up a picture of the condition, many people don't feel very satisfied with the diagnosis. They feel that it doesn't tell them exactly what is wrong with their body – for the simple reason that science doesn't yet understand exactly what is wrong. Some even say that they would feel more relieved if they were told that they were suffering from inflammatory bowel disease, which seems illogical because inflammatory bowel disease is far more serious than IBS. But this irrational reaction highlights the human need for understanding and the uncertainty of IBS, which leaves many feeling as though they don't have a real disease. We discuss the diagnostic process in detail in Chapter 7, but right now we consider what functions may be faulty in IBS.

Gut reactions: Dealing with dodgy digestion

Cast your mind back through the centuries to speculate about what your ancestors' guts got up to. Until recent times, humans ate a fairly standard sort of diet – lots of basic vegetables (particularly root veg), nuts, grains, berries, and, for the celebrities of the day, roast meat (mostly chicken, mutton, and venison, although nothing beat a spot of starling or hedgehog). Dairy products have been a part of our diet (depending on where you live) for several thousand years, as have bread and pies, which used to be about as close as things got to processed or fast food. So did Henry VIII and his subjects have IBS? Plenty of sources describe how their stomachs ached after a huge banquet, but we have no detailed medical reports from the time to help establish if IBS may have been to blame.

Fast forward to the 21st century. Our guts, which evolved gradually over millennia to a staple diet, suddenly contend with thousands of different chemicals. Fast food, chocolate bars, ready meals, and other modern interpretations of nutrition contain additives and preservatives that our ancient relatives never encountered. It doesn't take much imagination to guess how your gut may react when it comes across such delights.

Once school of thought considers that IBS is caused by a reaction to modern processed foods or chemicals within them. They suggest that the condition is a type of food allergy (where your gut wrongly identifies food as a dangerous invader and launches an attack on it by the immune system) or intolerance to food (where your gut simply doesn't have what it needs in the way of enzymes to properly digest the food). Strictly speaking, neither situation is IBS – food allergies and intolerance constitute conditions in their own right, and your doctor can do tests to rule them out. But even then, many people with IBS can pinpoint certain foods that are more likely to trigger symptoms. So although we don't understand how the food can upset your gut, dodgy digestion of certain foods may be something you want to look into carefully. We examine more ideas about the role of food as a trigger in Chapter 4.

Getting food moving through the gut

A different sense in which digestion may be faulty in IBS is in the way that your gut moves to churn up food and push it through your system. Scientists have found distinct abnormalities in the movement, or *motility,* of the small and large intestines in people with IBS.

Altered gut motility may be the result of differences in the electrical activity within the nerves and muscles of the colon or large intestine that can be detected in people with IBS. Differences in electrical signals may mean that the muscles in your gut get the wrong messages about what to do and so they don't contract in the normal way to push food through the gut. An abnormal pattern of electrical activity is more often seen in people prone to diarrhoea rather than people who tend to get constipation.

Abnormal gut motility may speed up or slow down digestion. A reduced transit time through the small intestine, for example, means food whooshes through, resulting in that urgent dash to the loo with diarrhoea. For the slow-coaches whose transit time is frankly no more than a leisurely ramble, the result is constipation.

Scientists have not identified why the gut gets its timetable in a twist, but current theories centre on the idea that the smooth muscle in the walls of the bowel is super-responsive to the signals in the nerves (whether those signals shout 'Stop!' and slow down your transit, or yell 'Go! Go! Go!' and increase your gut activity). These factors may account for why some people with IBS have urinary symptoms too: The smooth muscle in the urinary system may be hyper-responsive too, causing frequent and urgent trips to the toilet.

Talking about trapped wind

In 2004, a group of Italian doctors pulled together all existing data on IBS in an effort to define it clearly. Here's what they concluded:

> *IBS is a functional, multifactorial condition characterised by abdominal pain and irregular bowel habit.*

A *multifactorial* disease is a condition with several different causes or contributing factors, such as genetics and environmental influences.

The Italian doctors also determined that IBS happens when the muscles of the intestines act erratically. They point out that IBS is more likely to assault people whose intestines, completely without their owner's permission, get rather overexcited when a little bit of gas builds up and starts to stretch or bloat out the bowel. The doctors also point out that people with IBS may pick up more than their share of stress from their environment, which can also cause the intestines overreact.

The Italian group added a twist to the mystery of IBS with a new finding of their own. The researchers were excited to find that people with IBS cannot expel intestinal gas, which may therefore be a cause of IBS. You're probably not as excited as the doctors especially if, like many people with IBS, you feel that you're one of nature's own gas producers and bloating is a particular problem for you. Apparently, people with IBS have a special attachment to their gas and don't like to let it go. Most people produce up to 2½ litres of gas a day, although some people can produce as much as 4 litres. And if a portion of that gas gets stuck in your system, you're going to be uncomfortable.

Gas with no way out causes bloating and stretches your bowel, creating the most frequent symptom of IBS – abdominal pain. The Italian researchers say that when gas stretches the rectal area of your bowel, the pain activates certain areas of your brain, which makes you feel yet more symptoms of IBS. What the researchers don't yet understand, however, is *why* this problem occurs – what causes an inability to expel gas in the first place?

Here's our two pennyworth about the researchers' theory: Many people with IBS are fully aware of the phenomenon of explosive farting, where intestinal gas is expelled with such fury that a small amount of faeces is forced out at the same time. When you experience this really embarrassing problem, what's your natural reaction when you feel the need to pass gas? Of course you do your best to hold everything in until you know you're safe! And who wouldn't?

In Western cultures, passing gas in public is simply not polite. Loud farts may be a giggle among small children but as we get older we are conditioned to refrain from farting in public and many people feel a degree of shame if they happen to let one rip. And despite the increasing equality between men and women in modern society, girls still tend to be more inhibited than boys when it comes to giving free rein to their bodily functions. Research shows that women can tolerate higher pressures within their intestines than men, and are more able or willing to suppress the urge to pass wind or open their bowels. The social conditioning that tells girls that farting is 'unladylike' persists even today.

Does this theory fully explain why IBS is more common among women than men? Probably not, but we'd love to see further research on this topic!

Looking at the leaky gut

Another important idea about the cause of IBS is that the lining of the gut becomes leaky, allowing all sorts of chemicals that ought to be flushed away to stay in your body. However, controversy exists between conventional scientists (who don't really rate this idea) and complementary therapists (who like this concept). We look at this topic in more depth in Chapter 4, where we singe our fingers getting to grips with the heated debate about whether the yeast candida acts as a trigger for IBS symptoms. For now, we talk more generally about the triggers that may damage the delicate mucosal surface of the gut and make it leaky.

The leaky gut is far from proven as a theory. The idea is a useful way to demonstrate the mechanisms and symptoms of IBS, but scientific evidence to back up the concept doesn't exist. In the UK, most conventional doctors, probably including yours, may raise an eyebrow or three at the theory. The best we can suggest is to keep an open mind and see if taking a 'leaky gut approach' to your IBS helps you; if you don't get results, you may not want to pour your heart and life savings into pursuing the concept.

The list of factors that some people suggest may irritate the gut and allow undigested food molecules, bacterial toxins, and other chemicals to percolate into the lymphatic system and bloodstream is long. Factors include the following:

- **Alcohol:** A well-known irritant of the delicate tissues that line the gut, too much alcohol can cause nausea, vomiting, and diarrhoea as we discuss in Chapter 18. Severe alcohol poisoning can cause gastrointestinal bleeding. If you have a vulnerable gut, just small doses of alcohol may cause one or more of the above symptoms.

- **Antibiotics:** Like many medicines, antibiotics contain chemicals that can irritate the gut – we discuss antibiotics in Chapter 4. One theory is that antibiotics can lead to the overgrowth of yeast, which themselves cause leaky gut (see the bullet point on yeast, later in this list).

- **Bacteria:** *Pathogenic,* or disease-causing, bacteria contaminating the food or water you consume can harm the cells of the gut and cause symptoms of IBS.

- **Caffeine:** This bitter, toxic substance from the coffee bean stimulates bile production. Many people even use caffeine as a laxative. If you have IBS with diarrhoea, caffeine may be too much for your sensitive bowel.

- **Chemicals in air and water from industry:** Scientists have not done toxicology testing on even a fraction of the 60,000 chemicals used in industry, and so we don't understand their effects. Many industrial chemicals end up in our water supplies, the air we breathe, and the food we eat, especially in industrial areas. Some of the chemicals may have the potential to cause clinical symptoms, including IBS.

✔ **Chemicals in processed food, such as preservatives, colourings, and trans fats:** Chemicals in our food have the potential to cause physical symptoms in people in IBS. One of the symptoms of irritation caused by a chemical is diarrhoea.

✔ **Corticosteroid drugs:** Drugs used in the treatment of many disorders such as asthma and diseases of the immune system. They can weaken the gut lining, making it more vulnerable to yeast invasion (which we enlarge upon in the yeast bullet, later in this list).

✔ **Hormone replacement therapy:** Hormones can change the intestinal pH and cause an imbalance of organisms in the intestines – reducing levels of good bacteria.

✔ **Mould and fungus hidden in nuts, grains, flour, and fruit:** Tiny amounts of moulds and fungi may irritate the gut lining and cause allergic reactions.

✔ **Non-steroidal anti-inflammatory drugs (NSAIDs):** All NSAIDs, which are widely used for aches, pains and muscle strains, irritate the gut to a certain extent. One of the main side effects (even with good old aspirin and ibuprofen) is gastrointestinal bleeding. Bleeding is a sign of irritation of the lining of the gut, and irritation may mean the gut wall becomes leaky.

✔ **Wheat-based foods:** A number of complementary therapists, especially those working in food allergy, are of the opinion that the proteins in wheat can cause the gut to become leaky. But there's little scientific evidence to back up such a claim.

✔ **Viruses:** Our bodies are constantly exposed to viruses – from other people, from not washing your hands before eating, and even just by breathing them in. In the gut, viruses may irritate the lining cells just as bacteria can do.

✔ **Yeasts:** A theory suggests that when yeast cells, a natural inhabitant of the gut, are encouraged to thrive (for example by eating a high-sugar diet, or taking antibiotics or hormone treatments), the yeasts change from a round 'budding' stage to a thread-like, tissue-invasive stage. The threads can bore into the small intestine, making tiny holes in the lining and providing a microscopic super highway into the blood and lymphatic system for large molecules, allergens, and toxins. The end result, so this highly contentious and unproven theory goes, is symptoms from head to toe.

Understanding What Happens When Your Gut Goes Wrong

So what do the warning sirens of your sensitive gut sound like? What sort of symptoms can you expect if your gut malfunctions? The IBS symptoms you experience depend on which part of your system is problematic.

Reflux and heartburn

When the stomach phase of the digestive process goes amok, a whole host of symptoms can make your life miserable. Many of the following symptoms are associated with IBS:

- If your oesophageal sphincter – the band of muscle that forms a valve between your oesophagus (gullet) and stomach – isn't tight enough and doesn't work properly, acid reflux and heartburn are the direct result. As the muscles of your stomach contract fiercely to pulverise your food, the contents of your stomach (consisting of food mixed with acid) escape northwards and rise into your oesophagus – known as *reflux* – and cause a burning sensation that we call *heartburn*.

- If your oesophageal sphincter is very loose, food can rise all the way up into the back of your throat. In severe cases of acid reflux, you can inhale food into your lungs as it travels up the oesophagus and falls back down into the trachea or windpipe, which can result in pneumonia.

Nausea and vomiting

Got that unmistakable queasy feeling somewhere between your head, throat, and stomach? Around a third of people with IBS say that nausea is a major feature of their condition, and IBS is one of the most common causes of recurrent nausea. It can be difficult to pinpoint where that feeling is coming from, but the sensation is actually a message sent by your brain to tell you that things are not right at all – teetering on the disaster of vomiting, in fact. Not only do you feel terrible but you get a cold sweat, go pale, salivate, and lose interest in the people around you – hardly a great party trick! Meanwhile, deep inside, your stomach muscles become floppy, your *duodenum* (the upper end of your small intestine) starts to contract, and intestinal contents may reflux back up into your stomach.

Tracking what triggers vomiting

A number of nerve pathways, chemical messengers or *transmitters*, and receptors are involved in nausea and vomiting. Receptors in the stomach and small intestine detect mechanical and chemical factors that lead to vomiting. Mechanical factors include distension or swelling of the bowel, and powerful intestinal contractions, especially if pressure is rising behind a blockage. Chemical receptors respond to toxins, drugs, and even certain foods.

Receptors send signals that pass to an area of the brain called the *vomiting centre,* along with signals from other sources – other areas of the brain itself can generate nausea signals as a result of fear, bad memories, or simply anticipating that you are going to be sick.

Another brain centre – the chemoreceptor trigger zone – analyses blood and *cerebrospinal fluid* (the fluid that surrounds the brain) to check for problems and then feeds its results into the vomiting centre. When triggered, the vomiting centre stimulates your salivary glands, respiratory centres, and the muscles in your throat, gut, and abdominal wall to initiate vomiting.

If you're fortunate, the nausea passes without working the stomach up into a real stew. But if things get worse, retching may follow: The muscles of your abdomen, chest wall, and diaphragm contract fiercely. At the same time the muscles towards the top of the GI tract, including the oesophageal sphincter and the entrance to the airway, shuts tightly to hold stomach contents in and protect the lungs from vomit that may be forced up from the gut and overflow into the breathing tubes. So the contracting muscles are pushing against a closed door, increasing pressure inside the body while you hold your breath – it causes an extremely unpleasant sensation, which some people describe as a feeling of suffocation. At least the contents of your stomach are staying put for the moment. However, as the pressure inside the abdomen builds, retching ultimately leads to vomiting. Most people say that retching (sometimes called dry heaves or just heaving) is so unpleasant they'd rather just get the inevitable over with, and vomit.

If the muscular walls of your abdomen and chest contract long and hard enough, your diaphragm pulls down, the sphincter between your stomach and oesophagus opens, and your last meal returns rapidly and forcefully upwards to say hello. Vomiting often happens in waves, as sensations settle and then build again. Vomiting is a reflex activity, and not usually under voluntary control, although some people can suppress the urge to vomit to a degree and others can induce it.

People with IBS commonly feel nauseous, but the contents of your stomach returning to the surface for general inspection doesn't tend to be a feature. We all have different thresholds when it comes to vomiting, however: Some people, no matter how nauseous they feel, manage to keep things locked down firmly, whereas others just let it all go. The intensity of the pain and cramping alone may be sufficient to make someone sick.

If you vomit more than very occasionally, talk to your doctor. He or she needs to rule out a few other problems that can cause vomiting (see Chapter 7 for other things that cause IBS-like symptoms) and check that the diagnosis of IBS is correct. For example, some people relate their vomiting to eating certain foods, in which case the vomiting may be a feature of a food allergy rather than IBS.

Prolonged or repeated vomiting can cause serious health problems, including dehydration and loss of salts, and always needs medical attention.

Finding what reduces nausea in IBS is a very individual thing. What is useful for one person may be useless for another. Try the following:

- **Deal with your diarrhoea:** People who have diarrhoea as a feature of IBS often find their nausea settles when they manage to control their diarrhoea (see the section 'Diarrhoea', later in this chapter, for suggested treatments, and Chaper 8 for more detail on dealing with diarrhoea).

- **Follow your fibre intake:** Many people with IBS are particularly sensitive to dietary fibre – but some feel better with more fibre and others need to avoid it. Most people with IBS tend to do better with a reasonable amount of soluble fibre (for example from root vegetables and fruit) in their diet. Meanwhile those who tend to constipation may find that a regular dose of insoluble fibre (the tough plant fibres from grains, cereals and seeds) helps to get things going in the gut and reduces nausea – try eating a bran muffin every day for example.

- **Grab some ginger or munch on some mint:** Ginger can reduce nausea, but beware strong doses, which can irritate the gut – try ginger tea, ale, or biscuits as a simple way to get small amounts. Some people also find peppermint, taken as tea, in sweets or in more concentrated peppermint oil capsules, helps.

- **Keep a food diary:** Try to pinpoint if certain foods trigger nausea. Then try to exclude them from your diet (we talk about exclusion diets in more detail in Chapter 10).

- **Skip to the loo:** A bowel movement can relieve nausea for some people, but of course you can't always arrange this to order.

- **Talk to your friendly pharmacist:** You can buy a number of medicines in your local pharmacy to treat nausea. Most of them work by blocking a few of the chemical signals that pass to the vomiting centre in your brain. They include antihistamines, anticholinergics, dopamine blockers, and serotonin blockers. If you want to use them on anything but an occasional basis, talk to your doctor first.

Belching and Flatulence

In certain civilisations, a loud belch during or after dinner is perfectly acceptable – a sure sign of appreciation of a good meal. And in a few societies, farting (more formally known as flatulence) is considered so essential to normal bodily function that the wearing of trousers raises eyebrows because the garment blocks the dissipation of gas. Sadly, burping and farting just aren't the done thing in Western cultures, where most people expect us to keep our gas to ourselves. That makes life tricky for people with IBS for whom problems with intestinal gas are a major feature.

A survey by the IBS Research Appeal at the Central Middlesex Hospital in London found that *flatulence* (gas passed out through the rectum) ranked fourth as the worst inconvenience of the condition, taking 21 per cent of the vote after abdominal pain, impaired social life, and inability to travel.

A small amount of gas can be reabsorbed into the body, especially in the small intestine, but the rest must go one way or the other. Just about all the gas that heads upwards and pops out as a burp or belch is from the stomach. Very little stomach gas passes south into the small intestine.

'Top end' gas mostly comes from air swallowed with food or saliva (the salivary glands in your mouth constantly make saliva to keep your gut lubricated, although they produce even more when you eat).

Try the following to reduce the amount of air that you swallow:

- ✔ Chew your food slowly, with your mouth shut. Swallow food only when it's thoroughly soft and mashed, to reduce the amount of air trapped within the food particles.

- ✔ Don't talk as you eat (didn't your mother always tell you?).

- ✔ Don't drink too much fluid during a meal. Take gentle sips, not huge great gulps.

- ✔ Check for mouth breathing. If catarrh frequently blocks up your nasal passages, you probably breathe through your mouth and draw lots of air into your stomach. Talk to your doctor about mouth breathing – you may need expert advice from an ear, nose, and throat specialist.

- ✔ Tackle stress. Anxiety can cause changes in your breathing, meaning you draw more air into your stomach. People with IBS tend to be vulnerable to anxiety and need to work extra hard to keep on top of stress.

'Bottom end' gas (also known as flatulence, flatus or farts) is generated within the large intestines as food is digested in the gut and fermented by bacteria. It is normal to pass some flatus as many as 20 times a day.

Flatulence only becomes a problem when the gas smells foul, or when it emerges loudly, at inconvenient times or under high pressure, sometimes bringing faecal contents with it.

The following may reduce the amount of flatus that you produce:

✔ Eating a more varied diet to avoid large amounts of gas-producing foods.

✔ Avoiding foods particularly renowned as a cause of flatulence. Many such foods have undigestible or excess carbohydrates, which are not absorbed when they get to the colon. They include vegetables such as beans, cauliflower, peas, Brussels sprouts, broccoli, cabbage, dried fruits, and sugar substitutes such as sorbitol.

✔ Checking that you're not lactose intolerant (we discuss this condition in Chapter 4 and how to look out for it in Chapter 10).

✔ Eating at least 2 pots a day of 'live' yoghurt or similar food products containing friendly bacteria. They help to ensure good levels of beneficial bacteria in the gut, which improve the efficiency of digestion.

Indigestion

Indigestion is a common complaint. Stop anyone in the street and ask them what they mean by indigestion and – after they've checked for hidden TV cameras – you get a different answer every time. Those answers may include heartburn, reflux, abdominal pain, nausea, bloating, just about any symptom relating to the top end of the gut, and a few symptoms relating to the bottom end as well, such as seeing undigested food pass out in the stool.

The technical term that doctors use, *dyspepsia,* is no more useful because translated from its Greek origins it means 'abnormal digestion' – suitably vague and actually not always true, as digestion itself may be quite normal.

Most people mean a sense of discomfort somewhere between fullness and heartburn. When you describe your symptoms to your doctor, try to specify what you mean by indigestion, so that your doctor can target treatment accordingly.

Abdominal distension and bloating

Bloating and distension can be particularly hard to assess because their symptoms are difficult to measure. People usually use the word 'bloating' to describe how they feel – a sense of swelling out of the belly. Abdominal distension is more to do with an objective, practical measurement that demonstrates an increase in girth than with your subjective feelings.

Bloating is common – 16 per cent of people without IBS or other intestinal conditions experience it at least once a month (we're ruling out those afternoons where you've just eaten too much of your mother's delicious steak pie). As many as 75 per cent of people with IBS report bloating, even though it's not one of the current Rome III criteria used to diagnose IBS (discussed further in Chapter 1). Bloating is especially common in people who have a form of IBS known as midgut motility disorder (which we describe in the section on constipation, later in this chapter). Bloating tends to worsen as the day goes on and after eating. Women report bloating more often than men, especially just before and during their menstrual period. People who have constipation with their IBS are more likely to experience bloating – as many as 90 per cent do. But other research suggests that just as many people with diarrhoea and IBS get bloating. So we can say that pretty much everyone gets it.

A few experts have got out their tape measures and confirmed that the abdominal girth increases when people feel bloating. More sophisticated devices can directly correlate the severity of symptoms with the degree of distension. In some people with bloating, the abdominal girth increases by 10–12 centimetres by the end of the day – but the big question is why?

Most people blame gas for their bloating, and is yet another aspect of IBS that experts can't agree about. A number of detailed studies failed to show any excess gas in IBS, whereas other studies have shown excess gas when a person reports increased passage of wind, but not with bloating. Another suggestion is that for people with IBS, the bowel handles gas in a different way; yet some other bright spark proposes that the physical component of a meal may induce the sensation of bloating and the chemical component actually cause the gut to swell, resulting in distension. Research in which abdominal muscles were tested, suggested that they may be weak in IBS, relaxing too much after a meal and allowing the belly to distend.

Bloating is notoriously difficult to deal with, but you can try some of the following:

✔ **Check your diet:** The culprit may be hiding in your larder:

  • Reduce your sugar intake, especially after a gut infection. Damage to the lining of the bowel may disrupt its ability to break down sugars. Undigested sugars in the intestines provide a feast for bacteria, which scream 'Party time!' and whip up a whirl of fermentation that creates gas, bloating, and even diarrhoea – all symptoms of IBS.

  • Beware a high fibre intake. Doctors often used to recommend that people with IBS eat lots of fibre, but now they realise that too much fibres aggravates bloating and distension for many people.

  • Try withdrawing wheat from your diet. Look for foods based on other grains and oats instead.

- Limit your fat intake.

- Avoid fizzy (carbonated) drinks.

- Avoid artificial sweeteners, or try using a different one from your usual choice.

✔ **Head to your pharmacy:** A number of medications are worth trying (but remember to talk to your doctor if you plan to use any medications for a prolonged period of time):

- Treating constipation or diarrhoea may reduce the sensation of bloating, but go carefully because certain laxatives (for example lactulose) make bloating worse.

- Simethicone can, in theory, help to shift gas bubbles, but research doesn't show much more benefit than a *placebo* (dummy) treatment.

- *Beano,* a natural sugar-digesting enzyme, can reduce the amount of gas lower down in the intestines, but not a lot of evidence exists to show that *Beano* helps in bloating. This medication is no longer manufactured in the UK due to low demand, so if you want to try it you may have to look abroad.

- Antispasmodics drugs (we talk about these in the section on tummy ache, later in this chapter) sometimes make bloating less uncomfortable.

✔ **Move your abs:** Exercises that strengthen your abdominal muscles may help to reduce distension – and give you a great six-pack into the bargain.

✔ **Try a psychological therapy:** Various therapies can help with a lot of IBS symptoms – hypnotherapy, for example, has been shown to improve bloating.

Tegaserod is a drug known as a 5-HT$_4$ partial agonist. The drug stimulates the 5-HT$_4$ (also known as serotonin type 4) receptors in the enteric nervous system – the special nervous system of the gut – to increase movement of contents through the intestines. Tegaserod was marketed in the United States to relieve bloating and discomfort, but it was withdrawn in 2007 because of concerns about the risk of heart attack and stroke in people taking it. If nothing else, the drug shows how science is focusing on trying to modify the brain–gut axis (we talk about this in the section 'Sussing Out Your Sensitive Gut' at the beginning of this chapter) to make the gut less sensitive. So watch this space for more on the 5-HT front.

Tummy ache

Tummy ache, or abdominal pain, is top of the IBS charts. In the IBS Research Appeal survey, over 50 per cent of people with IBS said tummy ache was the worst inconvenience of their condition. But what one person is trying to describe when they say they have tummy ache may be completely different to what another person means. Some are referring to a sensation of soreness and burning behind the breastbone (as you may get when acid stomach contents rise up and irritate the lining of the gullet) whereas others mean a churning colicky pain coming from a very active colon. Such inconsistency makes it difficult to be sure of the significance of this finding. Many possible causes of abdominal pain exist, including the following:

✔ Too much fat in the diet can cause very strong contractions of the gall bladder, which then causes pain. Gall stones forming in the gall bladder can trigger abdominal pain when the gall bladder contracts.

✔ Irritation or inflammation from infection and exposure to acidic digestive contents in the small intestine can make the gut wall raw and may allow undigested food molecules and bacterial by-products to be absorbed into the bloodstream. This is called leaky gut, which we discuss in the earlier section 'Looking at the leaky gut'.

✔ One of the main causes of pain in IBS comes from the colon (large bowel). When you have IBS, your intestines do not contract normally, as you can see in Figure 3–1. Instead of contracting smoothly in a rhythmic fashion, the involuntary intestinal muscles seem to be disorganised and even violent. Like a muscle spasm, they contract in an exaggerated way and may cramp up for hours at a time. When the bowel is locked into a cramp, the faecal matter does not move along as it should. The intestinal wall continuously absorbs the water in the faecal matter, causing constipation. Gas can become trapped inside a section of cramping, causing swelling, bloating, and abdominal pain.

The pain tends to vary in nature depending on the other symptoms of IBS that occur. When pain occurs in association with constipation or diarrhoea, the pain tends to be relieved by opening the bowels. When pain is accompanied by bloating, nausea, and distension, it doesn't tend to be linked to abnormal bowel habits. In such a case (a type of IBS sometimes called midgut motility disorder, which we describe in the section on constipation in this chapter), the pain is more generalised and harder to pinpoint to one area of the tummy – pain of this type is not relieved by opening the bowels.

Diarrhoea

One of the odd things about IBS is that it can cause diarrhoea or constipation. The researchers have a theory that a specific subtype of IBS called *diarrhoea-predominant IBS* exists. We use this term (or *IBS diarrhoea* for short) because we feel it more clearly demonstrates what the problem is.

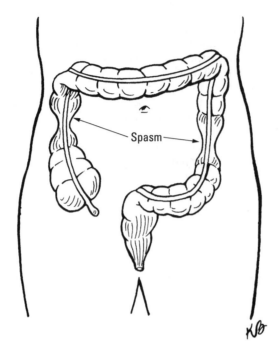

Figure 3–1:
The colon in
IBS.

Diarrhoea-predominant IBS typically includes the following symptoms:

- ✔ Bowel frequency (diarrhoea) that is particularly associated with pain (which is relieved by bowel action), rectal passage of mucus, and a sensation of incomplete evacuation.
- ✔ Abdominal pain.
- ✔ Visible abdominal distension (bloating).

Before you worry that we are trying to pigeonhole different people with IBS, and that you don't fit into any one compartment, researchers accept that the different types of IBS overlap and that some people have a combination of different symptoms.

The usual pattern is frequent and particularly urgent bowel movements. Someone with diarrhoea-predominant IBS may pass several stools in rapid succession, usually first thing in the morning. The first stool may be fairly well formed, but they become progressively looser. Some people call this the 'morning rush'. At its worst, diarrhoea-predominant IBS can keep you confined to home, terrified that if you leave the safety of your own loo you won't be able to find a toilet fast enough. Even people who manage to get out describe the uncertainty, anxiety, and exhaustion of the condition.

Inside the bowel, everything is in a hurry. The contents race through the small intestine and the right side of the colon. The first function of the large intestine is to remove excess water from the waste that ends up there. In the case of diarrhoea-predominant IBS, the waste moves through so quickly that the large intestine doesn't have enough time to grab that extra water, and watery diarrhoea results.

Medical treatments aim to slow the activity of the bowel, and include loperamide (taken regularly) and codeine (beware – one of the commonest side effects of codeine is constipation. Your IBS can simply change its form to become constipation-predominant IBS). Some antidepressants have also been shown to help – not because they make diarrhoea a cheery business, but because they may have an effect on the enteric nervous system, which combats the urgency and frequency, especially of the morning rush. Scientists are developing drugs that stimulate serotonin receptors and which may hold promise for the future.

Constipation

The IBS Research Appeal researchers and their Mayo Clinic colleagues have described a form of IBS called constipation-predominant IBS (also known as spastic colon syndrome). Not everyone who suffers from IBS and is constipated suffers from constipation-predominant IBS – constipation is a problem at times for anyone with IBS. But if constipation occurs a lot, then it may be constipation-predominant IBS.

Symptoms of constipation-predominant IBS include abdominal pain, visible abdominal distension (bloating), constipation with pain (which is relieved by bowel action), and rectal passage of mucus. The pain is often very sudden and piercing, and typically occurs in the lower abdomen. The discomfort may pass quickly and, just to confuse you, may cause stools that are looser than normal, even though constipation is a major feature. You may also feel a recurring sense of needing to visit the toilet – a sensation of incomplete evacuation – even after you've just opened your bowels. We discuss this problem in the later section, 'Incomplete evacuation'.

The area of the large intestine just above the rectum suffers the most cramping. When this area doesn't move, the intestine walls extract all the water from the stool and squeeze the eventual bowel movements into small hard pellets. In addition to this involuntary action, certain factors within our control can lead the work of the large intestine astray. For example, constipation can occur because of:

- ✔ Lack of fibre in the diet
- ✔ Insufficient water intake
- ✔ Failure to observe the call of nature when it comes

If constipation occurs regularly, the intestines can secrete excessive amounts of mucus to help protect the lining of the large intestine from irritation.

Often adults with constipation link their condition with bathroom habits that they picked up as children. Constipation may manifest in a strict classroom environment, where teachers only permit bathroom breaks at scheduled times, or constipation may be the result of 'holding it in' during long journeys as a child. The body learns to conform but leaves behind a disruptive condition – constipation.

Treatments for constipation-predominant IBS aim to tackle the problem in a variety of ways:

- ✔ Fibre makes the stools bulkier which more efficiently stimulates the intestines to contract regularly and push the stool along. Fibre also holds water in the stool, making it softer and so more easily squeezed through the gut. Make sure you eat enough of the right sort of fibre – ideally a balance of soluble and insoluble fibre – combined with an adequate fluid intake. We advise on how to eat healthily for your IBS in Chapter 10.

- ✔ Avoiding eating large amounts of fatty food can prevent the intestinal spasms that may occur in constipation-predominant IBS. Too much fat causes the cells of your gut lining to release a hormone called cholecystokinin, or CCK. Cholecystokinin increases the contractions of the muscles in the wall of your large intestine which, if inefficient or excessive, aggravate the pain of constipation.

- ✔ Simple remedies based on peppermint oil may also help reduce painful spasms in the intestinal muscles. Peppermint oil contains a chemical called menthol, which is known to have an antispasmodic effect and also reduces flatulence.

- ✔ Laxatives are helpful, if you use the sort that draw fluid in and soften the contents rather than those that stimulate muscle contraction to empty the bowel, such as senna. But be careful, as the continual use of certain laxatives can make the bowel work less efficiently. Talk to your doctor before using laxatives long term.

Talk to your doctor if you constantly have to strain to open your bowels, because it can cause a number of complications. Pressure build-up from constipation, combined with straining to have a bowel movement, can cause tiny pouches called *diverticula* to balloon out from the wall of the gut. Known as *diverticulitis,* it can lead to a variety of problems, which we deal with in Chapter 7. Many people who have IBS and constipation also have haemorrhoids, or piles, caused by straining. *Haemorrhoids* are varicose veins surrounding the anus and rectum. They're caused by pressure from straining, which blocks the surrounding blood flow and causes veins to balloon out, creating a risk that the haemorrhoids may burst, leading to bleeding, which can be very serious.

In addition to diarrhoea-predominant IBS and constipation-predominant IBS, the IBS Research Appeal researchers and their Mayo Clinic colleagues describe a third type of IBS – *midgut motility disorder.* In midgut motility disorder, the motility, or movement, of the colon is normal, but problems occur in the small intestines, where motility and sensation are faulty. The disorder typically causes widespread tummy pain, bloating across the whole abdomen, trapped gas, nausea, and loss of appetite. Many people with this type of IBS say that their symptoms often become worse after eating, which raises the question of food allergies. But the real cause is more likely to be altered sensitivity of the nerves of the GIT.

Urgency and faecal incontinence

Ideally, your gut gives reasonable warning when it wants action – a few niggling gripes slowly grow in intensity until you realise that you need to excuse yourself from the office board meeting, the finals of the local tennis championships, or the multimillion-pound financial deal you're negotiating, because more important business lies ahead. Usually, you have at least a few minutes (if not longer) to make a calm exit and take a leisurely amble to the nearest bathroom.

But when you have IBS, your gut likes to put you through your paces and may set you a daring race – can you get to the toilet in time? An urgency to empty the bowels is a common symptom that can instil deep fear and anxiety into a person who, by definition, tends to be on the anxious side already. If you have IBS, you may have just seconds of warning when you experience the sensation that your rectum is filling and you need to go to the toilet. This sensation is rather delicately called 'the call to stool'. Some people can resist the call for considerable periods of time, but that call may be so powerful when you have IBS that your brain can't ignore it.

One in five people with IBS lose the race with their own gut: They don't make it to the loo fast enough and experience faecal incontinence on an occasional or regular basis. Incontinence, especially faecal incontinence, is one of the ultimate social humiliations, a terrible embarrassment that drives people to become frightened and reclusive. Many people with IBS rate faecal incontinence as the worst possible symptom.

Faecal incontinence is a disastrous chain of events caused by the increased sensitivity of the gut to signals that normally trigger defecation, along with a nervous system wound into overdrive. Together, these factors mean that the contents of the bowel can be moved at great speed into the rectum, where it demands to be let out. Although the structure of the rectum and anal sphincters may appear normal in IBS, and perfectly capable of holding on a little, the nerves get increasingly overexcited and send more and more furious signals to the brain, demanding that you take action. When the rectum is full, it is hard to ignore the signals. When combined with a fear learned from terrible experience, your anxiety levels soon reach fever pitch, which doesn't help you to calmly hold on. Almost inevitably on occasions you lose control.

If losing control has happened to you, it may seem like the end of the world and you may feel like your IBS can't get much worse. But take heart because this symptom can be tackled in a variety of ways. In particular, a type of psychological treatment known as Cognitive Behavioural Therapy has been shown to help.

Cognitive Behavioural Therapy or CBT aims to help a person understand their condition and how it arises, and then work out ways to change their behaviour to manage the symptom or disease better. Simply knowing why you're getting problems with faecal incontinence, and what is going on in your body, is an important first step. CBT can help you to recognise when your gut's nerves begin to jangle and then use effective techniques which keep the lid on anxiety and gain better control over your gut. CBT is recommended by the British Society of Gastroenterology's Guidelines for the Management of IBS and we discuss the therapy further in Chapter 12.

In addition to CBT, other medicines are available that can help to calm an overexcited gut – talk to your GP about the alternatives, or read about them in Chapter 8.

Incomplete evacuation

Most people get a certain sense of comfort and relief when they visit the toilet, do what they need to do, and then leave knowing that the business is over for a time. But some people with IBS become locked in a constant state of heightened alert, which can be extremely stressful. After opening their bowels they don't gain that sense of relief but instead feel that they need to do more, even when they just can't. They continue to experience sensations from the lower end of the gut that tell them that something inside needs to come out (even though tests show that when this feeling arises the rectum is usually empty). As a result they may become housebound, unable to stray far from the safety of their own bathroom.

Scientists are not clear why a sense of incomplete evacuation occurs. Some people who experience it fear it is 'all in the mind', but it is more likely the result of a fault in the sensitivity of the wall of the rectum, which sends confusing signals up to the brain through the gut–brain axis (we describe this axis in the section 'Sussing Out Your Sensitive Gut', earlier in this chapter). You're convinced that your rectum still contains stools, even though you've just emptied it.

CBT may be useful in coping with this symptom, especially because it is particularly good at dealing with anxiety, which plays a central part in incomplete evacuation, possibly by winding up the sensitivity of the nerves of the rectum. CBT can help you to find ways to overcome or at least put up with the sensation of incomplete evacuation without letting it take over your life. Other techniques that deal with stress, including rest and relaxation methods, may also help to calm the symptom.

Pain in the bum

If you've read through other bits of this chapter and discovered how your gut misbehaves when you have IBS, and perhaps experienced many of the symptoms yourself, you may be reflecting that you realise only too well that IBS is a right pain in the bum.

But pain in the rear end, also called *proctalgia fugax,* is also a real symptom of IBS. Severe, short-lived, stabbing pain almost at the surface of the anus or just inside can be extremely disconcerting and unpleasant.

The cause of such a pain isn't clear, but it may be due to spasm of the muscle of the anal sphincters and the rectum, possibly as a result of excessive activity in the nerves to these structures.

Stress and overtiredness tend to make proctalgia fugax worse, and so managing your stress levels is a first step to beating this unpleasant symptom. Medical treatments that relax muscle also help. The type of muscle found in the anal and rectal areas is known as smooth muscle and, interestingly, asthma also features spasm of smooth muscle, but in the airways. Treatments for asthma that relax smooth muscle, such as the drug salbutamol, may also be used for proctalgia fugax (we're talking tablets, not inhalers!).

Chapter 4

Considering Causes and Targeting Triggers

In This Chapter

▶ Investigating initial causes of IBS

▶ Pointing the finger at food and chemicals

▶ Seeing how stress affects the guts

▶ Keeping an eye on other culprits

*I*n Chapter 2 we look at how the gut normally works and then in Chapter 3 we talk about what happens when it doesn't work so well. In this chapter we ask, 'Why?' What's going on in the tissues of the gut to generate the symptoms of IBS and what makes these symptoms flare up and get worse?

In this chapter, we introduce you to all the things that we know may cause IBS and the factors that provoke the condition into action. But you may have your own theories, especially about the triggers for your own symptoms. As you know your body best, you may well discover a trigger that other people haven't yet spotted. Please forgive us for not putting it on our list – so many triggers exist that it's easy to miss a few out.

Defining Our Terms

Before we go any farther, we want to clarify how we use several key terms in this chapter (and the rest of the book, for that matter). Here's how we describe and distinguish amongst them:

✔ **Cause:** An accepted physical reason for why your body developed the symptoms of IBS in the first place.

✔ **Possible cause:** A possible reason for why your body first developed the symptoms of IBS – something that's still up for debate.

✔ **Mistaken identity:** A disease or condition that displays very similar symptoms as IBS but has a different cause, with a different sort of chaos going on in the cells and tissues, and which requires different treatment. Distinguishing between the two is very important, because treating the wrong disease would at best be ineffective and at worst be disastrous.

✔ **Trigger:** A stimulus that sets off an action, process, or series of events. The event in this case is an episode of IBS, or flaring up of minor symptoms, and the action may involve running to the bathroom.

✔ **Associated condition:** One of several conditions, such as fatigue or muscle pains, that seem to occur frequently in people with IBS.

Looking at What Makes the Gut Sensitive

The medical world doesn't know exactly what causes IBS. Many people with IBS appear to be abnormally sensitive to what goes on in their gut, feeling sensations such as pain and gassy rumblings more acutely than other people, and perhaps overreacting by sending signals back to the gut that stir the problem up. But researchers have not yet answered the question of why these people are more sensitive.

Doctors generally refer to IBS as a *functional condition,* which means a condition that's not caused by a discernible organic disease. But it may simply be the case that nobody has worked out the cause yet, perhaps because the cause is hidden among the endless nerve connections that link the body to the brain.

We think that a chain of events may result in IBS, starting with an underlying predisposition to the condition (possibly from birth) and ending, after one or more other insults to the gut, with the symptoms of IBS. The underlying predisposition may be thought of as an initial trigger. A combination of several factors – a special recipe designed for your own body – may then mount up to create IBS symptoms. Some of the triggers that can lead to IBS symptoms include

✔ A bowel infection.

✔ An inherited genetic fault that disrupts the nerves that control the intestines.

✔ Antibiotics taken at an early age that irritate the bowels (intestines) and set up abnormal overgrowth of bacteria or other gut inhabitants.

✔ Growing up with family factors such as bad diet and poor environment.

✔ Inadvertent psychological stress – for example, soiling your pants as a child at school – which alters behaviour patterns, for example by

> making you particularly anxious about visiting the toilet whenever you feel the slightest twinge from your gut.

✔ Severe psychological stress that puts the nervous system (including the enteric nervous system, the gut's own nervous system) on a state of high alert (we talk about this in Chapter 12).

Our theory is that whatever the initial trigger may be for you, after it's set in place in your bowel and in your mind, then a food, environmental, or other stress trigger can create the tipping point that leads to IBS. The process seems simple enough, but on an individual basis you may not be able to tell specifically what causes what.

Several different theories about what makes the gut sensitive deserve a little more attention – infection/inflammation, an over-excited immune system, or changes in the micro-organisms that live in the gut.

Investigating infection and inflammation

Gastroenteritis, or infections of the gut, are common and disrupt life for most people every now and then, especially if they travel abroad. Symptoms such as nausea, vomiting, diarrhoea, fever, and fatigue usually last a few days and then resolve. But a few people find that some of their symptoms persist for weeks and months, settling into a pattern that is highly suggestive of IBS.

If you have persistent fever after a bout of gastroenteritis, in addition to symptoms such as diarrhoea, you need to get urgent advice from your doctor. IBS does not cause a fever, so it is likely that you have inflammation or unresolved infection in the gut to explain your symptoms, and need treatment especially for these.

Evidence that IBS can follow infection

For some people with IBS, doctors can identify a bowel infection as the definitive event that starts symptoms even though the exact way such an infection causes long-term changes in bowel function (that is, how it actually causes IBS) is not known. The infection may be due to virus or other micro-organisms, and the IBS that results from the infection is called *post-infectious IBS (PI-IBS)*. Chronic bowel turmoil resembling IBS develops in a quarter of patients after infectious diarrhoea. In a study from Sweden, researchers investigated people who had an episode of gastroenteritis five years previously: 12 per cent said that symptoms persisted for three months or more, and 9 per cent still had symptoms at five years. The study found two particular risk factors for the development of post-infectious IBS – being female and treating the gastroenteritis with antibiotics (possibly because the antibiotics killed off the 'good' bacteria in the gut – we talk about these bacteria in Chapter 2).

No one particular gastroenteritis bug links to PI-IBS. Aggressive forms of the common gut bacteria *escherichia coli* (*e. coli*) were mostly to blame in a group of travellers from North America to Mexico who developed post-infectious IBS. But other research shows all sorts of micro-organisms may be the culprits, such as bacteria, viruses, and a type of tiny single-celled parasite called protozoa. In Canada, contamination of a municipal water supply led to a large outbreak of gastroenteritis due to the bacteria *e. coli* and *campylobacter jejuni*, with the result that one in three people had symptoms of IBS two years later.

An episode of gastroenteritis appears to be one important event that initiates IBS. However, many people with IBS can't track their IBS back to a specific illness. These people may have suffered a very mild infection, or their IBS may have started for some other reason.

How infection and inflammation can cause IBS

Research on why and how infection causes IBS focuses on three areas:

- ✔ How the inflammation that accompanies a bowel infection damages nerves in the gut lining and alters the way the gut nervous system works
- ✔ How a low-grade inflammation remains in the gut following the infection
- ✔ How the bowel infection can lead to changes that alter the activity of the micro-organisms that populate the intestines

In general, acute gastrointestinal infections cause inflammation of the mucous membrane lining the intestines. The infections initiate a cascade of events that don't settle down as they usually would. The inflammatory process seems to have a life of its own where immune cells infiltrate the intestinal lining and become a local irritant to the nervous system.

Severe gastroenteritis can cause the *mucosa,* or lining layers of the intestine, to break down. Lovely hair-like folds, called *microvilli,* cover the inner surface of the small bowel and are responsible for absorption of food particles. Gastroenteritis destroys the *microvilli* and it can be many weeks before they redevelop. During this time digestive enzymes (including lactase, which we talk about in the later section 'Looking at lactose') fall to low levels and food may pass into the large bowel undigested. In the large bowel the resident bacteria may ferment the undigested food, producing gas that triggers bloating and cramping. The bowel lining can take weeks to regrow, during which time the enteric nervous system may reset itself, changing the sensitivity of the bowel.

Consuming *probiotics* ('good bacteria'), in yoghurt or in capsule or powder form, is a worthwhile preventive measure when you have an episode of gastroenteritis. Replacing good bacteria that may be lost with continuous diarrhoea may help to avoid the future development of IBS. See Chapter 9 for much more on probiotics.

Bacteria in the small intestine

IBS affects the large intestine, yet no studies show inflammation or signs of abnormal bacterial overgrowth or bacterial infection in the large intestine. But going a little farther up the food digestion chain, researchers found an abnormal overgrowth of bacteria in the small intestine.

Researchers believe that bacteria that live in the large intestine may spread along to the small intestine, where the grass is greener. Away from their normal confines, these bacteria feed on the rich smorgasbord of partially digested food in the small intestine. And when more and more bacteria grow in the small bowel (known as *small intestinal bacterial overgrowth,* or SIBO), abnormal fermentation results. This fermentation may lie at the heart of IBS symptoms.

Diarrhoea is a well-known symptom in SIBO, but constipation may also be a consequence because the methane gas that the bacteria produces can put the brakes on intestinal motility. Hardly surprising, then, that whether a person suffers from diarrhoea-predominant IBS or constipation-predominant IBS, almost all share the symptom of bloating.

The mechanism that triggers IBS may be the arrival of the wrong things in the wrong place in the bowel. Undigested food may pass in to mix with the bacteria in the large bowel, or the bacteria may move back up into the small bowel to find undigested food for themselves. Let this serve as a warning to those of you who chew once and gulp: If not properly digested, that mouthful of food becomes something else's dinner.

Despite these findings, the treatment for IBS is not as simple as taking antibiotics. In fact, antibiotics can be a possible trigger of IBS, as we explain in the section 'Avoiding antibiotics', later in this chapter. Antibiotics wipe out good bacteria and allow less friendly micro-organisms to set up house in your colon. So before you run out and take antibiotics to wipe out the bacteria in your small intestine, be sure to consider whether you're trading one problem for another.

Sussing out your souped-up immune system

Some people suspect that the immune system may play a part in IBS. These people suggest theories around the idea of a 'leaky bowel', in which bacteria and yeast, or their breakdown products, can easily get through the bowel wall and into the blood stream, triggering the immune system to produce a range of antibodies and other chemicals that cause symptoms. But many scientists aren't convinced that any reliable evidence exists to show this.

Some of the latest research focuses on other ways in which the immune system may link to IBS. Some studies pin the blame on the cells of the immune system that may be pouring out chemicals called *cytokines,* which razz up the level of inflammation in the body. People with IBS have raised levels of some cytokines. The researchers have found different cytokines in different types of IBS and have suggested a possible link between cytokine production and some of the other problems that people with IBS know better than most, such as depression and anxiety.

Other researchers look at the chemicals that connect the nervous system and the *endocrine,* or hormone, system, and so link the brain and the gut. In particular, the spotlight falls on a group of chemicals known as *corticotropin-releasing factor* (CRF), known to play a key part in the body's reaction to stress and which it is now believed may trigger symptoms of IBS and provide links to associated psychological problems, such as anxiety and depression. When you're stressed, your brain releases CRF. These chemicals then whizz around, co-ordinating the body's immediate response to the stress.

Experiments in animals show that when CRF is injected into the brain (to mimic an episode of stress), the colon goes into overdrive, jumping into action in exactly the same way as it does when you stand on a stage in front of a vast crowd or sit a difficult maths test. If the colon distends, CRF increases the sensation of pain. Meanwhile, when CRF is put into the blood stream so that it travels all over the body (including to the gut), the colon becomes much more sensitive to distension and jumpy (motility increases). So CRF makes a normal bowel mimic an IBS bowel.

In the future we may see drugs that block the effects of cytokines and CRF on the colon as treatments for IBS. Drugs that prevent CRF acting in the brain may control the pain signals pouring in from the gastrointestinal tract and calm down the messages of stress.

Meeting the new neighbours: Changes in the bacteria that keep you company

Earlier in this chapter we talk about how the arrival of an unfamiliar species of bacteria in the gut – in the form of a dose of gastroenteritis – may be an important precipitating factor in IBS. But although a gut infection can act as an initial trigger in IBS, more subtle or localised changes to the occupants of your intestines may also stir up trouble, leading to flare-ups of IBS symptoms.

Researchers aren't sure how these new tenants cause chaos worthy of an ASBO, but make no mistake – they can! The problems these bacteria cause may relate to the challenge that they present, as strangers, to your immune system, which drums up chemical signals that increase motility in the gut. Alternatively the new bacteria may alter the way your body breaks down and digests food.

Healthy holidays

Between 30 and 80 per cent of travellers report at least one episode of diarrhoea when away from home, although much depends on where you go. The risk from a quick hop over the Channel to Brittany is far less than a backpacking trek staying in the jungle longhouses of Borneo. Exotic trips, tropical climates, and poor kitchen and personal hygiene are risk factors, but gastroenteritis can occur anywhere in the world – harmful bacteria such as *salmonella, campylobacter*, and *listeria* flourish in the UK.

When you travel, practise the following safe eating and drinking habits to reduce your chances of getting ill:

✔ Avoid drinking tap water or using drinking fountains.

✔ Brush your teeth with bottled water, not tap water.

✔ Don't eat watermelon, which may be injected with water to increase its weight.

✔ Eat raw fruits and vegetables only if you've peeled them yourself.

✔ Steer clear of food from street vendors.

✔ Stick to food that's been cooked thoroughly and recently.

The following factors increase the chances of introducing new bacteria into your intestinal life:

✔ **Antibiotic treatment:** Some antibiotics kill off or clear out the old friends in your intestines allowing other, less friendly, bacteria that lurk in the gut in small numbers, or in the food you eat, to multiply and take over.

✔ **Changes in your diet:** Natural supplies of important friendly bacteria cover certain foods. For example, carrots and other vegetables supply a very rich source of *lactobacillus plantarum* (as long as you don't scrub them too clean or cook them). Eating lots of veggies can improve the health of your bowel, and processed and packaged foods that haven't even sniffed the outside world may encourage less friendly bacteria to take root.

✔ **Illness:** Changes in the internal environment of your body may make it hard for your friendly bacteria to survive, rather like the effects of a bleak cold winter. Meanwhile, other micro-organisms that you're less able to tolerate may like the new look and feel of your sick body and decide to stay.

✔ **Travel:** Your body gets used to most of the bacterial visitors in your home country, but travelling abroad and meeting new bacteria can cause problems. The locals may be used to these bacteria, but for the freshly arrived holidaymaker they spell trouble. The anxiety of travelling in a foreign land, and the common tendency to not drink enough and thus become dehydrated while travelling, may add to the trouble. Check out the sidebar 'Healthy holidays' for more on taking a trouble-free trip.

Controlling Candida

Candida albicans is a yeast (a type of fungi) found throughout our environment. *Candida* lives naturally in the gastrointestinal tract. If the environment in one part of the body changes, *candida* may run wild and grow in overwhelming numbers, resulting in a yeast infection known as thrush.

Two or three decades ago some researchers pinned the blame for a number of chronic conditions – including IBS – on *candida*. However, hardly a shred of scientific evidence emerged to back up this theory and most doctors do not believe in the idea that *candida* as a trigger of IBS. Even so, many complementary therapists have continued ever since to suggest that *candida* lies at the root of their patients problems. Evidence or not, some people find that following a *candida*-free diet or using treatments aimed at eliminating *candida* leads to a degree of relief from their IBS symptoms.

Much of the advice given about *candida* is good general health advice – avoiding processed and high-sugar foods, eating a healthy balance of different dietary components, taking pre- and probiotics, and keeping hydrated. Some *candida* theorists also advocate a bread-free diet – this coincidentally means reducing wheat intake, which helps some people because a sensitivity to or intolerance of wheat can cause IBS-like symptoms. The same goes for avoiding dairy products, which may allow lactose-intolerant people to avoid a trigger of gut problems. So although you may have been hoodwinked about the basis of your IBS, the end result is positive.

Anti-*candida* diets can be restrictive and may deprive you of essential nutrients needed for health. Make sure that you choose foods carefully to get all the calcium, iron, and other nutrients that you need – if you're worried, consider taking multivitamin and mineral supplements.

Finding Out Whether Food's a Factor

Many people with IBS, especially those who've had the condition for a few years, can tie in their symptoms to things that they eat or drink. But is food a trigger for symptoms or an innocent bystander that gets dragged into the problem by a sensitive gut that isn't working properly? And if food is the problem, how do you go about finding which of the hundreds of ingredients you eat every day are to blame?

Getting the terms straight

People with IBS think about food all the time. 'What can I eat?' and 'What can't I eat?' are big questions if you have IBS.

Before we discuss specific food triggers that affect many people with IBS, we want to be clear on how we use various terms associated with how people respond to food. Below we explain the difference between food allergies, food intolerances, and food sensitivities, all of which can be triggers for IBS. People who have problems with food sometimes use these terms interchangeably, but they aren't the same thing.

- ✓ **Food allergy:** Many people use the term *food allergy* when they notice their body reacting badly – for example, with a sudden gush of diarrhoea – to certain foods. The medical community is much pickier in its use of the term and relies on seeing evidence of a reaction by the body's immune system, in the form of an immediate and specific physical reaction – such as hives, asthma, shortness of breath, or swelling – or by finding a change in levels of certain immune cells or antibodies on blood tests. The most common food allergies relate to shellfish, nuts, and strawberries.

- ✓ **Food intolerance:** The medical definition of *food intolerance* is an inability to digest certain constituents of food, usually lactose or gluten. Lactose intolerance and gluten intolerance are usually inherited but can be acquired – for example, as a result of a bout of gastroenteritis. The conditions involve a deficiency in the enzymes needed to break down these foods. We talk about these two conditions a little later in this chapter and reveal that people often mistaken them for IBS. In the sidebar 'Feeling the force of fructose', we feed you the fruity facts about fructose – another natural sugar that can cause problems.

- ✓ **Food sensitivity:** Some people have food reactions that are neither allergies nor intolerances . These reactions are usually jumbled up under the heading *food sensitivity.* Some foods can simply be hard to digest and cause gas and bloating. A plateful of broccoli, Brussels sprouts, or onions produces a lot of sulphur in the intestines because these healthy vegetables contain large amounts of this mineral. Sulphur-containing foods can produce a very odorous result, and the gas can trigger an episode of IBS. (Sulphur is essential in the body, so don't avoid these vegetables but chose carefully the time, place, and amount that you indulge.)

Some people react very negatively to pesticides, herbicides, artificial dyes, colours, sweeteners, and other additives. We talk about some of the worst offenders, such as aspartame and MSG, in the section 'Focusing on food additives', later in this chapter. Your best defence against food additives is to read the labels and not eat anything that you don't know about.

We also point the finger at fats. Because fats in the diet trigger a flood of bile from the gall bladder, and bile can have a strong laxative effect on the intestines, fat is the enemy for some people with IBS. The same goes for spicy foods: The heat and irritation they produce can be too much for a sensitive IBS bowel.

Feeling the force of fructose

Fruit packs a great nutritional punch, so most of us assume that eating fruit and using sweeteners made from fruit sugar (fructose) must also be good. Not necessarily. Have you ever overdosed on juicy, mouth-watering peaches or plums only to find yourself running to the bathroom? Although not as well-defined as lactose intolerance, fructose intolerance affects some people with IBS, triggering diarrhoea, bloating, and cramps.

Other fruit sugars such as sorbitol and mannitol can also stir up symptoms of IBS, but you shouldn't confuse this with an intolerance. The bowel doesn't absorb these fruit sugars, and as they pass through the intestines they draw fluid into the colon, dilating the bowel, keeping the stool runny, and increasing gut motility.

You find fructose and sorbitol in many products labelled 'sugar-free', where they're added as sweeteners. Take too much of them (a tube of sugar-free mints does the trick) and even a person who doesn't have IBS is likely to be making a frantic dash for the toilet.

Scientists implicate fructose, sucrose (cane or beet sugar – table sugar), and high-fructose corn syrups in fructose sensitivity. Avoiding cane and beet sugar may be difficult but is probably going to improve your general health. Fruit, however, is an important source of vitamins and minerals. If you need to avoid fruit entirely, head to Chapter 10, where we talk about following a healthy diet to help your IBS.

Watching what and how you eat

Food contributes so much to IBS that it can make your head – or your bowel – spin. People with IBS obsess about food, because even the act of eating can turn on the valves and gears in your gut and make things move way too fast.

In the following sections, we discuss foods that may trigger IBS. Eliminating one or more of these triggers from your diet may alleviate your IBS symptoms. One study found that a group of people with IBS who strictly followed an elimination diet of potentially allergic foods had an 88 per cent reduction in painful abdominal cramps, a 90 per cent elimination of diarrhoea, 65 per cent less constipation, and a 79 per cent improvement in miscellaneous symptoms. In various surveys and studies, on average half of people with IBS report having one or more food intolerances.

Different triggers affect people with IBS in different ways and to different degrees. Get to know *your* triggers and then make every effort to avoid them. Don't let anybody tell you that something should or shouldn't trigger your IBS: You're the expert on what happens in your body.

Looking at lactose

Lactose is a *disaccharide,* or a sugar comprising two simple molecules – sucrose and galactose. Lactose occurs uniquely in milk from lactating mammals and other dairy products (up to 6 per cent of cow's milk is lactose). Many other foods and some medicines also contain lactose to increase their calorie content without making them unpleasantly sweet, or as a bulking agent.

For the body to absorb and use lactose, the natural enzyme lactase must break lactose down into its constituent sugars. This happens primarily in the *jejunum,* a part of the small bowel. But with insufficient levels of lactase are present, the breakdown of lactose is incomplete and some of it passes into the large intestine. Here, the effect is osmotic, which means that it draws water into the colon. Intestinal bacteria ferment the lactose, producing lactic acid and other chemicals such as short-chain fatty acids. The process creates some very gassy by-products – carbon dioxide, hydrogen, and methane gases. Dilation of the large intestine by fluid and gas, acceleration of the passage of food through the intestines, increased pressure within the colon . . . you can almost feel the symptoms of IBS rumbling. Lo and behold, within 30 minutes to two hours of ingestion of lactose, flatulence, bloating, abdominal pain, and diarrhoea burst forth.

These may be so familiar that you're probably already be wondering whether you have a lactase deficiency rather than IBS. An inherited deficiency of the enzyme lactase is common in late childhood and adult life in most populations around the world – most babies are born with lactase because they need it to survive on their mother's milk, but levels fall naturally after weaning. Lactase deficiency (which is the same as lactose intolerance) is least common in white people, and affects about 15 per cent of northern Europeans. But as many as 60 per cent of black people may have lactose intolerance, and in the Far East the condition affects more than 90 per cent, so it may even be considered normal there.

Lactose intolerance can also follow any condition that damages the lining of the intestines or significantly increases transit time through the jejunum. This is called secondary, or acquired, lactose intolerance. The most common cause is a bowel infection, where the delicate mucous lining of the gut falls away. That lining contains cells that manufacture lactase. The inability to make this enzyme causes an acquired lactose intolerance.

A lot of overlap exists between lactose intolerance and IBS, and unravelling the two can be difficult. People with IBS often report intolerance to food, particularly dairy products, and more than 25 per cent have lactose intolerance in addition to their IBS. In addition, restricting lactose can improve IBS symptoms, even when a lactose intolerance isn't diagnosed.

Your doctor may carry out tests such as a lactose tolerance test or a hydrogen breath test to see if you have a lactose intolerance (we describe these tests in Chapter 7), but by far the easiest way is to follow an elimination diet, which we explain in Chapter 10. Then, if necessary, steer clear of lactose or get in a supply of lactase enzyme (this comes as drops or tablets that you add to food to predigest the lactose) and wave goodbye to at least some of your symptoms.

To prevent future IBS symptoms or food intolerance when you have an episode of gastroenteritis, stop eating wheat, dairy, and fruit. Usually you can go back to eating these foods a couple of weeks after your symptoms subside.

Surveying sorbitol

Sorbitol is a sugar alcohol that occurs naturally in many stone fruits (such as plums) and some berries (such as Rowan berries), but your body can also make it from glucose. You find sorbitol in some laxatives that treat constipation, and it's often used as a sweetener in 'diet' foods and sugar-free chewing gum which can really play havoc with IBS.

The body only partly absorbs sorbitol. The unabsorbed part pulls water into the large intestine, causing distension that stimulates the muscles of the bowel and translates into the urge to have a bowel movement – sometimes at a moment's notice. Sorbitol also acts as a fuel for bacteria that create lots of nasty gas.

Some sorbitol-containing products carry a laxative warning, but the tiny labels on a one-serving dose of sorbitol don't have room to give you details about the gas, painful cramps, bloating, and diarrhoea that this two-timing sweetener can cause. Just two teaspoons a day of sorbitol achieves a laxative effect. If you buy a pack of sugar-free mints weighing 40 grams, about 20 grams may be sorbitol. Low-fat cake mixes, maple-flavoured syrup, toffees, and caramels can all contain enough sorbitol to make your life miserable. Even chewing sugar-free gum laced with sorbitol can be enough to trigger IBS. One doctor found that of seven adults who were given 10 grams of sorbitol, five experienced gastrointestinal symptoms.

Try cutting sorbitol out of your diet before you sign up for a doctor's appointment for your IBS. If you've gone sugar-free in an effort to control IBS or diabetes, remember other low-cal or no-cal options for sweeteners exist, such as aspartame or saccharin, so do some research and try them out.

Figuring out fat

Fat can be an IBS trigger because it stimulates the release of bile from your liver (for more on bile, check out Chapter 3). Bile can irritate your intestines if you have IBS. Fatty foods include

- ✔ Anything fried or cooked with lots of butter or oil
- ✔ Cheese
- ✔ Chicken and turkey skin
- ✔ Chocolate

✔ Egg yolk

✔ Full-fat dairy products

✔ Meat

✔ Oils and fats used in baking such as margarine or lard

Wondering whether wheat can make you wobble

As many as 1 in 100 people in the UK have a condition known as *coeliac disease,* sometimes also called *gluten allergy* or *gluten sensitive enteropathy.* If you're lucky enough to live on the beautiful west coast of Ireland, your chances of a gluten allergy are even higher – the condition affects many families here.

Gluten is a natural plant protein found in wheat, barley, and rye. Gluten triggers the immune system in some people to make antibodies that target the small intestine and damage the delicate lining. Researchers debate whether oats also have the same effect. Some people refer to the problem as a 'gluten intolerance', but this is not strictly correct as (unlike lactose intolerance) the problem lies not with an inability to digest gluten but directly to an immune reaction brought on by gluten.

We talk about coeliac disease more in Chapter 7, but meanwhile contemplate the symptoms:

✔ Abdominal bloating with wind

✔ Constipation

✔ Depression

✔ Extreme tiredness

✔ Pale offensive diarrhoea

Some people undoubtedly think that they have IBS but actually have coeliac disease. The only way to be absolutely sure is to check a blood sample for antibodies to gluten, but you can also try an elimination/challenge diet, getting rid of wheat for a few weeks to see if symptoms improve and then reintroducing it to see if symptoms return. For more on following an elimination diet, head to Chapter 10.

Rather inexplicably, a number of people find that even if they don't have anti-gluten antibodies, they feel better on a wheat-free diet. So it may be worth seeing whether cutting wheat out helps your IBS. Remember to be careful to keep your diet balanced and nutritious.

Focusing on fantastic fibre

There's no doubt about it: Fibre is good for your health. But if you have IBS you need to look on fibre as friend who has the potential to blow a gasket every now and then.

Doctors traditionally recommend a high-fibre diet for IBS, often with an emphasis on wheat fibre (bran) – this fact alone may be enough to get some people with gluten intolerance churning, as we explain in the previous section 'Wondering whether wheat can make you wobble'. People attribute fantastic powers to fibre – in the constipated bowel it bulks the stools and has a laxative effect and in diarrhoea-predominant IBS it can firm up the stool and slow it down. But doctors increasingly recognise that a blanket recommendation for fibre is not always the best advice for some people, and can make the symptoms worse.

If you tend towards the squittier end of the range, a lot of fibre can simply makes matters worse. But strangely, it can also make people with constipation-predominant IBS worse too. However, although fibre may give people with constipation-predominant IBS a big dose of bloating, abdominal distension, and farting, it does sometimes improve pain – and, of course, opening the bowels tends to be less hard work. So fibre may do more good than harm for people with constipation-predominant IBS. But if you have other kinds of IBS, you may want to be cautious.

Some fibres may be more likely to cause problems than others. Plant foods mostly contain a combination of two types of fibre – soluble and insoluble – although food manufacturers often classify fibre-containing foods more simply by which type of fibre is predominant.

Each type of fibre effects the gut in different ways. Soluble fibre, such as ispaghula, dissolves to form a gel that thickens loose motions and so helps diarrhoea, and softens the hard motions of constipation. So soluble fibre seems to be effective as a treatment to reduce symptoms for all types of IBS.

Insoluble fibre, such as bran, is a strongman that drags water into the stool and holds on tight to it (it holds up to 15 times its weight in water). The body doesn't absorb insoluble fibre but passes it through the bowel, pulling water and everything else with it – some people have even called it 'nature's broom'. In this way insoluble fibre may be helpful in getting constipation-predominant IBS moving, but can clearly aggravate diarrhoea-predominant IBS.

So according to current thinking, constipation-predominant IBS benefits most from a combination of fibre types, both soluble and insoluble, whereas diarrhoea-predominant IBS is best treated with just soluble fibre.

What you need in the way of fibre, and your particular balance of soluble and insoluble, is likely to be different to the person sitting next to you at the next

IBS conference you attend. Get it wrong at your peril because the line between healthy fibre and – whoooa! – too much fibre is very narrow. A very average sort of recommendation is a total fibre intake of 20 – 35 grams per day, of which about 6 – 10.5 grams should be soluble fibre. But you may have to tinker with different amounts and ratios of soluble to insoluble in order to find the correct combination that meets the individual demands of your innards.

Just to make your job harder, studies show that the bacteria in the gut quickly discovers how to recognise specific types of fibre foods and, within just two weeks of adding or changing your fibre intake, can up their waste disposal activities to break down the fibre and counteract your efforts to help your bowel function. You may want to dodge these so-called friendly bacteria by changing your fibre sources at regular intervals.

Just as Rome wasn't built in a day, so your bowel can't adapt to fibre in an instant – you need to add fibre to your diet at a snail's pace to give your sensitive bowel a chance to progressively adjust. If you suddenly start gnawing plants at every opportunity your gut may rebel with those old stalwarts of pain, cramping, gas, and diarrhoea, so take a few days or even a week or two to make changes.

Being coy about soy

Soy milk is a well-known substitute for dairy products. But for some people with IBS, soy isn't a happy choice. Beans in general, whether soy, black-eyed, or good old baked beans, can hold a sensitive gut to ransom because they all contain a sugar called raffinose, which some people don't have the digestive enzymes to break down. As a result the raffinose passes to the large bowel, where bacteria leap on it in glee as a source of food and ferment it, producing gases such as carbon dioxide, methane, and hydrogen that swell your belly and rip out into the wide world.

If you take soy as a dairy substitute or as a source of protein, consider eliminating it and then doing a challenge test to see if it suits you. You can find out more about elimination and challenge testing in Chapter 10. If you find that soy isn't your friend, you have many other dairy substitutes to choose from. Most health food shops and supermarkets sell rice, almond, hazelnut, and oat milks.

Keeping blood sugar on an even keel

Your blood sugar needs to stay within a certain normal range, and if it doesn't, lots of bells and whistles go off at central command in your brain. If the glucose (sugar) level in the blood goes too high, your body produces insulin that drives the glucose from the blood. If you eat toast and jam and gulp a coffee saturated with sugar, your blood sugar shoots up like a firecracker and your body rapidly deploys insulin to push all that sugar into your body's cells to use as fuel for energy production. As a result of the surge of insulin, your blood sugar suddenly plunges. If it drops a little too far, not enough sugar goes to the brain and you begin to feel dizzy and even nauseous, you see little stars, and you may even faint.

When your blood sugar levels drop, the body then releases adrenaline to keep itself going while sugar levels balance out. This is a normal response but can trigger a full 'fight or flight' reaction as your body gets confused and thinks it faces a deadly foe. As a result, your heart pounds, your palms become clammy, your skin sweats, and your bowels go into a clench as they clamp down in a hyperactive spasm.

At the same time, the adrenaline response causes the tight muscle sphincters that keep your bowels shut to relax, giving you a desperate urge to get to the toilet – this may be a survival mechanism; if your body senses a threat it may be helpful to eject any possible poisons in the food that you've eaten. But if you have IBS, especially diarrhoea-predominant IBS, it just serves to stir up your symptoms.

It's very important to keep your blood sugar levels on an even keel. However, people with IBS can get in a vicious cycle with low blood sugar because they tend to avoid eating in order to avoid symptoms. When you don't eat for more than three hours, your blood sugar levels may fall. And if you eat food that's high in sugar, you can get a rebound lowering of blood sugar levels afterwards.

We tell you more in Chapter 10 about the foods to eat and snack on that tend to be soothing for the bowel. Knowing what to eat and what not to eat is the first step in regulating your blood sugar. The second step is to eat frequent small meals to keep your blood sugar in balance.

Seeing the sense and sensitivity of allergy testing

If you haven't got the time or inclination to painstakingly work through a food elimination and challenge diet, which we describe in Chapter 10, or if you can't make sense of the results, you have another option: Allergy testing. This may involve the discomfort of giving blood samples or having small injections in the skin, or the emotional stress of parting with your hard-earned cash because not all allergy testing is available on the NHS.

Skin-prick tests are often the first step. Your doctor puts a liquid extract of the suspect food on a small patch of skin (usually on your forearm or back) and then makes a tiny scratch with a needle in the skin so that the liquid comes into contact with tissues below the skin. Your doctor may test several different foods in a number of patches at the same time. If redness and swelling develop around one of the patches, the test is positive for that particular food allergy.

Skin tests aren't totally reliable – you can develop a positive reaction without having allergic symptoms when you eat the food. (Some doctors feel very doubtful about skin testing for this reason and may advise you not to use it.) So it's important that a positive test matches the history you give about which foods seem to upset you.

Another test is a *RAST* (radioallergeosorbent test), which involves taking a blood sample. This is often a second stage after skin testing. Although RASTs may produce false positive results, they're more useful if you have severe food allergies: Unlike skin testing, they don't expose you to a sample of the potentially dangerous food, and you don't face the risk of an anaphylactic reaction.

The ELISA test is a simple blood test that detects an antibody that may cause delayed allergic responses to food. An ELISA test is much quicker than working through an elimination diet and can help you work out which foods to avoid. Some people find that after avoiding the villainous foods and letting symptoms settle for a year or two, they can re-introduce the problem foods without symptoms returning.

Not all doctors agree that ELISA testing is a reliable procedure. ELISA tests are rarely available on the NHS, so you may need to find a private practitioner – maybe a doctor working in nutritional medicine or a complementary therapy clinic. Some laboratories advertise a service directly to the public: They send you a kit to collect your own blood and return it to the lab. We thoroughly recommend that you talk to your GP before you go ahead. Not only can he advise you on whether he feels such a test is appropriate, but if you want to go ahead he, or the practice nurse, may be able to help you take blood for the test.

Many companies offer a scale of charges depending on how many foods they test you against. A simple test of the five most common troublesome foods may cost £50 or more, but testing for 100 foods may cost several hundred pounds. If this sounds like a fearful sum, don't forget that an elimination diet is free.

Another group of food allergy tests includes hair testing, electro-acupuncture, and various blood tests, available by mail order and through health food shops, sports centres, and complementary practitioners. No proof exists that these tests diagnose and help you to manage a food allergy. These tests may give false results, perhaps leaving you unnecessarily worried about a certain food, or lulled into a false sense of security, and they're often very expensive. The UK Royal College of Pathologists recommends that you do not use them, and we agree.

Stamping Out Stress

What if you eliminate all the other triggers that we describe in this chapter and you still have symptoms? Does that mean you haven't addressed an underlying trigger?

Many people argue that stress is the biggest culprit for people with IBS, but does stress itself cause IBS? Researchers and doctors do a lot of dancing around this question. People are understandably wary of saying that stress alone causes IBS, but on the other hand any excess stress in the life of someone with IBS can cause increased symptoms, and scientists can now clearly demonstrate the chemical and nerve links between stress and gut motility, or movement (we describe these links earlier in this Chapter).

We need to factor in many things when we talk about stress: Our nerves, our adrenal glands, and the games we play in our heads that go by many names – worry, fretting, agonising, obsessing. The gut and mind share so many of the same hormones, immune system cells, and neurochemicals that you may say that your head and bowel share a brain.

Letting your head rule your gut

Your head is at the controls of your body: If you eat or do something that you think may make you ill, then it just may. If you expect pain, you're more likely to feel pain. If somebody tells you something may make you feel nauseous, chances are you feel unwell after eating that something.

When you have IBS you may expect to get ill because you're out of the house for several hours without a handy bathroom. By expecting the worse, you may experience more symptoms than if you stayed at home.

The mind is a powerful tool. In Chapter 12 we suggest how to use positive thinking to stimulate good responses from your bowel instead of generating bad ones with negative thinking. If you think that we're saying IBS is all in your head, be assured that we aren't. We just think that the mind–body connection is stronger than many people like to admit, and when you have IBS you need to know how to use it to your advantage.

Linking your emotions and your gut

Many people think of the mind and body as separate entities, but we think that they're inextricably linked. In a healthy person, the enteric nervous system (the 'brain' of the gut) and the central nervous system (the real brain) work in harmony and influence the emotions we experience. Emotions are something that we instinctively perceive as going on in our brain, but they also result in changes in the body. When you feel sad, you may tense your muscles more, gulp deep breaths of air, and shed tears. When you feel excited, your heart beats faster and you breathe more rapidly. And when you feel frightened, you start to sweat and your pulse races.

On the other side of the connection, feedback from events elsewhere in the body can generate emotions. For example, an abnormally fast heart rhythm may make you feel anxious, and releasing muscular tension may make you relaxed and happy.

These links also involve events in the gastrointestinal tract: Constipation is a well-known feature of depression (and conversely, being constipated can make you feel down) whereas diarrhoea often occurs when you're anxious or excited.

There is another collection of nerves that helps to make the links between your mind and your body – the *autonomic nervous system* (ANS). The ANS controls bodily functions like heart rate, digestion, and breathing patterns. We don't have to think about making our heart beat, releasing enzymes for digestion, or remembering to breathe. The ANS does all that for us.

In a perfect world, the central, enteric, and autonomic nervous systems work in balance by reacting to what's going on. But if you have IBS, the balance may be lost. Your body may misinterpret signals from your gut and generate aberrant emotions or symptoms. Anxiety, for example, is a biological warning system that tells your body to react mentally and bodily to threatening or dangerous situations – but you don't have a control system to ensure that your interpretation of the situation is correct. If you interpret every physical symptom as a sign of serious disease (a danger), you experience more anxiety reactions than people who don't see the world in this way. This *catastrophising,* as doctors call it (see Chapter 12 for more about this), can switch the ANS into a heightened state that stimulates the enteric nervous system and leads to exaggerated gut reactions – IBS.

Anxiety also alters your perception of pain: The more anxious you become, the more pain you feel. This may explain why people with IBS, who tend to be worried about what is happening in their bowels, feel especially sensitive to the discomfort of distension in the gut. *Visceral hypersensitivity* – an exaggerated experience of pain in response to mildly painful or even normal sensations from the internal organs – is a classic feature of IBS. This suggests that undue anxiety about sensations from the gut may play a part in the development of IBS.

Counting on stress

Your nervous and immune systems directly connect your mind to your gut, so that stress and emotional upsets almost immediately become apparent as griping spasms or an episode of diarrhoea. How many times have you worried yourself into running to the bathroom? A phone call from someone special or someone you don't want to talk to can create the same effect. The connection of the mind to the bowel makes it all happen.

People with IBS have a unique relationship with stress that can lead to a physical reaction. Therefore, being aware of the numerous stressors in your environment is important. Here's a list of some common stressors:

- **Biological:** Bacteria, viruses, fungi and moulds, parasites, foods, animal hair and skin cells, dust, and pollen.

- **Chemical:** Chemicals derived from gas, oil, and coal, pesticides and herbicides, mercury, lead, aluminium, asbestos, chlorine, copper, nickel, illegal and legal drugs, and tobacco smoke.

- **Physical:** Heat, cold, weather cycles, noise, and X-rays.

- **Psychological:** Family stress (alcoholism, sexual abuse, family disruption, prolonged illness of a family member), psychological stress within your relationship (arguments, affairs, break-ups), stress at work (overwork, poor relationships, job loss), and a death in the family.

If you need some instant relief after reading this list, turn to Chapter 12 where we talk about stress and how to deal with it.

Weighing Up Nature and Nurture

Ask someone with IBS to pull out their family tree and they can probably point out another family member with IBS – or at least they would if everyone talked about having the condition but many people don't even feel comfortable to tell their nearest and dearest about their suffering.

Scientists believe that IBS has some sort of inherited tendency, or *genetic predisposition*. For example, studies show that IBS is twice as prevalent in identical twins as in non-identical twins, which is usually a sure sign that something genetic is going on – share the genes and you share the disease. More research shows that people with a close relative with a history of abdominal pain or bowel disorder have more than double the odds of having IBS compared with people without such a family connection.

The bad habits you pick up from your parents may be even more important than what's in your genes. If your mother or father had IBS when you were a child, you may have picked up how to have the disease by observing it in them. It can be a simple matter of seeing your mother holding her stomach and running to the bathroom following a meal or hearing your father complain of bloating. An unassuming child can come to think that this is a natural response to eating. On outings, a parent frantically searching for a toilet can create anxiety in the whole family. Such behaviour can't help but trigger a sensitivity to bowel issues.

Several studies show that children whose parents have IBS visit the doctor and hospital more than other children. These doctor's visits can be for any condition, not just for gut issues. That means environment and social conditioning contribute to the development of IBS. We don't know yet whether these children learn to place their stress in their guts or are just more aware of and sensitive to gut symptoms. In addition, people who use the same family recipes and have the same eating patterns have similar habits.

So genetics can't shoulder all the blame for a condition that runs in a family. Our home life and the meals we share also trigger IBS – we inherit the bad recipes and bad habits. People share much more than genes; they share the same foods, the same water, the same indoor and outdoor air, and the same cigarette smoke (which may be a trigger for IBS – as we discuss in the section 'Sounding out smoking, later in this chapter). Ultimately, whether we develop IBS or not is determined by a combination of both genetics ('nature') and the environment in which we grow up ('nurture').

Making the Chemical Connection

You may not realise that every breath you take, every bite you eat, and every drink you swallow is potentially laced with approximately 60,000 chemicals in common use. And these aren't just chemicals produced in your own home. We now have reports that vicious dust storms that originate in Arab countries and China become mixed with petrochemicals and heavy metals and show up on our doorsteps. In fact, the science of dust is worth a moment or two of awe-inspiring contemplation, for if you wipe over a surface or two in your house you collect a microscopic treasure trove of human skin cells, particles of insect bodies, diamond molecules from some lost planet across the galaxy, and many other more modern earthly chemicals. A barrage of chemicals constantly bombards our bodies – the chemicals are in the air we breathe, the dust we touch, the food we swallow, and even the water we drink – when scientist test any body of water for chemicals they find medications, pesticides, herbicides, and heavy metals.

So are all these 60,000 chemicals in daily use potential threats to our health or possible triggers of IBS? Science can't tell us for sure. Many probably have no, or very little, significant effect on our wellbeing. Some may even make us feel better – medications are chemicals, of course, as are food additives and even cigarette smoke (most of us enjoy tastier food and smokers feel better in the short term for a cigarette, even if the long-term implications may be devastating).

But some chemicals may have an adverse effect on us, sometimes without us even knowing it. At least we think that these chemicals may be harmful – scientists have done precious little research into many chemicals and haven't got a good grip on what they can do in the long term. When you're struggling to manage your IBS it may pay to be on the suspicious side and play the detective game with chemicals that comes your way. Even the fluoride in water and the high amounts of fluoride in tea (both green and black) may trigger IBS.

In the following sections, we discuss some of the chemicals that stand in the dock most often, accused of triggering IBS. In many of these cases expert witnesses from the world of science and the world of complementary medicine face each other in battle. With so little research to back up the arguments we must leave you, in many cases, to judge for yourself whether the chemical is guilty.

Avoiding antibiotics

Antibiotics kill one-celled organisms. When you take antibiotics to stop a bacterial infection, however, the drugs don't distinguish between the good and the bad guys and they wipe out the good bacteria along with the nasties.

The cells that form the delicate membrane lining the intestines depend totally on the friendly bacteria that normally live there. These cells get their energy and food supply directly from food that the good bacteria breaks down into tiny molecules. Without the good bacteria the cells starve and die. This can cause diarrhoea and difficulty absorbing food from the intestines.

Friendly bacteria also play an important part in maintaining the lining of the gut because they prevent harmful bacteria from entering the body through the wall of the intestines. They also help make vital vitamins and keep the digestive system working as it should. So you have an increased risk of infection when you lose your gut bacteria. More widespread disruption of gut mechanisms, for example transit times or speed of movement of food through the gut, leading to IBS.

Analysing other medications

Some other medications can trigger IBS symptoms, including antihistamines, antibiotics, antacids containing magnesium, laxatives, diuretics, sedatives, medications containing caffeine, antidepressants, and mineral supplements containing excessive amounts of magnesium.

Antidepressants such as fluoxetine and other selective serotonin reuptake inhibitors (SSRIs) can cause nausea, vomiting, dry mouth, constipation, and diarrhoea. In fact, any medication that you swallow possesses the potential to cause gastrointestinal symptoms. So, if you're on a new medication and you experience increased bowel movements, ask your doctor whether that drug may be to blame.

The irony is that some doctors prescribe antidepressants for people with IBS (see Chapter 8 for more on medications in IBS). Make sure that you and your doctors are completely aware of the drug's side effects in case your doctor prescribes something that actually increases the risk of diarrhoea and constipation.

Focusing on food additives

Some people report IBS-like symptoms of nausea, diarrhoea, and abdominal pain after eating the food flavouring monosodium glutamate (MSG) or the sweetener aspartame.

Aspartame occurs in hundreds of food products, including many low-calorie and 'diet' options. You can find it on the label if you look closely. You find MSG in all sorts of products, including stock cubes, barley malt, canned soup, flavourings, and seasonings, but sometimes you won't see it listed on the label as such – instead the European Union food additive code, or 'E' number E621 is used. MSG is also reputedly used as a flavour-enhancing ingredient in Chinese food, although many good Chinese restaurants now avoid using MSG.

Over the years MSG has been very heavily investigated, leading to a general agreement among scientists that it is safe for the vast majority of people. A similar conclusion has been reached with aspartame – despite previous controversy, most authorities believe that it is not a health risk to the normal population. In the UK, the Food Standards Agency recommends an acceptable daily intake of 40 milligrams of aspartame per 1 kilogram of body weight per day – that's 125 sweetener tablets or 14 cans of low-calorie drink a day!

Moving away from mercury

Mercury is a naturally occurring, highly toxic metal. Natural sources of mercury include contaminated ground water, fish and seafood, dental fillings, and some vaccines. Some researchers point out that mercury is a powerful antimicrobial agent and when you ingest mercury, such as from eating contaminated fish, the mercury kills off friendly bacteria in your intestines. This may be a mechanism for stirring up a sensitive bowel, but that's as far as the hypothesis goes.

Limiting mercury in your own environment is something you can begin today. Here are some positive steps you can take now:

- ✔ Avoid mercury thermometers: They're an unnecessary health hazard. Other types of thermometer, such as the digital variety, are far safer, so invest in one now, and properly dispose of the ones that contain mercury by returning them to your pharmacy.

- ✔ Ask for a single-dose vial when you have vaccinations that's not preserved with the form of mercury called thimerosol.

- ✔ Go to www.mercurypolicy.org to read more about mercury and its effects.

- ✔ Talk to your dentist about the risks if you have mercury amalgams in your teeth.

- ✔ Visit to www.epa.gov/ost/fish to find out which fish are safe to eat. The safest fish tend to be smaller deepwater fish. Larger fish, like tuna, have eaten far too many smaller fish and accumulated all their mercury.

Sounding out smoking

In the 1800s, people used tobacco tea as a purgative. Yep, it's as bad as it sounds: 'Hey, let's go down to the new health spa by the creek, drink down some tobacco tea, and spend the rest of the day vomiting and evacuating our bowels!'

Many of you probably remember the first time you had a secret cigarette with a friend. You probably felt nauseous and sweaty, and you may well have ended up in the bathroom vomiting or with diarrhoea. Tobacco contains several poisons, and the body tries to purge them if you keep on taking it. Nicotine, the main addictive chemical in tobacco, is a drug that irritates and stimulates the gastrointestinal tract, causing heartburn, reflux, and IBS. One of the common outcomes of quitting smoking is constipation. If you're a smoker and have IBS, a little constipation may sound like a great idea right about now.

If you have IBS and want to quit smoking, you may not be able to use nicotine patches, because nicotine causes bowel irritation. Join a group for support or try acupuncture or hypnosis to help you quit and to help decrease your stress, which is probably why you smoke in the first place.

We've heard of people with constipation-predominant IBS using nicotine patches to get their bowels moving. Do not try this! Not only is nicotine an addictive drug, but far gentler ways exist to deal with constipation (we discuss these in Chapter 8).

Finding out about fluoride toxicity

In the 1970s researchers in Holland showed that some people's gastrointestinal symptoms got better when they omitted fluoride from their diet. Without the patients knowing, the researchers then gave them fluoridated water and – lo and behold! – their symptoms relapsed. Because the patients didn't know that the water was fluoridated, the researchers weren't able to blame the symptoms on worry or anxiety about this chemical. Other research shows similar results.

In the UK, the Medical Research Council concludes that fluoride can be intensely irritating to the stomach but that, for most people, the amount of fluoride found in drinking water is not likely to cause gastrointestinal effects. However, the level at which fluoride becomes toxic isn't far above that found in drinking water – add in a daily dose of fluoride from toothpaste and fluoride from dietary sources and you may begin to swallow enough of the chemical to trigger IBS symptoms.

So what can you do if you want to try cutting down on fluoride to see for yourself if it helps you?

- ✔ Add tamarind paste or concentrate to your cooking – it can help eliminate fluoride from the body.
- ✔ Avoid tea and other dietary sources of fluoride, such as seafood, gelatine, and kelp.
- ✔ Be aware of fluoride in dental products – most toothpastes contain fluoride.
- ✔ Contact your local water board to check fluoride levels in your water supply. Only about 10 per cent of the UK's water supply contains fluoride, although natural fluorine occurs in many other areas.
- ✔ Check any medicines you're taking, as some – such as fluoxetine – contain fluoride.
- ✔ Give non-stick cookware a miss.
- ✔ Use bottled water that's fluoride-free.

Managing magnesium levels

Magnesium is an important mineral involved in the transmission of nerve signals and the activity of muscles, especially in the gastrointestinal tract. When absorbed into the bloodstream magnesium whizzes around to relax the muscles of your bowel. But if your body doesn't absorb it properly and it remains within the bowel itself (as some magnesium salts do), your gut may start dancing because the magnesium increases the amount of fluid retained in the faeces, distending the bowel and irritating the lining. This isn't usually a problem with foods containing magnesium, as levels of the mineral in food aren't very high. But it can occur with magnesium supplement or magnesium-based digestive aids and it explains why several laxatives contain magnesium. But although it may be good for constipation-predominant IBS, it can be a trigger for diarrhoea-predominant IBS.

Homing in on a Holistic Theory of IBS

We spend most of this chapter trying to pick apart IBS and find individual factors that may trigger or cause the condition. But this doesn't take into account the complexity of human life – the individual mix of a person's genetic make-up, biology, psychology, environment, social life, exercise routines, diet, and every other ingredient that makes you *you*. Not only has your individual mix made you the person you are – it has also made your bowel sensitive.

You're unlikely to stumble on just one factor that you can magically right to restore your bowel to glorious health. If you change one aspect of your life, you may well push another out of balance and so put your sensitive gut under a different sort of stress.

Instead, the path forward is likely to involve considering the whole. How is your home–work balance? (In Chapters 14 and 15 we talk about living your home and work life with IBS.) What combination of exercise, activity, and rest is right for you? (We focus on exercising with IBS in Chapter 11)What is the best balanced diet that suits you? (Nibble on Chapter 10 for more on diet.) Pay attention to the whole of your life and how you pull it all together. Think about how you can adapt every part of your life to encompass the needs of your body.

Leaving No Trigger Unturned

As if the rest of the information in this chapter weren't enough, we need to fill you in on a few additional known triggers for IBS symptoms:

✔ **Drinks:** Alcohol (which we discuss in Chapter 10), coffee, tea, and carbonated drinks can contribute to IBS, mostly because of irritating chemicals in these liquids.

✔ **Gas and bloating:** Someone with a cast iron gut may have no reaction to a bit of gas, whereas the same amount of gas can trigger a bout of pain or diarrhoea in a person with IBS.

✔ **Hormones:** As we explain in Chapter 5, women experience more symptoms of IBS than men. Some men do get IBS, and so female hormones clearly don't shoulder the entire blame for IBS. But female hormones stir up the bowel just enough to be a real problem for many women.

✔ **Laxative use:** A history of laxative overuse can lead to chronic bowel irritation and the loss of the body's normal reflex to move the bowels.

✔ **Low fibre in the diet:** Low intake of fibre can cause constipation that scrapes and irritates the intestines. A full intestinal load can then trigger an episode of IBS diarrhoea.

Chapter 5

Who Gets IBS and Why

In This Chapter

▶ Finding out who has IBS

▶ Focusing on women

▶ Thinking about cultural influences

▶ Coping with what life throws at you

*A*t some time or another, everyone suffers from bowel upset, which may be due to overeating, overindulging in alcohol, too much excitement, flu, food poisoning, or a parasite infection. IBS is diagnosed only when the upset becomes a permanent fixture. (We focus on different diagnoses in Chapter 7.)

Everybody is susceptible to IBS. For example, a severe bowel infection at any age may be a cause of IBS. In Chapter 4, we explain how a bowel infection can lead to IBS.

Fifty per cent of people with IBS began having symptoms in childhood, and most people with IBS develop the condition before age 35. If you develop symptoms of IBS after age 40, the chances of the problem being inflammatory bowel disease (which we talk about in Chapter 4) or cancer are greater. Your doctor, quite rightly, wants to rule out these other conditions before diagnosing IBS. IBS very rarely develops in old age.

Stating the Statistics

The harsh fact is that as many as one in ten people may have IBS. The number is probably even bigger, as many people, especially those with milder symptoms, don't seek medical advice or get a proper diagnosis. IBS is much more common in women than men: 65–70 per cent of people diagnosed with IBS are women. But researchers admit that most of the studies and surveys done on IBS focus mostly on women, so current statistics may be biased. Maybe men just aren't great at admitting they have a problem. In the section 'Singling Out Women', later in the chapter, we discuss some of the theories that attempt to explain the female predominance of IBS.

Wishing for a cure

As we discuss throughout this book, IBS has a significant negative impact on schooling, work, and the social life of people with the condition. Doctors admit that they don't have enough tools (by which they mean medications) to treat IBS properly. And people with IBS agree: One of the most vocal complaints from people with IBS is that no drug exists to make the condition go away.

We talk about the pharmaceutical treatments for IBS in Chapter 8, where we discuss the pros and cons of treating a condition that has no definitive cause with medications that are often designed to suppress symptoms. In Chapters 9–13, we give you an array of non-drug tools and remedies to help alleviate your symptoms.

Up to 12 million British people have IBS. Surveys show that about 10 per cent of the population of Western countries admit to the condition, but there may be even more people who keep their symptoms to themselves.

About 80 per cent of people with IBS-like symptoms never go to a doctor about their symptoms. Doctors and researchers refer to these people as *mild cases,* but that description may not be entirely true. Although a number of the sufferers probably do have only mild symptoms, others carry on in silence, read books like this one to try to get help, haunt Internet chat groups (sometimes getting questionable advice), and still don't get any better.

Only about 20 per cent of people with IBS actually pick up the phone, make an appointment, and show up at their doctor's surgery. Of all the patients who are referred to gastrointestinal specialists, a very large number (an estimated 20–50 per cent) have symptoms of IBS. Just imagine how that percentage would grow if more people with IBS symptoms actually went to their doctor.

Here's another statistic worth chewing on: In economic terms, diagnosing and treating IBS in the UK may cost the NHS more than £1.5 billion per year. The costs due to time off work and lost productivity greatly increase that total.

Singling Out Women

The female bowel and the male bowel are essentially identical. Yet in the Western world, twice as many women as men admit to having IBS, and women go to the doctor four times as much as men for their IBS symptoms. Men with IBS symptoms often won't even admit to having the condition when presented with a health questionnaire. We know from personal clinical experience that many men under-report their health symptoms. The discrepancy between the occurrence of the condition and reporting makes it difficult to identify the reasons why one gender may be more vulnerable to IBS.

Grappling with the gender gap

You may wonder why more women than men get IBS, but we have a few even bigger questions: Why are more women than men diagnosed with diseases such as depression, chronic fatigue syndrome, and *fibromyalgia* (a condition that causes chronic muscle pain and tiredness)? Why do surveys show that women take more medication and get more surgery compared with men? And when you look at the pattern of visits to doctors in general, why do women seem to go far more often than men?

Here is what we think:

✔ Women are generally more interested than men in their health. Women's interest is fostered by a society that accepts that women worry about health. Despite the gender equality debates of recent decades, the macho image persists. Men who show concern about the health of themselves or their family are often viewed a little suspiciously, as though they should merrily laugh off pain and be as unbothered by a lump or bump as they are by a broken fingernail.

✔ Women's interest in health is bolstered by the huge amount of information on health targeted at women as the 'gateholders' of family health, through magazines and other media. Health campaigns often ignore men as a target.

✔ Women have far more opportunities to talk to health professionals when they access services such as:

• Family planning: Women usually see a doctor or nurse to discuss contraception. But for men the most widely used family planning method – condoms – can be purchased in pharmacies and even petrol stations, where men aren't likely to chat with health professionals.

• Cancer screening: All women of a certain age in the UK are called up for NHS cervical smear tests and mammograms, but no routine, countrywide calls take place to screen men.

• Antenatal care: Although an enthusiastic husband or boyfriend may accompany a woman attending antenatal appointments, as the child grows it is often the mother who sees a raft of healthcare professionals when she takes her child for vaccinations and development checks. In the UK women still tend to be in charge of their children's health.

With these points in mind, you're probably not surprised to discover that more women than men tend to know more about, and are more likely to be diagnosed with, conditions that take time to pinpoint.

Women have many more opportunities than men to receive services from healthcare professionals. When you're lying on the examination couch, awaiting a smear test or a check for breast lumps, your doctor is bound to ask how you feel. If you mention you have gas and bloating and several bowel movements a day, you increase your likelihood of being diagnosed with IBS and (we hope) of getting treatment.

Meanwhile, your partner may be sitting in the waiting room – or the surgery toilet – with the very same symptoms, but chances are he doesn't make a special visit to the surgery to talk about his bowel habits.

Our analysis may be a bit simplistic, but we believe that if men had to go to the doctor every time they wanted to buy condoms, they may talk more about how they're feeling, take more medications, have more surgery, and be diagnosed with a lot more diseases.

The incidence of IBS in men remains about the same from age 20 to 70 years. In women, IBS peaks at around 20 to 30 years of age and then drops as low as in men when women reach menopause – providing they don't take hormone replacement therapy (which we discuss in the section 'Cycling symptoms of IBS', later in this chapter). The drop is an indication that a woman's hormones have an impact on her bowel. At menopause, when the surges of hormones finally stop, so do some of the symptoms of IBS. We discuss the IBS–hormone connection in the section 'Honing in on hormones', later in the chapter.

Realising that the gender gap starts early

Before puberty, girls and boys experience the same incidence of IBS. After puberty, the numbers change, and girls start to visit the doctor more often with symptoms of abdominal pain.

Why the change? After puberty girls quite naturally tend to be more sensitive about their body and its functions (or malfunctions) and less willing to discuss the nitty gritty details with parents. If your daughter has a painful abdomen, it can be hard to work out whether the problem is intestinal or gynaecological. You can't just toss a coin, and so you go to the doctor – and your daughter's cycle of doctors' visits begins. If your son has the same complaint, you at least rule out the gynaecological problem; in fact, you probably give him an over-the-counter medication for a tummy upset and assume he'll be fine.

Children with IBS often experience weight loss because they stop eating in an attempt to reduce their symptoms. Some children avoid talking about their symptoms, especially if their family frowns upon 'bathroom talk'. IBS can be very frightening for children, as they generally do not have access to the medical information that adults have. We discuss IBS in children in more detail in Chapter 16.

Putting up with pain

Studies show that women tolerate more pain compared with men. For example, women tolerate thrusting their hands into ice-cold water better than men do. Perhaps this isn't a big surprise: After all, women can force an 8-pound baby through an opening that before and after the event is no wider than a few millimetres. Challenge a man to think about shoving something that size down the urethra of his penis and he almost passes out at the thought of it.

Despite being more used to pain (many women have to deal with menstrual pain every month, after all), and perhaps being more able to put up with pain compared with men, women report a lot of pain with IBS – all evidence of what a severe condition it can be.

An American survey of 700 general practitioners and gastroenterologists and 1,000 women with IBS found important information on how big an impact IBS has on women's lives: As many as 40 per cent of women experienced significant abdominal pain that was intolerable and not relieved by any treatment they tried. Their pain made them miss days from work and meant they had to curb social activities and limit their travel.

Another piece of research found that abdominal pain was the symptom of IBS that women rated as causing the most disruption to their normal life. The women in the study said that abdominal pain occurred at least minimally on 62 per cent of days.

Although these are US studies, the statistics are probably very similar for women in the UK. In other words, more often than not women with IBS have to find ways to get on with all the activities we need to do every day – working, cleaning, organising – while coping with a certain degree of pain.

Women with IBS take three times as many sick days as their female co-workers who don't have IBS. They also find that IBS can limit the sort of activities they can manage at work, IBS can even make a difference in a woman's choice of career – for example, having IBS can make it very difficult to hold down a job as a cab driver or a police officer.

Homing in on hormones

Why, then, do women have more IBS and, apparently, more sensitive bowels than men? During evolution, did having a sensitive bowel (called *visceral hypersensitivity*) somehow offer a woman a greater chance of survival ? Or is there something different in a women's bowel that causes the greater sensitivity?

The symptoms of IBS are often worse during a woman's menstrual period. So perhaps IBS is related to hormones. However, 40 per cent of women with IBS report having painful periods, and 50 per cent have PMS – not very different from the statistics for women who don't have IBS. Researchers agree that hormones are not the cause of IBS. After all, men don't have periods, but some men certainly do have IBS. But the hormonal fluctuations of the monthly menstrual cycle may still influence IBS, for example by altering the pain threshold or aggravating other symptoms.

Linking hormones and constipation

The two major female hormones are oestrogen and progesterone. Research shows that oestrogen slows down the gastrointestinal tract, which translates into food travelling at a slower rate. A slower transit time means constipation and bloating, especially if you don't take in enough fibre and liquids. Men have very little oestrogen on board, have a faster gastrointestinal tract, and seem to suffer less from constipation compared with women.

Progesterone, which is more dominant in the second half of the menstrual cycle and produced in massive amounts during pregnancy, also makes the bowel more sluggish. Anyone who has been pregnant can vouch for that (although other factors at work during pregnancy cause constipation too). The question is: Do oestrogen and progesterone make the gut more sensitive? Researchers don't have an answer to this question, but the speeding up and slowing down of the bowel due to fluctuations in levels of oestrogen and progesterone may certainly be enough to make an already sensitive bowel react.

Cycling symptoms of IBS

To make a woman's period start, oestrogen and progesterone drop naturally and dramatically, in unison. This major shift in hormones marks the onset of the worst phase of IBS symptoms in women. Diarrhoea, gas, bloating, and pain are much worse during this time of the month.

Postmenopausal women on hormone replacement therapy (HRT) experience twice as much IBS as women not on HRT. Women on HRT experience IBS much like women who are still having their periods.

Holly believed she'd suffered mild IBS for at least ten years. She was aware of her trigger foods and avoided them. She was also aware that her symptoms worsened around the time of her menstrual cycle. As menopause approached, she went to see her general practitioner for advice and decided to try HRT, which she took religiously. Within a month, Holly was experiencing more urgent diarrhoea and increased cramping. She attributed the change to starting HRT and stopped taking it, making particular efforts instead to follow a soya-rich diet and get plenty of exercise. She was greatly relieved that her IBS symptoms settled down again, and her mild menopausal symptoms also seemed to settle.

With or without IBS, most women admit to increased constipation and bloating the week before their period. Then, with the period comes several days of looser bowel movements. For women who have PMS and severe menstrual cramps, the bowel and hormones seem to create a conspiracy of discomfort and pain. Women with IBS have symptoms all month, but their IBS constipation symptoms are worse the week before the period and jumbled up with their PMS symptoms, whereas their diarrhoea symptoms are worse during their period – mixed in with period pain and cramps.

Fifty per cent of women who visit their doctors about the combination of abdominal pain, pain during intercourse, and painful periods also have symptoms of IBS.

Planning for your period

Research tells us that women are more likely to have worsening IBS symptoms before and around their periods. Some people suggest that women on the contraceptive or birth control pill have fewer symptoms of IBS, but so far no studies prove this association.

The good news is that if you know that you're more susceptible to IBS symptoms immediately before and during your period, you can use that information wisely. You can make plans based on knowing your menstrual cycle and knowing that you don't want to be stuck on an long train or plane journey, or looking after a houseful of visitors, in the middle of the worst week in your month. Sometimes you have no choice but to cope with symptoms in difficult situations. Check out our suggestions for managing the demands of family and friends, and ideas for IBS-friendly travel in Chapter 14.

Avoiding misdiagnosis

Misdiagnosis can occur when IBS causes severe abdominal pain that is easily confused with other very serious conditions. Earlier in the chapter we pointed out that women can find it particularly difficult to unravel which symptoms are caused by IBS and which are gynaecological in origin. The difficulty may explain why one study found that women with symptoms of IBS are often referred to a gynaecologist rather than to a gastroenterologist. Another study that researched women at a gynaecology clinic who experience pelvic pain found that more than half of them showed symptoms of IBS. After the clinic completed all the necessary testing and investigations, the study found that only 8 per cent of the women with IBS also had a true gynaecological problem.

For example, women with IBS can have pain during intercourse, which makes them (and everyone else, including their doctors) think that they have gynaecological problems. If you have this problem and your gynaecologist doesn't remember their training in gastroenterology, they may miss a diagnosis of IBS and send you off to surgery. The result, according to concerned health advocacy groups, is that surgeons are more likely to perform unnecessary operations – usually gynaecological – on women with IBS. For example, hysterectomy and ovarian surgery occur more often in women with IBS than in women without IBS, but may do little to calm symptoms.

Penny's GP referred her to a gynaecologist, who found she had ovarian cysts. The gynaecologist believed that the cysts may be responsible for the pain that accompanied Penny's diarrhoea. Penny had experienced IBS symptoms for several years and was hopeful that the removal of the cysts would bring an end to the IBS. The surgery was deemed successful, but to Penny's dismay, her diarrhoea symptoms worsened, as did the cramping and bloating. She also developed *vaginal thrush,* or yeast infection.

Convinced that something had happened during the surgery, Penny quizzed her doctor about the steps in the procedure. Penny discovered that she'd been given a strong antibiotic during surgery to prevent infection, and she realised that the antibiotic had destroyed the friendly or 'good' bacteria in her gut and vagina, allowing *candida* yeasts to take over and cause vaginal thrush. Penny's doctor recommended a course of *lactobacillus.* Penny was amazed that her IBS symptoms actually improved, but it took ovarian surgery to find an effective treatment for her IBS – a dose of gut-friendly bacteria!

The most effective way to take adequate doses of *lactobacillus* and other friendly bacteria is to swallow prepared capsules or powders known as *pro-biotic supplements,* which you can get from health food shops and pharmacies. You can also take in *lactobacillus* by eating plenty of vegetables (especially root veg such as carrots) and fruit, and yoghurts or pre-packaged fruit drinks containing the bacteria. The bacteria live on the surface of the veg and fruit, so gently wash your veg but don't scrub or peel them. You need several large portions of fruit and veg every day to get an adequate dose of friendly bacteria, so if your symptoms don't respond you may want to try a course of probiotic supplements to top up levels.

People with IBS have higher rates of surgery than the general population. Researchers examined almost 90,000 patient records, which showed that patients with IBS suffered three times the normal rate of gall bladder surgery and twice the rate of appendicectomy and hysterectomy. Patients with IBS also underwent a 50 per cent higher rate of back surgery.

Remember how modern medicine works: specialists tend to recommend the sort of treatments that they've been trained to use. If you have abdominal pain and go to a surgeon, you have a greater chance of being offered an operation, whereas if you see a dietician you're more likely to get a thorough analysis of what you eat. If you don't want to end up in surgery – and who does? – we recommend that you talk everything through very carefully with your GP first. Ask her if you can be referred to a gastroenterologist, dietician, or nutritionist who knows about IBS. If you do end up in the clutches of a surgeon, check the surgeon's advice back with your GP and even consider asking for a second opinion if you still have any doubts about going under the knife.

Linking IBS and Your Upbringing

Sometimes drawing the line between symptoms that are mild IBS or a variation of normal is tricky. Similarly, what one person considers to be a severe illness another may consider a minor disruption. Each individual gauges his or her condition in a different way and comparisons are difficult.

One of the strongest influences on how we feel about our bodies, and the way they function or go wrong, is the culture in which we are brought up. Our families teach us as children (often subconsciously by their actions) what to accept as normal. Perhaps as a child your parents insisted that you open your bowels once a day, at a set time every morning. Or perhaps in your household everyone accepted that you went to the bathroom whenever you needed to go, even if that meant several times a day and interrupting whatever you were doing.

Whatever you grow up with as 'normal' affects how you react when IBS gets its grip on your daily routine. A person with a set 7 a.m. appointment with the toilet may be more disturbed by a frequent need to open their bowels or days of constipation than a person who is happy to respond to their gut whenever nature calls.

School routines also play a part. Many teachers insist that you visit the toilet only at set times. Luckily, our bodies generally learn to work to a timetable and to a degree you train your bowel into certain habits. But IBS can play havoc with the classroom routine: If a teacher doesn't understand the needs of a child with IBS, the child soon believes that an urgent need to visit the loo is abnormal. Some unkind teachers even make the child feel that he's deliberately causing trouble. A child may believe that IBS is socially unacceptable and that by having the condition he's 'bad' or a nuisance; conversely, those with an understanding and flexible teacher may not think too much of frequent loose motions.

Whether we perceive sensations as abnormal or just a nuisance depends on what we discover from those around us. Pain is a good example. No one is arguing here about severe pain, but think about those little bumps, bruises, and niggles that are a part of everyday life. Although some people seem able to brush aside tweaky muscles or minor trauma without stopping for breath, others are deeply distressed and howl in agony at the tiniest scratch. How you see others around you react and what your family considers acceptable determines, at least in part, how you react. If you grow up with your dad or granny screaming and weeping when they stub their toes or get a mouth ulcers, then it is likely that you too howl at the slightest trauma. But if you're surrounded by the 'stiff upper lip' sort of family role models, you're more likely to swallow hard and hide your agony.

IBS affects people around the world but you may have problems if you try to swap notes with someone who has IBS on the other side of the globe, because their culture may give them a very different perspective on their condition. A study recently compared IBS sufferers in Crete, Greece, and in Linköping, Sweden. It found that although individuals were troubled with the same disease, their different cultural environments meant that they thought their everyday life was affected in very different ways. The Cretan people, especially the women, reported that IBS had much more effect on their mental health (causing depression or anxiety, for example) and everyday activities, than on the Swedish people.

Everybody's IBS means different things to them. Pain is totally subjective – as are many other symptoms. You need to interpret symptoms against a background of the individual's life and culture. No one other than the person with IBS can really know what their symptoms are like, or how important they are.

You may find it helpful to bear in mind a famous definition of pain, made by a specialist nurse Margo McCaffery a few years ago. She said that 'pain is what the person experiencing the pain says it is, and is as bad as the person says it is'. A similar definition can be made for many IBS symptoms. If only all health professionals listened to, and believed in their patients' views as sympathetically.

People who have experienced severe psychological distress have a higher rate of anxiety and depression, as well as a higher rate of IBS. Bottling up problems, because you have understood that in your society these things ought to be kept quiet, may just add to your stress and make your IBS worse. We focus on stress in Chapter 12, where we give practical and useful tools to help you deal with emotional and stressful issues.

Ananya developed IBS after a trip to Kerala in India for her cousin's wedding. When she asked her GP why she'd got IBS, her GP suggested that it may have been triggered by the episode of gastroenteritis she experienced when out there. However, when the doctor questioned Ananya more closely, Ananya admitted that she'd suffered from bloating and excessive gas for years. Her symptoms got worse whenever she stayed with her parents, who cooked all her favourite spicy foods and curries. Although she loved going home, she found the visits especially stressful because she had to entertain distant relatives and often share a bedroom and toilet with people she didn't know well. Ananya's GP explained that although the exact cause of her IBS was a mystery to medical science, she need look no farther than the family around her to understand why her symptoms were bad.

Although many causes of stress can aggravate IBS, one cause you shouldn't have to deal with is the stress of leaving the house when you have IBS. When you plan an outing, call ahead to find out about the toilet facilities available, or do an Internet search to see if a branch of a well-known cafe or coffee shop exists in the area – they almost always have a customer toilet, so you can pop in to use the loo if necessary. If you can feel assured that your destination has easily accessible facilities, your stress about leaving the house may diminish. We provide lots more tips for getting out of the house in Chapter 14.

Taking Action

Although understanding how our environment and culture influence IBS is vital, humans do have the less than helpful habit of only looking outwards and blaming events on things around us when we become ill. Scientists don't fully understand the cause of IBS, but they generally agree that events in life – whether a major exam, a nasty infection, or a small argument – can and do make symptoms appear or get worse.

Seeing yourself as a victim, out of control, and damaged by outside events won't help you get on top of your IBS, but taking a look at how your personal beliefs and attitudes shape your experience of IBS may. As soon as you understand the ways in which your own actions or thoughts may be making the symptoms worse, you can start to make changes. Reading this book can help you to do so and as a result, gain control over your IBS.

In 2000, a study of 239 women with gastrointestinal problems looked at how they coped with chronic pain and if they actively worked on solving their problems. It may seem like common sense, but the researchers proved that the better your coping skills, the better the outcome. Using a series of question-naires, the researchers rated the women as having good or poor coping skills. Those who coped well made fewer visits to their doctors and experienced less psychological distress and pain. The women rated as having poor coping skills felt helpless and powerless in the face of their condition. Those women experienced more psychological distress, visited their doctor more frequently, and were bedridden more often.

You can do a lot to improve your own coping skills, and in Chapter 12 we offer a few suggestions to help you take charge of your problems.

Part II
Getting Medical Help

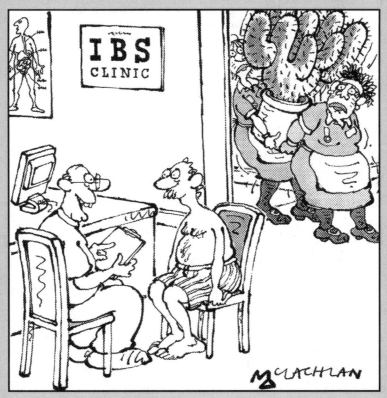

'The good news is we have discovered the most _amazing_, herbal suppository for IBS relief, but the_re_ is one slight drawback . . .'

In this part . . .

Although IBS is not a disease managed on a day-by-day basis by a doctor, it's important to find a doctor you can work with to make sure you have the right diagnosis. In this part, we guide you in what questions to ask your doctor to help you work out if he or she will really be able to help you.

We then explain the various tests your doctor should run to ensure a proper diagnosis. These tests are designed to rule out conditions whose symptoms may resemble IBS, such as gluten intolerance, lactose intolerance, and inflammatory bowel disease.

To treat the symptoms of IBS, you may wonder about the benefits and drawbacks of prescription and over-the-counter medications. We offer an in-depth look at the pros and cons of these options so you and your doctor can decide what's best for you.

Chapter 6

Working with Your Doctor

In This Chapter

▶ Knowing when to see your doctor

▶ Asking the right questions

▶ Dealing with embarrassment in your doctor's surgery

▶ Helping your doctor help you

Maybe you've been worried about your symptoms for a long time but have been too scared or embarrassed to get help. Perhaps you suspect that you have IBS and want a diagnosis. Or maybe you've searched the Internet for information and already tried simple remedies. You've been trying your hardest to do what you can but now it's time for teamwork. In this chapter we look at how your doctor can help you.

Your doctor should take the time to explain IBS, the treatments available, and the impact of triggers on your symptoms. A good relationship with your doctor doesn't just make you feel warm and fuzzy; it actually translates into needing fewer visits to the surgery. The words you really want to hear from your doctor are: 'I know about IBS and I think that I can help you'.

In Chapter 7, we show you how your doctor diagnoses IBS. That chapter assumes you have a good doctor to go to who understands IBS. In this chapter we help you find that good doctor.

We actually think that the most important step you can take in managing your condition is to take charge of your own body. If you've read all of this book, you may know more about IBS than most doctors. You understand how to read your body signs, and you know what pulls you into IBS symptoms and how to avoid those pitfalls. A knowledgeable and independent patient is actually what most doctors want. So in this chapter, we also encourage you to take charge of your own health.

Knowing When to Get Medical Help

The main reasons people with IBS go to a doctor are much the same as with other conditions:

- For an initial diagnosis
- For advice on managing their condition
- For a second opinion
- For emergency care
- For prescriptions

In this section, we explain the symptoms that often compel someone with IBS to seek medical attention, as well as the importance of being proactive about your health.

 In an ideal world, you get support and advice as soon as any unusual medical symptoms arise, and definitely by the time you're aware that your IBS symptoms are ongoing rather than a short-lived effect of some acute illness. But in the real world, for a variety of reasons, people often delay seeing a doctor. Some people don't get the help they need until their symptoms become unbearable or frightening, or both. In this situation they often go, or are sent by their GP, straight to hospital in a panic that they have a life-threatening condition which needs powerful drugs.

We must stress that this is *not* the way to address your symptoms. Although it may be important to rule out other more dangerous diseases, the basic way to manage IBS is through diet and lifestyle changes. The more severe your symptoms at the time of your first visit to your GP, the more likely you are to be treated with drugs in the hope that these may suppress your symptoms, instead of calmly looking at possible triggers such as the stress in your life or the food you eat, or trying simpler therapies. Drugs for IBS, as we explain in Chapter 8, aren't very effective in IBS – they may help in some instances but can also bring their own side effects to add to your problems.

Sussing out your symptoms before you see a doctor

People are often uncertain, at least at first, whether the gastrointestinal symptoms that we describe in Chapter 3 warrant a trip to the GP. The simple answer is that as soon as your body's functioning gives you cause for concern, or seems different to usual, feel free to talk it through with your doctor.

If your symptoms are mild, or you can relate them to explainable events (indigestion after a blisteringly hot curry, for example), then you may choose to wait a little and see whether the symptoms settle. Alternatively, you may want to read up on your symptoms or explore simple remedies. Remember that symptoms typical of IBS can occur now and then for everyone. Many aspects of daily life, from what we eat to how hard we exercise, can contribute to episodes of loose motions, constipation, bloating, discomfort, and similar problems.

But when symptoms persist or make you feel particularly anxious, the best action is to explore them with your GP. Try not to worry that your GP thinks that your symptoms are trivial or that you're wasting his time (if he does give you this impression, you may want to ask yourself whether he is the right doctor for you, which we consider later in this chapter). If your symptoms are enough to concern you then your GP wants to help. The answer may not be IBS, or any other identifiable condition, but checking is better than fretting. Talking to your GP also helps him to build up a picture (and a written record) of the sort of symptoms you're experiencing. Like pieces in a jigsaw puzzle, this picture may, over time, start to resemble a particular pattern that leads to a clear diagnosis.

Sounding the alarm

Some symptoms do need to be dealt with more immediately, because they are a clue that your problems may not be IBS at all but something more dangerous, like a cancer or a serious infection.

So what should make you seek urgent help? The following alarm symptoms, many of which are *not* actually symptoms of IBS, signal that you need to book an appointment with your GP sooner rather than later. In some instances, such as bleeding, you may even need an emergency appointment.

- ✔ **Abdominal bloating that does not get better overnight:** IBS bloating is usually due to gas, which dissipates overnight. Symptoms that seem like bloating but don't ease at night may be caused by something other than IBS and needs to be checked by your GP.

- ✔ **Bleeding from the rectum:** Rectal bleeding indicates that something other than IBS is going on. As we note in Chapters 3 and 7, rectal bleeding may indicate an inflammatory bowel disease. Some people experience rectal bleeding if they have eaten lots of roughage, such as nuts, seeds, or popcorn; they scrape open a capillary on the wall of the intestine or at the anus. Haemorrhoids may also cause rectal bleeding. Any amount of bright red blood, or dried blood that turns your bowel movements black, is a special cause for concern; it may indicate rapid blood loss from a growth in the bowel or a burst blood vessel in tiny weaknesses in the gut wall known as diverticuli.

✔ The bottom line: If you're bleeding from your rectum, seek immediate medical attention. Don't try to guess the cause for yourself. There may be a simple explanation for what you think is bleeding – for example, eating beetroots can turn your stool red, whereas indigestion remedies that contain the metal bismuth (such as Pepto-Bismol) can turn stools black. But it is vital that you get this important symptom checked by a doctor.

✔ **Difficulty swallowing and food sticking in the oesophagus:** This symptom is usually related to a growth or tumour in the oesophagus and is not the same as feeling that something is in your oesophagus but still being able to easily swallow food, which can be a result of extreme stress or intense emotions.

✔ **Fever:** If you have IBS symptoms and develop a fever, it's not a sign of IBS. Instead, fever is a sign of infection or inflammation. It may indicate inflammatory bowel disease (IBD), diverticulitis (inflammation of tiny out-pouchings of the gut wall), or a bacterial infection in the abdomen or pelvis which needs urgent treatment with antibiotics. Your GP can help you identify the cause of your fever. .

✔ **Night-time diarrhoea:** Diarrhoea that wakes you at night is not a symptom of IBS and must be further investigated. It can indicate inflammatory bowel disease or cancer.

✔ **Stomach or abdominal pain that wakes you up at night:** Although there are many causes of abdominal pain at night that disturb sleep, IBS is not usually one of them. This symptom needs to be checked by your doctor.

✔ **Tenesmus:** this is the feeling that you haven't finished a bowel movement and still need to go, even though all your stool has emptied out. This can be a sign that your rectum and perhaps your large intestine are inflamed, for example as a result of inflammatory bowel disease.

Reviewing red flag symptoms

Some symptoms, which may seem less urgent to you than those on the previous list, are a signal to your doctor that he needs to investigate a little more closely because something serious may be going on. Doctors call these 'red flag' signs.

✔ **Anaemia (low levels of blood in the body, which may show as paleness):** In a patient with symptoms of IBS, anaemia may indicate a slow blood loss from the gut that may not show up visibly in the toilet. It may point to an ulcer or tumour in the intestines and needs investigation.

✔ **Sudden onset in someone over age 40:** Without a history of recent travel or recent use of antibiotics, IBS in a person over 40 is rare and symptoms imply another cause such as a tumour.

✔ **Unexplained weight loss:** Suddenly losing more than four kilograms can be an indication of something much more serious than IBS. Cancer is often the cause of such sudden weight loss. However, a serious infection in the gut can cause such a sudden drop in weight as well through loss of fluids.

Finding the Right Doctor for You

When you have a chronic problem such as IBS it's particularly important that you feel comfortable with your doctor and are happy to work with him. In the UK, you're able to get care on the NHS from any GP you choose, as long as he has space on his list and is willing to take you on. And if you need help from a specialist your GP must give you a choice of which hospital to go to.

So you can 'shop around' a little and find a doctor that is right for you (although the only way to be absolutely sure of seeing the specialist of your choice may be to go privately, which can be very expensive). Even GPs have areas of specialty – ask at your surgery about each of the doctors special interests. Don't panic if your current GP doesn't seem very experienced – IBS is so common that most GPs know about treating it.

Ask your GP directly if he has particular experience of, or interest in, gastrointestinal medicine – he'll be happy to tell you. Or ask the practice manager if any other doctors in the surgery specialise in IBS. If you want to look farther afield, ask friends or colleagues about their doctors and whether they recommend them, or gather practice leaflets from other surgeries and health centres to see what they have to offer.

You don't have to tell your old GP that you're leaving, or give a reason. Simply find a new practice that is able to provide care and the staff there can sort out transfer of the paperwork. But don't make the decision to change doctors lightly – your old GP may have built up a good understanding of you and your medical issues.

Believing in IBS

We talk in Chapter 1 about the way that attitudes to IBS have changed. In the past the lack of scientific evidence to show changes in the gut meant that some health professionals doubted that IBS was a real condition with serious physical manifestations. Fortunately, modern science is slowly providing hints and clues about what is going wrong in your body and IBS has much more credibility than it used to, even if we don't yet have all the answers. These days there's a good chance that your doctor is going to believe everything you tell him about your misbehaving gut. But there may be a few doctors who haven't kept up to date with new knowledge, and if your doctor is one of them he may not put a lot of stock in your symptoms of gas, bloating, pain, and changes in bowel movements.

You want a doctor who is on the same side of the table as you are. You want someone to believe what you say about what you're experiencing. If your doctor discounts the existence of IBS, focusing on your concerns becomes difficult.

If you've any doubts about your doctor's stance on IBS, take your doctor a copy of the Rome III criteria that we show you in Chapter 1 and a completed symptoms questionnaire from later in this chapter. You may also want to take along a general article on IBS that shows the incidence of the condition, from one of the websites we recommend in Chapter 20, as well as a copy of this book, Bringing these solid pieces of evidence about IBS helps persuade your doctor that you're a knowledgeable patient with legitimate concerns about your health. The attitude you want to develop is one of teamwork where you tackle this problem situation together.

Don't be surprised if your doctor doesn't immediately write out a prescription for medication for your IBS – this doesn't necessarily mean that he doesn't believe in your problems. A growing number of doctors and other health professionals are very concerned about the way conventional medicine, with its focus on treatments such as drugs and surgical intervention, handles chronic illness. To help their patients, these professionals are incorporating other therapies into their practice, such as massage, aromatherapy or meditation. A name had been adopted for this type of practice – *complementary and alternative medicine,* or CAM. (We prefer the term complementary because we like to think that these therapies work alongside modern medicine, rather than as an alternative to it.)

Building a Partnership with Your GP

Your greatest chance of effectively managing your IBS comes from good teamwork between you and your doctor. You're the expert about your body, how symptoms affect you, and how different treatments suit you and your lifestyle. And your GP has a range of skills, including knowledge of the research into different treatments, and access to diagnostic and specialist resources, which are key to dealing with your symptoms.

You don't need to share his taste in ties or footwear, or even particularly like him, but it does help if your GP is someone you feel you can work with and trust.

Ask yourself the following questions about your doctor:

✔ Does my doctor really hear what I say and respect my view?

✔ Does my doctor seem to have my best interests at heart?

✔ Do I feel comfortable with, and able to trust, my doctor?

✔ Am I able to tell my doctor when I feel that his advice isn't right for me and I want to look at other options for treatment?

If the answer to any of these is 'No', then you and your doctor may not be able to work well together and you may want to consider changing doctors.

Some people feel intimidated when waiting in a busy surgery. They feel that the doctor has more important things to do than answer questions about strange bowel habits or a rumbling stomach, while dozens of other people (all, no doubt, with severe and imminently life-threatening diseases) queue up waiting for a few precious minutes of the doctor's time. But most GPs we know would be very sorry to think that one of their patient's was thinking this. Try hard not to feel unimportant or hurriedly play down your worries when you do get to see your doctor. Your doctor realises that in coming to the surgery you've something important to say, and he wants to work as hard as possible with you to find out what is troubling you.

Getting over the embarrassment

You may be surprised how often people go to see their GP and leave without asking about what was really worrying them. Many people never even get as far as the doctor's surgery. They're so embarrassed about their problems that they simply prefer to keep it to themselves and suffer in silence. This is especially true for people living with conditions such as IBS who find it diffi-cult to talk freely about their bowel movements. They let their emotions rule and feel weak, dirty, or unacceptable, instead of just seeing their symptom as a natural variation of a biological process. They may even feel guilty and believe that their symptoms are a result of something they have done. Maybe you bought this book because, like them, you want information about IBS but don't want to talk to anyone about it.

Although these are very common reactions, they aren't helpful. Your doctor isn't going to judge you – he is there to work with you. Although what is happening to you may seem horrible or gross, nothing you can say shocks, surprises, or upsets your doctor. The opposite is true – the more you open up to your doctor and spell out clearly what is going on, the happier your doctor is. And if you still can't overcome your awkwardness, why not come right out with it and tell your doctor that you're having problems explaining things because you feel embarrassed? That may diffuse your tension, and it certainly makes your doctor aware that you have issues that he needs to tread carefully through.

When you see a doctor for your IBS, it's very important to be specific, detailed, and yes, even graphic. Simply saying, 'There's something wrong when I go to the bathroom,' won't get you very far. If that's your approach, your doctor has to begin the detective work by first finding out whether your bowel or your bladder is the culprit. When that gets sorted out, a long list of questions begins with, 'What's wrong with your bowel?' If you answer, 'I go to the bathroom a lot,' you and your doctor are going to be talking for a long time before you get to the bottom of your problem.

Believe us when we say that your doctor has probably heard it all before, so you don't need to tiptoe around this topic. Just take a deep breath and let it all out. Imagine that you're talking to yourself and don't give it a second thought. Tell your doctor how often you open your bowels, what the motions are like and how long the problem has been going on.

The following sort of summary phrases may help to get you started – adapt them to match your symptoms:

- ✔ 'I have diarrhoea every morning – really loose and explosive stools. Its been going on for the past six weeks'.
- ✔ 'I've been constipated since my summer holiday more than two months ago. I only manage to open my bowels very few days and then the motions are very hard and cause a lot of pain'.

This gives your doctor lots of points that he can ask you to expand on.

Stating your symptoms

Your doctor's first goal is to diagnose your problem. In order to establish a diagnosis, your doctor starts by asking you to tell him all about your symptoms. Just give him your story, keeping in mind the Rome III Diagnostic Criteria for IBS that we list in Chapter 1.

Here's an example of how your speech may go:

> *On and off, but for about 12 weeks, my bowel movements have changed in frequency and appearance. I get constipated for a few days and have hard, lumpy stools. Then I have diarrhoea, which starts out soft then turns watery by the end of the day. I have about six movements a day for a few days. I have bloating and abdominal pain after I eat, and often the abdominal pain goes away when I have a bowel movement. I also pass mucus in my bowel movements, but I haven't seen any blood. The pain and the bowel movements sometimes keep me from going to work or out at night.*

Your doctor probably then asks a lot more questions that probe into:

- How often the symptoms occur
- Whether you can relate the severity of your symptoms to any other events in your life
- Whether you've tried any simple remedies and how the symptoms respond to these treatments
- Whether you've any other medical problems at the moment
- Whether anyone else in the family has had bowel problems

In asking these questions, your doctor tries to build up a pattern and match this to the typical patterns of symptoms found in a variety of diseases. This is how doctors go about making a diagnosis. They don't look for a 100 per cent match with the textbook description of IBS, because everyone's IBS is slightly different. Instead, they search for enough of a pattern to make IBS likely and guide which tests and investigations may help.

As we explore in Chapter 3, the common symptoms of IBS are very variable.

Ready, steady, flow! Noting when symptoms started

When your IBS symptoms started is an important piece of your story. It's one thing if you've had these symptoms on and off since childhood and quite another if your symptoms followed a camping trip or a holiday to India which gave you a dose of gastro-enteritis. IBS can follow such an infection but this 'post-infectious IBS' is a category all of its own and is a lot easier to nail down than symptoms that just seem to come out of the blue. (See Chapter 4 for a discussion of post-infectious IBS.)

Mike's case helps us see that sometimes, just by telling your doctor specifically when your IBS symptoms started, the two of you can identify what may have caused or triggered them. We discuss possible causes and triggers of IBS in Chapter 4. Following is a brief overview of the reasons why IBS symptoms may occur:

- **Bowel infection:** Food poisoning, travellers' diarrhoea (bacteria or parasites), and other infections of the gut including viral infections like gastric flu can irritate the bowel, causing incomplete digestion of food and symptoms of IBS.
- **Symptoms after taking antibiotics:** Diarrhoea and/or constipation are common after taking an antibiotic, which can alter the types and numbers of bacteria living in the gut, wiping out the 'friendly' bacteria and leading to overgrowth of harmful micro-organisms.

✔ **Radical change in diet:** Eating lots of dairy, wheat, or fruit when you aren't used to it can overburden your enzymes and lead to symptoms of IBS.

If you're able to tell your doctor that your symptoms began after any of these situations, diagnosis may be much easier.

Asking questions

You're bound to have a long list of questions that you want to ask your GP, especially if it's early days and you haven't yet been diagnosed with IBS. Bear this in mind before you even make the appointment. Draft out a list of questions, and try to put them into order of priority, but remember that you may not have time to ask them all on your first visit.

Most GPs schedule no more than ten minutes (sometimes only five) for each consultation – hardly enough time to say hello properly. If you know that you've a lot to say and many questions to ask, find out from the receptionist whether your doctor accepts double appointment bookings, to give you twice as long. Most GPs are happy to do this because they prefer to plan in advance for a longer appointment than find they run over schedule.

As morning or afternoon surgery progresses, and emergency cases are slipped into the schedule or problems take longer than anticipated to sort out, your doctor may run late. If you don't want to spend lots of time in the waiting room, try making an appointment first thing in the morning or in the early afternoon as soon as the doctor returns from lunch, before delays have built up.

When you ask questions, your goal is to keep the conversation friendly and not confrontational. The last thing you want is a doctor on the defensive. Having said that, some doctors don't like to answer questions – mainly because of the time constraints they work under. If you have a lot of questions to ask, you may want to ask the surgery receptionist if you can book a double appointment. Or ask your doctor if he can refer you to a good source of information in IBS. If your GP is reluctant to give you the time you need, you may want to think about whether he is the right doctor for you.

The following questions may help you work out whether your current GP is the right person to help you with your IBS:

✔ **Do you have patients with IBS?** This may be the only question you need to ask. If the doctor says that he doesn't have patients with IBS, his answer doesn't make sense when you consider that up to 20 per cent of the population suffers from IBS. If your doctor says he sees nobody with IBS, he may have selective vision and you may want to consider changing GPs.

✔ **What do you think causes IBS?** By reading this book, you're gaining great information about the causes, triggers, and conditions associated with IBS. You probably know more than your doctor, so go easy here. A simple answer like 'We don't know the actual cause, but many triggers involve diet and stress' lets you know that your doctor is on the right track.

Be very wary of a doctor who insists that a specific cause of IBS exists. If you've read Chapter 4, you know that identifying the cause of IBS isn't that simple. Don't be intimidated into believing that *this* doctor is the *only one* who knows the true cause. When it comes to IBS, no absolutes exist.

If your doctor tells you that he knows the specific cause, ask where he got his information or whether that is his personal opinion. He may have observed certain common triggers but these are different from the cause of IBS.

✔ **How do you diagnose IBS?** You've hit the jackpot if your doctor says he goes by the Rome II criteria (see Chapter 1) but investigates alarm symptoms. That statement alone lets you know that your doctor is well informed (and has probably read this book from cover to cover). You also want to know whether he helps to sort out food triggers and food intolerance.

✔ **Do you check patients with IBS for lactose intolerance?** If your doctor says no and that lactose intolerance doesn't cause IBS, you're back to square one. True, lactose intolerance doesn't *cause* IBS, but it's easy to mistake the two conditions for each other. The best way to find out whether you have lactose intolerance is to follow an elimination challenge diet, which we explain in Chapter 7. Other tests such as the hydrogen breath test may also be useful.

✔ **Do you check patients with IBS for gluten enteropathy (coeliac disease)?** If your doctor gets uncomfortable and says he has to leave the room for a minute, you may have a problem. It may mean he is going out to consult his medical dictionary to remind himself what coeliac disease is all about. If he says that coeliac disease occurs in children only and requires a small bowel biopsy to diagnose, you know he is living in the Dark Ages. (We explain the test for this disease in Chapter 7.)

Sometimes, to spare the patient an intrusive test, doctors minimise the importance of coeliac disease. And sometimes, to spare themselves the embarrassment of not knowing about a disease, doctors minimise its importance.

✔ **What do you know about fruit intolerance and IBS?** This subject is not taught in medical school. Many doctors say that fruit is very good for you and does not cause adverse reactions. But as we note in Chapter 4, fruit intolerance can be a very real problem for people with IBS.

✔ **Does *candida albicans* have a role in IBS?** This is a controversial issue which we explore in detail in Chapter 4. Some doctors believe that over-growth of *candida* yeast after gastrointestinal infections and antibiotic use sets up irritation in the gut that leads to symptoms of IBS. But other doctors believe that *candida* plays little or no part in IBS, and focus instead on other triggers and causes. Doctors on both side of the fence may be able to give you what they believe is reasonable scientific evidence to support their view. You must choose what feels right for you. Even if your GP doesn't believe in a role for *candida,* he can support you while you explore this possibility and see for yourself whether taking action against *candida* helps.

✔ **Do food allergies play a role in IBS?** You may be looking for a discussion about leaky gut (see Chapter 3) and the absorption of undigested food molecules into the bloodstream, which are then treated like allergy-causing substances. This is not mainstream medicine, and your GP may not follow this theory. This does not necessarily mean that he is not the doctor for you, but that there remain many unknowns in IBS and not everyone holds the same views. So don't immediately storm out of the surgery and declare your doctor to be an ignoramus. If, after reading this book, you want to find out more about leaky gut and food allergies and your GP can't help you, you may want to get extra information from a naturopath, a CAM practitioner, or a nutritional therapist.

✔ **How do you rule out Crohn's disease and ulcerative colitis?** If you have any of the signs or symptoms of these inflammatory bowel diseases, your doctor explains that a colonoscopy by a gastroenterologist is in order (this test is explained in Chapter 7). He may also say that blood tests are available to help rule out these conditions based on immune factors.

✔ **How do you treat IBS?** The answer you want to hear is that your doctor is willing to work with you to determine what's best for you. What you don't want to hear is that drugs are the only answer.

Your doctor's answers to these questions lets you know whether you can work with him to help diagnose and manage your condition.

Having a physical examination

How thoroughly your doctor examines you depends on how concerned he is about your symptoms, and sometimes how much time he has for the consultation. As a basic minimum he should ask you to lie down on the couch while he makes a brief superficial check, looking at your hands, eyes, and skin, and examining your abdomen.

A physical exam can actually be a very reassuring experience, giving you confidence that every effort is being made to make sure that there's nothing sinister causing your symptoms. Most doctors are comfortable with performing this procedure and strive to make patients feel comfortable as well. What your doctor discovers from very simple physical signs may surprise you.

When your doctor examines you, he looks out for certain physical signs in the following list. Very few GPs have specific training in nutritional medicine, but if yours does he looks out for signs of nutritional deficiency. You can assess your own body and see if the following physical signs apply to you:

- ✔ **Dry, rough, and bumpy skin on the backs of the upper arms** is associated with vitamin A and essential fatty acid deficiency, which may indicate coeliac disease or a problem with the absorption of nutrients from the gut into the body, in leaky gut syndrome (which we talk about in Chapter 3).

- ✔ **Jaundice,** or yellowing of the skin, is not a sign of IBS but may be a clue to a different cause of abdominal pain: liver disease (for example due to gallstones or obstruction of the liver's normally drainage).

- ✔ **Lack of small blood vessels in the whites of the eyes** is a sign of anaemia. This is common in coeliac disease due to problems with absorption of the nutrients such as iron and certain vitamins needed to make blood, and sometimes in severe inflammatory bowel disease where the inflamed lining of the bowel loses blood. Anaemia may also be a sign of dietary insufficiencies when someone follows a very restricted diet in an effort to manage their IBS.

- ✔ **Pale complexion** can be another sign of anaemia.

- ✔ **Rashes** may be caused by fungal infection or food allergies.

- ✔ **Swelling of the abdomen** can be down to many different factors, from the more innocuous such as constipation to the more sinister such as tumours or liver disease.

- ✔ **Tender areas over the abdomen** can indicate trapped gas in the intestines, or inflammation in the gut or surrounding tissues (for example, in Crohn's disease).

- ✔ **Thinning, dry, and brittle hair** indicates a deficiency of essential fatty acids and fat-soluble vitamins such as vitamins A and D.

- ✔ **White spots on the nails** are a sign of mineral (especially zinc) deficiency, which can occur in malabsorption due to leaky gut syndrome (see head to Chapter 3 for more on this syndrome).

The final part of the physical examination is the rectal examination. Many people feel apprehensive about the rectal examination, and it's not a pleasant experience, but it's a very important for ruling out the most ominous cause of a change in bowel habit – cancer of the bowel. It also reveals haemorrhoids (or piles), fissures of the anus, and other reasons to explain how bright red blood may appear on the surface of a bowel movement (people often notice this as bright red blood on the toilet paper after opening their bowels). For men, the rectal exam also gives the doctor the opportunity to examine the prostate gland for size and tenderness.

You can make the rectal examination much easier on yourself if you relax. Your doctor asks you to lie on your side facing away from him and to curl your knees up in the fetal position. You take a deep breath as your doctor slips a lubricated, gloved finger into your anus. Tensing up your anal sphincter just makes the whole experience more uncomfortable. Don't forget that you pass stool much wider than the doctor's finger all the time, and you do it by relaxing the anal sphincter.

A routine physical examination may not reveal any noticeable signs of IBS. As we explain in Chapter 1, IBS is a syndrome without any specific physical manifestations, except maybe some abdominal tenderness or pain on deep pressure. Even bloating, which most people with IBS complain about, is often not really evident to an observer. *You* know that your trousers are much tighter since you ate your last meal, but you'd have to bring before and after measurements to prove it to your doctor.

As your doctor examines you, all the signs of various types of bowel disease race through his mind. For example, weight loss and the paleness of anaemia may be signs of coeliac disease or a cancer of the colon. A very tender abdomen may be a sign that the intestines are inflamed as a result of Crohn's disease or ulcerative colitis. The skill of medicine involves weighing up the possibilities and deciding which diagnoses need to be considered further, possibly with tests or special investigations.

Seeking specialist help

In the previous section, we focus on GPs. In the UK, most people with IBS are looked after entirely by their GPs, sometimes with the help of other health professions in the surgery such as a practice nurse or dietician.

But occasionally a GP may decide to refer someone with suspected or diagnosed IBS to a hospital specialist, usually a gastroenterologist but sometimes a pain specialist or a general physician (hospital doctors who use drugs and other medicines – but not surgery – to treat people with a wide variety of illness from heart attacks to pneumonia to gut problems). Situations that may prompt your GP to refer you include when:

- The diagnosis is in question
- Symptoms don't fit a typical pattern
- Further exploration of triggers and food factors is needed
- Symptoms are particularly severe
- Red flag symptoms exist (we explain these earlier in this chapter)
- Symptoms don't improve despite intense efforts to manage them

Under the NHS 'Choose and Book' system, your GP can help you choose which local hospital specialist or clinic you would like to see. When you've chosen a particular hospital, you may find that you see any one of the doctors working in the gastroenterology team there. Although the consultant usually sees the new patients in clinic, you may find that you see a junior member of the team.

Even if your GP doesn't suggest referral, you can ask your GP to send you to a specialist if you want. But your GP is not under any obligation to comply with your request on the NHS if they don't think that it's necessary or appropriate. In this situation your only options are to seek a second opinion from another GP, or to ask your GP to arrange a private referral to a specialist of your choice.

Most gastroenterologists know about the Rome III Diagnostic Criteria, from hearing about them at conferences, reading medical journals, and discussing the topic with colleagues. Although most people with IBS are looked after in primary care, gastroenterologists do see a lot of people with IBS. Quite often, they're asked to confirm the diagnosis when the GP is uncertain, and initiate management.

Gastroenterologists have access to the latest tests to help diagnose the full range of gastrointestinal diseases and distinguish them from IBS. But they tend to take a fairly conventional approach and may pooh-pooh ideas such as fruit intolerance, food allergies, and *candida albicans*. So you may choose to seek out the view of a CAM therapist at the same time as seeing a gastroenterologist.

Seeing a dietician or nutritionist

You may ask your GP for a referral to a dietician or nutritionist who is knowledgeable in the treatment of IBS to help you sort out your diet. If you're a junk food eater and your fridge is mainly stocked with beer and condiments, you're going to need a lot of handholding. There's a lot of overlap between the work of a dietician and a nutritionist but as a very general rule dieticians tend to work with both the well and those with illness to help them make food choices that improve their symptoms and keep them healthy, whereas nutritionists are more involved with using micronutrients to prevent disease.

Many general practices and health centres have only limited help from dieticians or nutritionists, and you may find it very difficult to get the advice you need unless you're able to pay for a private consultation. Your GP should be able to recommend a dietician and refer you, or you can do some research yourself to find one locally and make an appointment yourself.

A registered dietician is specially trained up to university degree level, particularly to work in hospital and clinical settings, and can advise patients on all aspects of diet. The title 'dietician' is protected by the UK Health Professions Council (HPC); check out their Web site at www.hpc-uk.org. This means that dieticians must be fully qualified and registered with the HPC in order to use the title *dietician,* and must also show that they've kept up to date with their knowledge and skills.

Your GP can recommend a local dietician or the British Dietetic Association (BDA) can supply you with a list of registered dieticians working in private practice in your area. Take a look at their Web site (www.bda.uk.com).

The term 'nutritionist' is not currently protected by the HPC, and so anyone can call themselves a nutritionist, no matter what qualifications, experience, and skills they have. Nutritionists tend to work in a broader range of settings, including health promotion, research, the food industry, and the media. Unless they've undertaken training in dietetics, they aren't specifically trained to provide individualised dietary advice to people who are unwell.

The Nutrition Society is the major scientific and professional organisation for nutritionists in the UK. Members must have a minimum of three years relevant postgraduate work experience in nutrition and hold a university degree in nutrition or a closely related subject.

 A dietician who is also a nutritionist is probably the best person to look for when seeking help with your IBS diet, because he can look both at suitable food choices to control your symptoms, as well as the micronutrients (such as vitamins and minerals), which can help to keep you well. If you haven't ruled out lactose intolerance, celiac disease, food allergies, and *candida* overgrowth, such a person can help you create an elimination diet. In Chapter 10, we talk more about the elimination and challenge diet, which involves avoiding possible offending foods and then reintroducing them to see whether your symptoms return.

A dietician/nutritionist can also talk with you about necessary supplements to help boost your immune system, heal your leaky gut, and eliminate a possible imbalance of bacteria in your intestines.

Seeing a CAM therapist

A wide range of complementary medicines may have something to offer in your efforts to manage your IBS. What you try is up to you, but keep an open mind about how much help they really give you. Only limited scientific evidence exists about the effects of most complementary therapies, and the cost of repeated consultations can soon add up. After all, few GPs refer you for any sort of CAM on the NHS. We give lots more detail about complementary treatments in Chapter 13.

Re this line above, this is very true, but likewise there's only limited data on the effects of conventional treatments for IBS. The medical community can't even agree on whether IBS is a real condition!

Preparing for Your First Appointment

Elsewhere in this chapter, we describe the situations that may prompt you to see a doctor about your IBS symptoms.

If you suspect that you have IBS, you'll probably benefit greatly by taking some responsibility for helping your doctor make a diagnosis. We don't suggest you waltz into the doctor's office and announce, 'I have IBS!' Your doctor may not take kindly to that approach and may even try to prove you wrong. Instead, when you visit your doctor, be prepared to provide concise and complete information about what you're experiencing. Instead of assuming that your doctor is going to ask all the right questions to elicit the right information, take time before you arrive at the surgery to consider what the right information is. In the following sections, we offer our suggestions.

Filling out a questionnaire

Arriving at your doctor's surgery with a completed IBS questionnaire, such as the one we provide in this section, can be very useful. The questionnaire can be a real time-saver in your appointment because your doctor doesn't have to go fishing for information. Instead, he can spend more time telling you what to do for your IBS.

Describe your symptoms by ticking all the points that apply to you.

❑ Abdominal cramping

❑ Abdominal pain on the left side

❑ Diarrhoea

❑ Bloating

❑ Constipation

❑ Straining with a bowel movement

❑ Feeling like your bowel movements aren't complete

❑ Gas

❑ Other _____

How long have you had these symptoms?

❑ A few weeks

❑ About 12 weeks

❑ About six months

❑ Less than one year

❑ Less than five years

❑ Five to ten years

How often do you have these symptoms?

❑ Once a month

❑ Once a week

❑ Every day

❑ Several times a day

❑ Constantly

Do your abdominal cramping and pain subside after a bowel movement?

❑ Yes

❑ Yes, but not completely

❑ Yes, but only after several movements

❑ No

Describe your stools

❑ Mucus in your stools

❑ Blood in your stools

❑ Hard, lumpy stools

❑ Loose, watery stools

❑ Undigested food in your stools

❑ Black colour in your stools

Have you missed time from school or work because of your symptoms?

❑ Yes

❏ No

If yes, approximately how much time? _____

How are you managing your IBS symptoms?

❏ Prescription medication

❏ Acupuncture

❏ Hypnotherapy

❏ Over-the-counter laxatives

❏ Over-the-counter muscle relaxants

❏ Herbal remedies

❏ Other _____

Which of the above have helped your symptoms? _____

Charting your symptoms and diet

In addition to filling out the questionnaire we provide in the previous section, we recommend keeping an IBS diary. Your doctor is unlikely to have time to read your diary in full, but by keeping a diary you can find out a tremendous amount about your symptoms and the possible triggers (which we discuss in Chapter 4). In your IBS diary, try keeping a record of your symptoms, your diet, and your sleep habits. You can also create a list of questions to ask your doctor. Then, before your appointment, you can transcribe your notes into a useful brief summary for your doctor.

The questionnaire is helpful so the doctor can see at a glance the types of symptoms you're experiencing, whereas the diary gives you the opportunity to provide more detail. You can create a daily chart in your diary that lists your major symptoms on the left side and lists the days of the week across the top. For example, you may keep track of the following:

- ✔ **Abdominal pain or discomfort:** For each day, note your level of pain on a scale of 0 to 5.
- ✔ **Bloating:** You can take waist measurements before and after meals and list those on the chart.
- ✔ **Constipation:** Simply note if you have no bowel movements on a given day.

> ✔ **Diarrhoea:** Record the number of episodes each day and describe your diarrhoea (from completely watery to soft).

Save some space to make notes about the type of stool you're having – loose or hard – as well as any other information you think may be helpful.

In addition to your symptoms, write down everything you eat and drink. Pay particular attention to your alcohol intake, and the amount of sugar, dairy, wheat, and processed foods you eat. You may discover connections that you'd rather deny, but if after every Saturday night pizza party with the neighbours you have an attack of IBS, that tells you something.

It may help you to realise that the local Health Protection Units (HPUs), works the same way. Along with local Council Environmental Health Departments and regional Food, Water and Environmental Microbiology Laboratories, these units monitor complaints about food poisoning; if they get enough reports about the same place, they can be fairly certain that the restaurant is serving contaminated food. A similar thing may be happening to you, but in your case, food that is perfectly safe for someone else may be toxic to your body.

Perusing previous test results and family history

If you've seen other doctors in the past about your symptoms, take copies of previous laboratory tests and the results of investigations that have been done (if you have access to these). These results can help your doctor develop a picture of you and your condition.

You may want to ask your parents and grandparents whether they've had bowel problems. These problems may be all too evident, but some people hide their symptoms very well and you need to ask them. As we mention in Chapter 4, IBS is not necessarily passed along in the genes, but it can be triggered by the dietary habits of a family.

Really think about your family gastrointestinal history before going to your doctor. Your parents or family members may have experienced a gastrointestinal disorder but never had a formal diagnosis. So find out about any signs, symptoms, and suspicions of IBS or an inflammatory bowel disease (see Chapter 3) in your family. Give your relatives a call. And if your father's bathroom visits assault your senses on a regular basis, realise that he may be experiencing IBS symptoms. Even if he's not diagnosed, let your doctor know about your dad's habits.

Packing for your appointment

Okay, we've given you lots of assignments to complete before you see your doctor. Here's a handy checklist of the things you need to bring to your doctor's surgery for your appointment:

- ✔ A completed symptom questionnaire
- ✔ A list of questions to ask your doctor
- ✔ A list of medications, supplements, and herbs you are taking (bringing the actual bottles is usually the best way for your doctor to see the dosage and ingredients)
- ✔ Your symptom and food journal
- ✔ A notebook
- ✔ A friend for support and to make sure that you don't forget anything

Chapter 7

Looking into the Problem

• •

In This Chapter

▶ Bringing on the blood tests

▶ Scrutinising scans

▶ Studying your stools

▶ Ruling out other diseases

• •

*W*ith most health problems, your doctor starts the diagnostic process by asking about your symptoms and looking for signs. A *symptom* is something that you say is happening to you – it's a subjective experience you have. A *sign* is something objective that a doctor observes or finds in a physical examination. With knowledge of the symptoms and signs, the doctor conducts *investigations* – she uses certain processes and procedures to diagnose a condition.

But getting an accurate diagnosis for IBS is hard because, like a number of other chronic conditions, IBS is not a disease but a *syndrome* – a collection of symptoms that varies from person to person that doctors (based on current knowledge, at least) can't attribute to a single defining thing wrong with the body. In other words, you don't have the solid lump of a cancerous tumour or the high blood thyroid hormone level of *thyrotoxicosis,* which doctors can easily test for to pinpoint the diagnosis.

Instead of showing a clear identifiable image, the picture that the results of IBS investigations provide is blurry: When you look at it you may think that it's one of several different pictures – there may be a strong hint of bowel disturbance and a suggestion of distension of the bowel, but your doctor may still confuse the overall image for a number of diseases or other syndromes. The more tests you have, the more familiar the picture may become, but this is usually because the tests slowly rule out the subtle details of all those other diseases, syndromes, and conditions. Eventually, nothing else but IBS explains the blurry image, so your doctor rules the condition in.

Sometimes, your doctor can make a diagnosis very easily if you're able to provide a complete picture of your symptoms and medical history. In addition to your current symptoms and past medical problems, a physical exam may be all that is necessary. But in other cases, you may need blood tests, stool tests, a fibre-optic endoscopy, and/or X-rays and other scans, all of which we talk about in this chapter.

Considering Key Investigations

In Chapter 6, we describe the situations that may prompt you to see a doctor about your IBS symptoms, the typical symptoms you may experience, how much your GP can help you, whether your doctor may refer you to a specialist, and which symptoms may need particularly urgent assessment. Now we look at the sort of tests that your doctor may offer.

But first, bear in mind that GPs work in very different ways. How quickly and how far your GP investigates your symptoms and which tests she orders depend on her own experience and interest in the field, the accessibility of gastroenterology services at your local hospital, and the particular interests of the specialists there. Your GP may not know much about IBS, for example, and may swiftly pass you on to the local 'one-stop bottom shop', the cheeky name given to a new NHS service set up by a few enthusiastic gastroenterologists around the UK who promise to carry out all necessary investigations for a bowel problem in just one visit to their clinic – the idea is that you walk out with a diagnosis. St George's Hospital in London and Blackburn Royal Infirmary were among the first to set them up, and their good results have inspired others although these one-stop clinics aren't yet run in every hospital – check with your GP as to whether you can access such a service.

But in other areas you may encounter lengthy waiting lists to see a specialist. However, some GPs who have a special interest in gastrointestinal problems (these 'GPs-with-a-Special-Interest' are sometimes called GPwSIs, or 'Gypsies') get the ball rolling with necessary tests very quickly.

So be prepared to go with the flow. If you're worried that investigations are taking a long time to arrange, talk to your GP and ask how investigations are normally managed locally – in fact, you probably want to ask her this the first time that you go to her to discuss your IBS.

Physical and rectal examination

A full physical examination is important for diagnosing IBS, but not because your doctor is looking for something that enables her to cry 'Bingo!' and instantly declare that you have the condition. The physical examination is normal in IBS so there isn't anything that the doctor can search for in order to identify the disease. Even bloating, which affects most people with IBS, is often not very evident to an observer. *You* know that your trousers feel much tighter since you ate your last meal, but you'd have to bring before and after measurements to prove it to your doctor.

The physical examination is part of the process of ruling out other causes for your symptoms. What your doctor can find out from very simple physical signs may surprise you. Signs such as paleness of the tissues in your mouth and around your eyes may hint at anaemia and blood loss, which is more likely to be a sign of inflammatory bowel disease or a gastrointestinal tumour. Or signs of muscle wasting and vitamin deficiencies may indicate poor absorption of nutrients into the body due to gluten intolerance (coeliac disease).

An essential, if unpleasant, part of the physical exam is the rectal examination. This involves your doctor examining the back passage or anus to feel the surfaces inside. See Chapter 6 for more on the rectal examination.

After taking a thorough history from you and conducting a physical examination, your doctor may be able to reassure you that your bowel symptoms aren't part of a serious disease. Because the condition is so common, most doctors see dozens of people with IBS symptoms, and reassure patients even on the first visit that the condition won't kill them, even if it may be tough going to get the symptoms under control.

Often people avoid going to the doctor to get a diagnosis because they worried they have something awful. However, the stress of *not* having a diagnosis can actually make IBS symptoms worse.

Faecal occult blood test

Another good source of clues about the state of the gastrointestinal tract is the stuff that empties out of it every day – faeces, stool, motions, poo, or whatever term your family likes to use. The faecal occult blood test provides an answer to one particularly important question about this stuff: Is there any blood in the stool? Bleeding into the intestines occurs in a number of conditions such as ulcers, inflammatory bowel disease (ulcerative colitis or Crohn's disease), benign growths in the intestines called polyps, and bowel cancer. Bleeding is not a feature of IBS, so looking for blood rules out other conditions in order to diagnose IBS.

Heavy blood loss from near the top of the gastrointestinal tract may turn the faeces into a black tarry slurry, and blood loss farther down the bowel may appear a fresher, bright red colour. But many of the conditions that cause bleeding cause only a trickle of blood that easily hides in the dark colour of the stool and so passes unnoticed. This is known as occult (or 'unseen') bleeding.

A faecal occult blood test can check for this hidden blood. You can buy faecal occult blood testing kits to use at home, or your GP may provide you with some to use (they may even test a sample for you in the surgery). The test involves scraping a small sample of faeces onto a piece of specially treated paper that contains a reacting chemical. If the chemical comes into contact with blood it changes colour, indicating that blood may be present and that the person may have a problem. You have the result almost immediately. However, make sure that you get help interpreting the results if you do the test yourself, because it may not be entirely reliable for a variety of reasons. For example, bleeding may be intermittent and so missed by a single test. Results from a series of several tests are usually needed to be certain. In addition, a negative result doesn't mean a positive diagnosis of IBS – it just means some other conditions are less likely causes of your trouble.

If the test is positive, your doctor may do further tests to find the source of the bleeding. These include a sigmoidoscopy or a colonoscopy. We discuss both of these tests in the section 'Sigmoidoscopy and colonoscopy', later in this chapter.

Having blood in your stool does not automatically mean that something is seriously wrong with you. You may get an episode of blood in the stool after eating a lot of nuts, popcorn, or other roughage due to a small tear in the lining of the rectum. Blood on the outside of a bowel movement is a common sign of haemorrhoids. However, always talk to your doctor to let her determine whether the blood is a sign of something serious or not.

Blood tests

No blood test can diagnose IBS, but a number of blood tests help in ruling out other conditions. Whether your doctor decides to do blood tests, and how many different samples are needed depends to some extent on your symptoms and what she found when examining you. She may take the blood samples from you herself or send you along to the local hospital to have them done. The blood tests that your doctor may request include some of the following:

✔ **C reactive protein (CRP):** CRP is test that checks the level of a protein that is produced during inflammation. A raised level points to inflammation somewhere in the body. However it doesn't tell you where or why inflammation is occurring because the protein is not specifically produced by just one condition or tissue of the body. So raised levels can mean any of a number of diseases.

✔ **Erythrocyte sedimentation rate (ESR):** The ESR test also indicates whether there's inflammation in the body.

✔ **Full blood count (FBC) and differential:** The FBC test measures the amount of haemoglobin (or oxygen-carrying pigmented protein in the blood cells) and the number of white blood cells zooming around the body. A low haemoglobin level (anaemia) may be a sign of blood loss from a tumour or inflammatory bowel disease. Anaemia may also be a sign of gluten intolerance, where there may be problems absorbing iron and folic acid into the body (these are necessary to build red blood cells). A raised white cell count indicates inflammation and infection as the immune system gears up to tackle an enemy, and the differential shows the proportions of different types of white cells (in particular, during infection a large number of a type of white cells called neutrophils are released).

✔ **Urea and electrolytes (U&Es):** This series of tests measures the levels of salts, such as sodium and potassium, and other chemicals in the body. The test is a good screen of how well your kidneys and liver are working and may occasionally show problems with the bowel (for example, when large amounts of salts are lost during diarrhoea), but should be normal in IBS. If the results are abnormal, your doctor does more tests to find out why.

Blood tests can also check levels of certain proteins that suggest bowel cancer, in particular levels of carcinoembryonic antigen (CEA). But these tests aren't very reliable and doctors don't usually use them as a general screening tool.

It can take a week or two for the results of blood tests to be sent back from the laboratory to your doctors surgery. Once they're available you should make an appointment with your GP so that they can explain to you what the results mean.

Pelvic examination

Being female adds an extra complication to the investigation of abdominal pains and related symptoms. The uterus, ovaries, and fallopian tubes lie in close proximity to the intestines and it can be difficult to be sure where pain is coming from. The pain and pressure from fibroids or ovarian cysts can be similar to IBS pain, may irritate the intestines, and may cause diarrhoea.

Your doctor may decide that it's necessary for her to examine the pelvic organs in order to check whether your womb or ovaries are enlarged or tender. The procedure is very like having a smear test, and although it shouldn't be painful, it can feel a little uncomfortable. The doctor then looks at the cervix and places two fingers into the vagina in order to palpate, or feel, the uterus and ovaries. She may also take a swab and send it to the lab to check for infections (results may take a week or two).

Sigmoidoscopy and colonoscopy

Sigmoidoscopy and colonoscopy are tests done using an *endoscope* – a narrow flexible tube with a mini camera and light source at the end that doctors use to peer deep into the body and look at the inside of the bowel. These procedures are often referred to more generally as *endoscopy*. Endoscopes were used in industry to snake around obstructions in drains and pipes before someone got the bright idea to use them to get a peek inside the human body. Endoscopes have now mostly taken over from X-rays in the field of bowel diagnosis.

Endoscopy of the bowel is usually carried out in a specialised hospital outpatient clinic known as an endoscopy unit but some experienced GPs can carry out these tests. In most cases you're given a sedative before the test to make you relaxed and sleepy but not unconscious, and you're allowed home later the same day. Occasionally a general anaesthetic is recommended.

After thorough lubrication, the doctor inserts the endoscope into your anus. In a sigmoidoscopy, the doctor uses a medium-length tube to view the sigmoid region of your colon (the region just above your anus and rectum). For a colonoscopy, the doctor uses a much longer tube to view the entire colon (see Figure 7–1).

Your doctor works the controls of the endoscope like a virtual reality game, looking directly through the scope or viewing the action on a video monitor, and moving the camera in on suspect sites. She can bend and twist the flexible tube to move around curves in the gut, and can even extend a pair of scissors that can snip off samples of tissue. If the doctor finds polyps – usually benign outgrowths of the intestinal wall – she can snip them off at their base. She can also take still pictures of areas of concern so that she can study them later.

These procedures don't specifically diagnose IBS but they help to rule out the three big Cs: cancer, Crohn's disease, and (ulcerative) colitis, all of which we talk about in the section 'Differentiating Your Diagnosis', later in this chapter. Endoscopy should be normal in IBS

During either type of endoscopy, your doctor looks for several things: polyps, *diverticula* (weak, tiny outpouchings of the wall of the intestine that can fill with debris and become inflamed and infected: see the section 'Barium enema' later in this chapter for more on these), ulcerations, and tumours. Your doctor also looks at the lining of the intestines to determine whether it's healthy or not, whether there seems to be equal blood flow to all sections of the colon, and (by taking samples from the intestinal contents) whether infection or abnormal bowel flora exists.

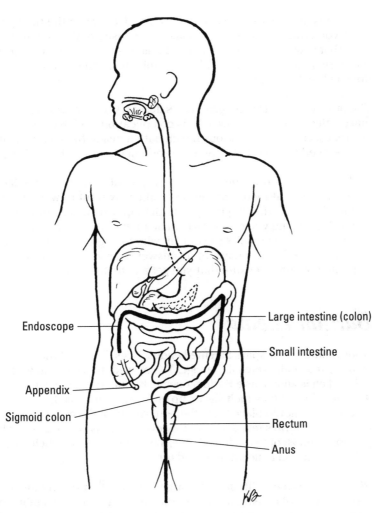

Endoscope

Large intestine (colon)

Small intestine

Appendix

Sigmoid colon

Rectum

Anus

Figure 7–1:
The route
of a
colonoscopy.

In order for your doctor to get a good look at the whole inner surface of the bowel, and not miss any odd little patches, the walls of your intestine must be as free from debris as possible. This means that to have an endoscopy, you must have a near squeaky clean colon. You accomplish this by what is known as bowel preparation. First, you follow a liquid or 'low-residue' diet for up to three days before the test. The night before the procedure you then take a powerful laxative drink. Alternatively, sometimes your doctor can place a medicine into the anal canal to induce the bowel to empty (such as a solid suppository or a liquid known as an enema). Doctors usually schedule endoscopy procedures for first thing in the morning because you can't eat before them either – your gut must be as empty as possible.

The endoscopy procedure itself isn't painful, but even the thought of it may make you cringe. Your medical team is very used to the embarrassment or fears that endoscopy can bring and should help to be able to help you through these. Sigmoidoscopy lasts only a few minutes, and colonoscopy is usually done in less than 30 minutes.

The procedures, although generally safe, carry a very small risk that they may make a tiny hole in the bowel. This complication, which occurs in about 1 in 100 cases, can cause a serious inflammation inside the abdomen and doctors usually need to operate to open the abdomen and sew the hole up again.

At the end of the procedure, your doctor probably knows immediately whether your colon is healthy or not. However, she may want to wait until you wake up fully from sedation (if given) or until biopsy results return from the laboratory before telling you exactly what she found. Some endoscopy services simply send all the results to your GP who then gives them to you. So you may have to wait a few days for an answer. This formality is not designed to frustrate you but to ensure that you get a definite answer.

Barium enema

Before some bright spark invented endoscopes, X-rays of the intestines coated with barium chalk were all the rage. The procedure which allows these X-rays to be taken is known as a Barium Enema. Barium is a metal which is available in a liquid form, and which shows up on X-rays, whereas the term *enema* refers to a chemical liquid placed into the bottom end of the gut. These days, doctors rely on these X-rays less and less. However, in areas where a specialist who performs endoscopies isn't available, a barium enema can help doctors to find polyps, diverticula, ulcerations, and tumours.

Diverticulitis is a condition of the large intestine that occurs mostly in people with a history of constipation. Spending too much time straining to go to the toilet can cause weakness in the wall of the intestine, and your body forms tiny pouches (*diverticula*). These show up on a barium enema as a series of little rounded white blips on the outer edges of the intestines. Diverticulitis occurs when the diverticula become inflamed and the condition can cause severe pain and constipation.

To prepare for a barium enema, you must clean out your colon by following a bowel preparation routine. This includes taking a strong laxative the night before, and then avoiding food or drink for some hours before the test.

Barium enemas are carried out in hospital X-ray departments. During the test, a doctor inserts a well-lubricated tube through the anus into the rectum, and pours in several hundred millilitres of a liquid metal called *barium sulphate*. The barium is white and shiny in your intestines and, more importantly is radio-opaque, which means that X-rays cannot pass through it, so the barium shows up white on an X-ray, contrasting against the black or grey of the tissues. That's why barium is sometimes known as a 'contrast medium'. Your doctor then takes several abdominal X-rays as you move your body into various positions.

Two types of barium study exist:

- ✔ **Single-contrast study:** Barium simply fills the intestines, and the shape of the white tubes outlines the intestines to show up narrowings, large craters formed by ulcers in the lining of the bowel, and other large abnormalities.

- ✔ **Double-contrast (air-contrast) study:** Your doctor drains out the barium, leaving just a thin layer on the inner wall of the bowel. Your doctor then pumps air in, and this provides a more detailed view of the inner surface of the colon, showing up polyps, cancers, and patches of inflammation. This procedure takes much longer but tells the doctor a lot more about your gut.

You may be given a light sedative to relax you, but you're usually awake throughout the barium enema procedure. You may feel the pressure of liquid going into your intestines, but you shouldn't feel any pain.

It can take up to two hours to perform a barium enema from start to finish. However, the test is often quicker than this and sometimes longer, depending on how fast your intestines fill up with the barium liquid and how many X-rays the doctor takes. After the barium study, your body soon gets back to normal although your stools appear white for some days – this is just the barium leaving your body.

Upper gastrointestinal series

As with the barium enema, this test isn't used as frequently as it was before the invention of endoscopes. But to specifically rule out Crohn's disease in the small intestine, your doctor may request an upper gastrointestinal X-ray known as a small bowel follow-through. You swallow a tall glass of chalky barium liquid, and a technician takes a series of many X-rays as the liquid passes through the gastrointestinal tract, to look for signs of ulceration that define Crohn's disease. In other words, the X-rays follow the barium through the upper part of the gut.

CT and MR scans

As *computed tomography* (CT) scans and *magnetic resonance* (MR) imaging become more sophisticated and widespread, doctors increasingly use them to examine deep inside the body. In expert hands, CT and MR scans can give a very good picture of the organs and soft tissues. Some radiology specialists predict that one day these tests may completely take over from X-rays. But for now, they're expensive and used only in difficult cases or where cancer is suspected. Your doctor probably won't offer these tests if she's fairly sure that you have IBS.

Tests for lactose intolerance

Doctors use two types of test to detect lactose intolerance (where the body cannot break down the milk sugar lactose): the lactose tolerance test and the hydrogen breath test. We discuss each in the following sections.

Testing sugar in the blood

The lactose tolerance test measures how well your body breaks down lactose in the intestines and absorbs it into the blood stream. When you have this test, you must not eat or drink for 8 to 12 hours before the test. After this, your doctor takes a blood sample to check the amount of sugar in the blood. Then your doctor gives you a dose of lactose, such as a milky drink, and takes a series of blood samples over a two-hour period.

The test is positive if intestinal symptoms occur and blood glucose levels don't increase very much above the fasting level. This shows that the body is not breaking down lactose or absorbing its sugar products. So the lactose passes through into the large bowel where it ferments, causing symptoms of abdominal pain.

A high rate of false positive and false negative results exists with this test, so many doctors prefer to use the hydrogen breath rest.

Testing hydrogen in the breath

The hydrogen breath test is more sensitive and specific than the lactose tolerance test. The test is based on the following principle: The body does not normally produce hydrogen, but the bacteria in the colon can generate hydrogen if it consumes sugars. So when lactase deficiency (the cause of lactose intolerance) occurs, undigested lactose gets through to the colon where the bacteria ferment it and produce gases including hydrogen. The hydrogen enters the bloodstream by absorption and then it passes to the lungs, from where you exhale the gas.

For this test, all you have to do is drink a lactose-loaded beverage and then exhale into a machine that measures the amount of hydrogen in your breath. If hydrogen is pouring out, you can spot colonic sugar fermentation.

In addition, this sort of test can also be used to screen for gluten intolerance (coeliac disease) and is much less invasive than a bowel biopsy – the definitive test for that condition. The presence of a sugar called *D-xylose* in your breath may indicate adult coeliac disease. (Most gastrointestinal specialists, however, feel that a bowel biopsy is still required for diagnosis.)

Tests for gluten intolerance

Gluten intolerance goes by several names, including gluten enteropathy, coeliac disease, and coeliac sprue. Whatever you call it, this disease can wreak havoc if it goes undiagnosed and your doctor may mistake it for IBS, as we explain in Chapter 4. Gluten is a mixture of two proteins, gliadin and glutenin, found in wheat, barley and rye. When someone who is susceptible to the condition eats these foods, the gluten sticks to the internal surface of the intestines and triggers the immune system to attack this delicate lining layer. As the lining is damaged, nutrients from food can no longer be absorbed and pass out of the gut, leading to diarrhoea, and vitamin and mineral deficiencies.

Doctors need to be as certain as possible of the diagnosis because the diet for gluten intolerance is so restrictive and can be difficult to follow in a way that ensures an adequate intake of all necessary nutrients. In this section we discuss the three tests that can detect gluten intolerance: blood tests that check for antibodies, a gut biopsy, and following a gluten free diet.

If you think that you may have gluten intolerance, discuss your symptoms with your doctor. Don't try a gluten-free diet yet, as this interferes with the results of tests that specifically identify coeliac disease. Continue to eat your normal diet – including bread, pasta, and cereals. If you have already eliminated gluten from your diet, you must re-introduce it for at least six weeks before your doctor can carry out any diagnostic tests.

Checking for antibodies

Your doctor may take a sample of blood for a simple test that detects endomysial antibodies (EMA) and/or tissue transglutaminase antibodies (tTGA). These antibodies are ammunition produced by the immune system when a person with gluten intolerance swallows the gluten found in wheat. Unfortunately, the target is the body's own cells, in particular the cells that line the intestines, which become damaged. But although a positive test for these antibodies may indicate gluten intolerance, you can get a negative result and still have the condition. Other blood tests may also be taken to check for anaemia and other signs of malabsorption.

Performing a gut biopsy

The best and most reliable test is a biopsy of the gut. A hospital specialist carries out this procedure by passing a flexible viewing tube, known as an endoscope, via your mouth down into the small intestine (this can be done using local anaesthetic on the throat and sedation). Doctors collect small tissue samples and examine them under a microscope to check for abnormalities.

Trying out a gluten-free diet

The ultimate test is to follow a gluten free diet. If you have a positive response to the diet – symptoms subside and the small intestine returns to its normal, healthy state – your doctor can confirm the diagnosis of gluten intolerance.

The fly in the ointment here is that you must initiate the gluten-free diet only after the first three steps. But many people with IBS symptoms eliminate sugar, wheat, and dairy because they're common allergens, and doctors do not usually send them for gluten intolerance testing until much later – if at all.

Cynthia had never heard of coeliac disease until she was trying to uncover the secret behind her gut-wrenching symptoms. Finally, following an intestinal biopsy, she was diagnosed with coeliac disease and discovered that it's a genetic disorder. Her mother had always complained of stomach troubles but never obtained a diagnosis. Naturally, Cynthia was concerned for the health of her own children but, at the same time, was not eager to put them through a biopsy. Cynthia's doctor banished her worries when he told her that most testing for coeliac is now done by a simple blood test to identify the presence of antibodies.

Food allergy tests

Tests that look for antibodies that have been produced by the immune system against certain foods can be helpful in identifying food allergies. Food allergy is often mistaken for IBS. These tests, which include blood tests and skin tests, are discussed in depth in Chapter 4. Some GPs carry out these tests but many doctors prefer to send their patients to a specialised allergy clinic, either in the NHS or, because allergy clinics are few and far between and have long waiting times, to a private service.

Food allergy tests can supply you with a list of foods that you have an immune reaction to. The test results can give you answers that take weeks or even months to find out with other methods (such as the elimination and challenge diet that we talk about in Chapter 10). Having this information gives you an opportunity to stop eating these foods for a time so that your body is no longer fighting them.

However, many doctors aren't yet convinced that there's enough evidence to show how accurate food allergy testing is, and still feel that the elimination and challenge diet is the gold standard of food allergy and sensitivity diagnosis.

Comprehensive digestive stool analysis (CDSA)

The CDSA is a panel of tests that looks for evidence that the gut is not digesting food properly, or not absorbing nutrients correctly. It also looks for abnormalities in the types of intestinal bacteria and other micro-organisms found in the gut.

A stool sample collected at home is sent to a special lab that conducts the CDSA. The tests then tell you, for example, if blood is present in the stool (which is undeniably important); the amount of fat (which can imply fat malabsorption); and whether certain digestive or fermentation products, and various types of micro organisms, are present and in what quantities.

CDSA is more often recommended by complementary health practitioners than conventional doctors, who are more likely to question just how useful the information from the tests are, and whether they're worth the cost. Because doctors doubt its worth, it's very unlikely that you would get this test on the NHS and therefore you may probably have to pay for CDSA testing. Those who believe that IBS links to bacterial or yeast overgrowth (which we suggest is something of an out-dated theory now – see Chapter 4) may place great stock in such a test. But doctors are more sceptical, and many worry that vulnerable patients may be swayed into stumping up large sums of money for a test that doesn't help in the long run.

Differentiating Your Diagnosis

Your doctor may ask you how long you've experienced IBS symptoms, how many bowel movements you have a day, what your stool looks like, whether you have blood or mucus in your stool, whether you have pain, and whether you have gas and bloating. Your doctor then sifts through the *differential diagnosis* – a list of diseases common to your age group – and matches your symptoms and signs. These diseases include the following:

 ✔ **Amoebiasis and giardiasis:** Amoebiasis, or amoebic dysentery, is an infection of the digestive system caused by a tiny organism called an amoeba, specifically *entamoeba histolytica*. You pick it up from food or water contaminated with human faeces. Although it doesn't cause symptoms in most cases, it can irritate the intestines to cause diarrhoea, abdominal pain, and fever, sometimes months after the initial infection. To diagnose this infection, doctors check a stool sample under a microscope for amoebae or take a blood test that looks for antibodies to amoebae.

Giardiasis is another gastrointestinal infection caused by microscopic parasites called protozoa, specifically *giardia lamblia*. This infection is the most common cause of diarrhoea throughout the world. Symptoms comparable to amoebiasis, with watery diarrhoea, foul-smelling faeces, stomach cramps, flatulence, indigestion, and nausea.

Doctors can treat both amoebiasis and giardiasis with a simple course of antibiotics.

✔ **Cancer of the colon:** Bowel cancer is a common cancer in the developed world – more than 36,000 new cases emerge each year in the UK. The cause is unknown but important factors include an inherited tendency; a diet high in animal fat and low in fibre; smoking; drinking; taking little exercise, and being overweight. Often, few symptoms emerge until later stages but the cancer can cause a change in bowel habit (diarrhoea or constipation), mucus production, bleeding from the bowel, and abdominal pain – symptoms that resemble IBS. Benign growths such as intestinal polyps can also cause IBS-like symptoms. Colon cancer is diagnosed using endoscopy or barium enema (which we discussed earlier in this chapter) and treated with a combination of surgery, radiotherapy, and chemotherapy.

✔ **Crohn's disease:** The main distinguishing features of Crohn's disease, which we talk about in more detail in Chapter 1, are blood in the stool and unrelenting diarrhoea. But in some people with Crohn's disease, symptoms fluctuate between constipation and diarrhoea, both with pain. There may also be mouth sores, anal fissures, fevers, weight loss, and generally more severe illness than in IBS.

✔ **Dairy allergy:** This is an immune reaction to a protein called casein found in milk. It occurs more commonly in children, where it may cause an immediate immune reaction (with symptoms such as facial swelling, vomiting, and diarrhoea), or a slightly slower reaction or delayed reaction (with symptoms such as eczema, vomiting, and diarrhoea). Most children grow out of dairy allergy by the age of four but some remain allergic for life. Occasionally, adults develop a dairy allergy, and have an immediate reaction or eczema. To find out if a dairy allergy is to blame for your symptoms, try keeping a dairy diary (we give you lots of great tips on this in Chapter 9) and follow a dairy exclusion diet (which we explain in Chapter 10).

✔ **Endometriosis:** Endometriosis is a common condition in women. Cells that normally line the uterus appear elsewhere in the body, especially in the pelvis or abdomen, where they may settle on the outer wall of the intestines. As these cells respond to the monthly cycle of hormones by growing and then regressing (just as the lining of the womb does), this can cause pain, swelling, bleeding, and scarring that can disrupt the intestines, producing symptoms similar to IBS. One clue to the diagnosis is the way that symptoms tend to wax and wane with the menstrual cycle, although some women have more constant problems.

✔ **Gluten intolerance (coeliac disease):** Coeliac disease is an autoimmune disease triggered by a protein called gluten found in wheat, barley, and rye. The distinguishing features of this disease, which affects as many as 1 in 100 people, include chronic symptoms of fatigue, weight loss, and anaemia, as well as symptoms such as bloating, diarrhoea, nausea, wind, constipation, skin problems, and depression. (Does this list ring any bells? – it's easy to see how IBS and gluten intolerance get confused.) Older patients in their thirties and onwards, can have osteoporosis because they don't absorb both iron and calcium properly, and fertility problems. Doctors often miss gluten intolerance in adults because the condition is most common in children.

✔ **Lactose intolerance:** This condition features long-term symptoms of alternating diarrhoea and constipation, gas, and bloating, related to the consumption of milk and milk-products. The most common form is due to an inherited inability to digest the sugar found in milk, due to a lack of the enzyme lactase. Lactose intolerance is much more common among people of African or Asian origins, where as many as 90 per cent of people may be affected. Some people can acquire lactose intolerance after a gastrointestinal infection, or as levels of the enzyme lactase fall with age.

✔ **Ulcerative colitis:** Like Crohn's disease, ulcerative colitis is an inflammatory bowel disease, and so the distinguishing features also include blood in the stool and unrelenting diarrhoea. However, the condition usually only affects the colon.

✔ **Wheat allergy/intolerance:** As we explain in Chapter 4, a food allergy differs from food intolerance. An allergy to wheat that triggers a serious response from the immune system is actually extremely rare, although some doctors believe that a more low grade allergy can occur (but this opinion is controversial). Wheat intolerance is much more common, where eating wheat or food containing wheat-based products triggers symptoms including diarrhoea, bloating, wind, and/or constipation. To find out if wheat intolerance is the culprit for your symptoms, you need to keep a food diary, go on a food avoidance programme, or have blood testing. (See Chapter 4 for more information on all of these approaches.)

Chapter 8

Treating IBS Symptoms with Drugs

● ●

In This Chapter

▶ Weighing benefits against side effects

▶ Focusing on medication for short-term relief

▶ Treating symptoms of diarrhoea and constipation

▶ Controlling the pain of IBS

● ●

*Y*ou can do a lot to manage IBS yourself. Some of the most important strategies include lifestyle changes, attention to diet, and dealing with stress – and this book is packed with helpful tips.

But most people also find that they can get some relief from their symptoms with treatments provided by health professionals. This chapter looks at some of the conventional drug treatments used in IBS, which your doctor may recommend. You may also want to try different complementary therapies, which we discuss in Chapter 13.

Keep all the practitioners you use posted on what you're doing with any other practitioner. Some herbal remedies can cause problems when taken at the same time as modern drugs, for example, making a drug more or less potent. And many complementary therapists adapt their treatments in the light of which drugs you take and what side effects you experience.

This chapter discusses the medicines that your doctor or pharmacist may recommend for your IBS, how these drugs work, and what the pros and cons of each of them are likely to be. However, we're not actively recommending that you try any particular one of the drugs that we discuss. You need to discuss all medication – and which specific treatments may be helpful in your case – with your GP.

Do not take any medicines without consulting your doctor or pharmacist first. Always follow the instructions on the packet label, never take someone else's medicine, and seek urgent medical advice if you have any cause for concern.

Trying Not to Expect Too Much from Drug Therapies

Although practitioners use a wide spectrum of treatments in IBS, each benefits a small proportion of patients only, and no single drug is effective in relieving IBS over the long term. Put simply, no cure for IBS exists – no remedy stops the condition in its tracks and holds it at bay for ever. That's not great news, we admit, but you can use medications to your advantage in short-term situations and look at diet, dietary supplements, and lifestyle changes for the long term.

Because drug treatments for IBS aren't particularly effective at dealing with symptoms (and often have side effects), having someone to listen to your worries, explain your symptoms, and reassure you that IBS is a benign condition that's not fatal, are some of the most important parts of treatment. But knowing that IBS isn't about to terminate your existence doesn't do much to detract from the undeniable misery and damage that it can do to your social, working, and personal life. And it doesn't stop most people from wanting to at least try medications that may – just may – make things easier.

Expert opinion suggests that when anxiety, panic attacks, and depression are prominent features of IBS, doctors should put psychological therapies first in the treatment line. Reliable evidence shows that specific types of psychological treatment, such as cognitive behavioural therapy (CBT), can develop the coping skills of someone with IBS; hypnotherapy can bring general improvements in symptoms; and relaxation therapy may also be beneficial. Treatment of associated anxiety and depression also often improves bowel symptoms.

That said, you're no doubt by now itching to find out more about the medicines on offer. But if you go to a doctor and ask for help with your symptoms, you may well expect to walk away with a prescription in hand, and your doctor may well feel under pressure to give you one. So expectations all round may not be matched by the reality of the available medicines. Before you get stuck in this situation, you may want to mull over the information in this section.

Waiting for better drugs

Every year specialist gastroenterologists and other interested health professionals from all over the world attend a number of major gastroenterology conferences and symposia. At these events, presentations on new treatments for IBS draw a large audience. Clearly, doctors want to help their patients with IBS symptoms and recognise the urgent need for better medicines. The question is: How far can the drug treatments we already have provide an answer?

Drugs therapies for IBS consist of:

- ✔ Laxatives for constipation
- ✔ Bulking agents for constipation and diarrhoea
- ✔ Antimotility drugs to slow the gut in diarrhoea
- ✔ Antispasmodics for pain
- ✔ Antidepressants for pain stress and possibly stress

Patients are often surprised to find that their doctor has relatively few options for treating IBS. Unfortunately, most of these treatments don't do much to help the majority of people with IBS. Although some get limited relief from certain symptoms, others respond initially, but their symptoms recur. A number of people with IBS don't respond at all to these medications. Prescribing for IBS can be distressing for both patients and doctors because finding the right combination of medications to help someone is such a hit-and-miss proposition.

A common complaint in the IBS community is that scientists do not do enough research into IBS to find a cure. Unfortunately, research is a slow and very expensive business, and in order to get it done, doctors and research scientists need to find funding from charities, government bodies, or the pharmaceutical industry. Limited resources mean it can be a nightmare to find the money because researchers working on hundreds of other conditions are also looking for funding. Understandably, everyone thinks that their own condition or study is most deserving.

But digging around for a cure is jumping the gun in IBS. We don't even know yet how the disease develops. The research most likely to eventually lead to a cure involves basic scientific investigation into the causes. Then, after we know exactly what is going on, it should be much easier to search in the right direction for a cure. But this means spending time and money getting the basics sorted.

With so much frustration surrounding drug therapies, it's worth giving a lot of time and thought to advice on lifestyle changes, such as improving diet. The problem is that most people with IBS symptoms tell their doctors that they have already tried dietary changes and that the changes didn't work. Therefore, their doctors quickly assume that medication is necessary. As we point out in several chapters of this book, diet is a rich field to explore. We encourage you to read Chapter 10 about diet before looking for medication.

Reviewing clinical trials

The way doctors try to relieve the main IBS symptoms of abdominal pain and bloating is changing. Drug treatments used to focus on relaxing the smooth muscle of the gut, but the aim now is to try to alter movement of food through the gut, and to influence the way the brain receives and perceives sensory information coming in from the gastrointestinal tract and related organs. However, the treatment of symptoms related to bowel dysfunction (constipation or diarrhoea) still mostly focuses on accelerating or slowing the passage of intestinal contents.

Treatments that research suggests are significant for IBS include the following:

- Dietary therapies (see Chapter 10 for the lowdown on diet)
- Hypnotherapy (head to Chapter 13 for hypno-info)
- Pharmacological, or drug, treatments:
  - Antispasmodic drugs
  - Antidepressants
  - Antidiarrhoeal drugs
  - Fibre and laxatives
  - Probiotics
- Psychological therapies (which we discuss in Chapter 12)

Dealing with Diarrhoea

Antidiarrhoeal medications take several forms:

- Bile salt inhibitors, such as colestyramine (Questran)
- Bulking agents, such as psyllium and polycarbophil
- Codeine and other mild opiate drugs
- Drugs that slow down the intestine, such as loperamide (sold as Imodium) and a combination of atropine and diphenoxylate (sold as Lomotil)
- Probiotics
- Serotonin blockers

Here, we offer details about the use and effectiveness of each one.

Co-phenotrope

Co-phenotrope (a combination of the two drugs diphenoxylate hydrochloride and atropine that's commonly known by its tradename Lomotil) has been around for decades. It stimulates the inhibitory nerves of the bowel's own nervous system – the *enteric nervous system* (see Chapter 2 for more), which slows down intestinal movements and reduces secretions. This means co-phenotrope stops the rush of intestinal contents that are still in their liquid state. This minor traffic jam means the contents stay in the intestines for longer and the bowel absorbs more water, making the stool more solid.

Researchers haven't studied co-phenotrope in IBS, so we can't state clearly just how effective this drug is. But co-phenotrope is widely used (which suggests it must work to some degree) and doctors understand its side effects well.

Only use co-phenotrope in the short term and not at all if you suspect you have a bowel infection. Diphenoxylate is a type of drug known as an *opioid analogue,* which means that it has an effect like an opiate and is classed as an opiate drug with addictive properties. It doesn't make you feel 'high' but some doctors have concern that in large doses this drug may cause physical and psychological dependence. In other words, if you use it daily for preventing episodes of diarrhoea, you may start to think that you need it all the time (although no evidence proves that people use more and more of it in the way they do with street drugs).

To lessen the possibility of addiction, the manufacturers add another drug called atropine to co-phenotrope as a deterrent. Atropine causes *antimuscarinic adverse effects,* which relate to the way the drug blocks the action of the neurotransmitter chemical acetylcholine in the central and peripheral nervous system. Common antimuscarinic effects adverse include (among many others) a dry mouth, blurred vision, unsteadiness, inability to pass urine, and confusion.

You don't want to use co-phenotrope all the time. In fact, although you can buy it without a prescription in the pharmacy, its licence states that it should be for short-term use only and so it is only sold in small amounts. It's far better to find out what triggers your IBS symptoms and just use co-phenotrope to get you through a plane ride or an evening out. The more you use it, the more susceptible you are to side effects of dizziness, drowsiness, dry skin, itching, nausea, and vomiting, especially if you're taking other medications that may interact with it, such as opiate pain killers.

Loperamide

Like co-phenotrope, loperamide (which most people know as the tradename Imodium) is an opioid analogue that works on the enteric nervous system to slow down the movement of food through the small and large bowel, allowing the reabsorption of water. So loperamide is recommended for urgency and diarrhoea in IBS. However, that's not the only story. Research shows that loperamide appears to enhance the resting internal anal sphincter tone. What does that mean? Loperamide keeps the anus tight when you're at rest. For that reason, it helps to improve stool leakage at night, which is helpful for certain people with IBS who have that problem. (For some people, leakage is such a problem that they must use incontinence pads, which we talk about in Chapter 14.)

Although studies show that loperamide significantly reduces diarrhoea and the BSG guidelines recommend the drug, it has little effect on abdominal pain or distention. Even so, many people with IBS rely heavily on loperamide to control their frequent trips to the toilet. Fortunately, loperamide is much less likely to be addictive than co-phenotrope because it doesn't cross from the bloodstream into the brain, and it doesn't cause confusion or antimuscarinic side effects like co-phenotrope can. So it can be safely used on a regular basis for diarrhoea without too much concern about these sorts of side effects.

Its also worth noting that loperamide works faster and lasts longer than than other anti-diarrhoea drugs such as diphenoxylate (Lomotil) or codeine.

You can buy loperamide from the pharmacy without a prescription. The dose you need varies from person to person – you need to follow the instructions on the packet and test it out on your own gut. There is no specific limit on how often you should take it and most people can use it as often as they need to. Many people take it long term – for weeks or months. Although you're very unlikely to come to much harm it is always wise to check your use of medication with a doctor at regular intervals, perhaps every three months or so. If you're taking large frequent doses of loperamide with no effect then you definitely need to talk to your doctor about it, and consider stopping.

Although generally safe, loperamide can cause problems. For example, it can worsen constipation. In fact, this medication can throw you from diarrhoea into constipation and can cause the type of IBS symptoms that involve alternating diarrhoea and constipation. In addition, loperamide can occasionally cause complications in certain types of bacterial gastroenteritis, so you need to check with your doctor before using it if you suspect you have a bowel infection. Other side effects include abdominal pain, dizziness, dry mouth, nausea, and vomiting.

You can give an extra hurrah to loperamide because it can be taken in a syrup formulation, which makes it easier for you to fine-tune the dose and so reduce the risk of constipation. You can also use loperamide as a preventative or *prophylactic* measure when diarrhoea is likely to be a problem (for example, before going out).

Colestyramine

Colestyramine (sold as Questran) is a drug known as a *bile acid binding agent* that is more commonly used in the treatment of high cholesterol. It prevents mops up bile acids in the gut and prevents them from stimulating the colon.

In this roundabout way, it slows down the movement of intestinal contents, allows the body to reabsorb water from the intestines, and relieves diarrhoea. It's not the first line of treatment for diarrhoea-predominant-IBS but doctors may try this drug if other treatments don't help.

The BSG guidelines point out that you're only likely to respond to treatment with a bile-acid binding agent if you've been diagnosed by your doctor as having a severe bile-acid *malabsorption.*(where the salts within bile aren't absorbed into your body as they should be, causing diarrhoea). About 10 per cent of people with diarrhoea-predominant IBS have problems with bile salt malabsorption, and may respond to colestyramine.

Colestyramine may also be effective when a person has acute diarrhoea that their doctor suspects is due to infection, or nocturnal diarrhoea.

Colesytramine can only be prescribed by a doctor and not bought directly in the pharmacy. It can be taken long term if necessary but, like all medicines, its use ought to be regularly reviewed. You mix colestyramine with water and may take it several times a day. It must be taken three hours before or after other medications so that it does not interfere with the absorption of those drugs.

The side effects of colestyramine relate how it interferes with bile. One side effect is a degree of malabsorption that occurs when the body binds up and removes bile. Other side effects, unfortunately, may be similar to the symptoms that your doctor prescribes the medication to treat: abdominal pain, bloating, constipation, gas, a feeling of fullness, and nausea. Many people have problems with these side effects of colestyramine and prefer other treatments such as loperamide.

Bulk-forming agents

The usual bulk-forming laxative agents such as unprocessed wheatbran and psyllium (sometimes called ispaghula) may help in both diarrhoea-predominant IBS and constipation-predominant IBS. The agents work by 'mopping up' water within the intestines. This absorption of water makes the contents less fluid (reducing diarrhoea) or it keeps the fluid content of the stool higher, making it softer and more bulky, so easing constipation and helping to move waste through the intestines.

Bulk-forming agents do tend to cause gas and bloating, so if your colon is hypersensitive to gas and bloating, they may not be the ideal treatment. However, judicial use of fibre can help absorb excess fluid, which is the main component of diarrhoea. The main bulk-forming laxatives for diarrhoea include psyllium and the synthetic substance methylcellulose (sold as Celevac).

Some guidelines take a look at dietary fibre and bulking agents, and point out that most research fails to show much benefit. One survey actually suggests that cereal fibre may make symptoms worse in 55 per cent of patients, with only 11 per cent reporting any benefit. A recent systematic review of 17 clinical trials concludes that the benefits of fibre in IBS are marginal and that insoluble fibre may make the condition worse. But all this research took place in hospitals rather than out in the community where people may be more successful at tweaking the fibre in their diet to help their symptoms.

Soluble fibre such as psyllium (also called ispaghula), and pectins and hemicellulose (found in fruit and vegetables) are probably the best choice (rather than insoluble fibre such as bran) for managing diarrhoea in IBS.

Serotonin blockers (5-HT antagonists)

Serotonin blockers are a type of medicine which, although not currently available in the UK, are used in a number of other countries and are also the subject of intensive research here. You may be interested to know a little about them.

The role of a chemical called serotonin (also known as 5-hydroxytryptamine or 5-HT) in the control of gastrointestinal motility, sensation, and secretion, is currently the topic of intensive research around the world. You can read more about this in Chapter 3 and Chapter 17.

Drug developers are now exploring the idea that chemicals that activate one type of 5-HT receptor (known as *5-HT4 receptor agonists*) may help speed up the bowel, and those that block 5-HT3 receptors (*5-HT3 receptor antagonists*) may slow gastrointestinal transit, so helping diarrhoea, and reduce sensations from the gut.

A number of drugs that work in this way have already been the focus of research and a few have come into general use for IBS. But there have been problems along the way. One drug called alosetron (sold as Lotronex), which is a 5-HT3 receptor antagonist, was approved for use in the USA in 2000. But within months it has been linked to a life-threatening gastrointestinal side effect called *ischaemic colitis* and was withdrawn. A couple of years later, it was again given approval in the USA but only for use by women with severe diarrhoea-predominant IBS who failed to respond to conventional treatment, under the direct supervision of a gastroenterologist.

Although neither alosetron nor any other 5-HT3 receptor agonists are available in the UK, some of these drugs currently in development may appear in the pharmacy (on prescription only) in the next few years. For example, two trials show that a new 5-HT3 receptor agonist called cilansetron adequately relieves abdominal pain/discomfort and abnormal bowel habit in both men and women with diarrhoea-predominant IBS.

Probiotics

Millions and billions of 'friendly' bacteria nestle in the warm cosy environment of your intestines. There are main different types or species of these bacteria, which we describe In Chapter 2 we describe the main different types or species of these bacteria, which are essential for the health of the intestines. They break down food to give energy to the cells that line the inside of the intestines, and they keep harmful bacteria at bay.

But sometimes overwhelming infections (tummy bugs or *gastro-enteritis*) or a course of antibiotics taken for other infections destroys our friendly bacteria. Without these bacteria the gut can go a little haywire and unwelcome micro-organisms can take over, triggering the symptoms of IBS.

So trying to replace or boost levels of the friendly bacteria by taking supplements known as probiotics seems to be a logical solution. Probiotics – a concentrated source of friendly bacteria –, when taken in large enough amounts reestablish the balance of micro-organisms in the bowel, stimulate the immune system, modify the acid/alkali balance of the gut, and protect and stabilise the barrier formed by the lining of the gut. It may also be important to take 'prebiotics' too – these are the basic nutrients in foods that probiotic bacteria thrive on.

There are now at least five carefully run trials of probiotics to show that they may help some symptoms, notably bloating and flatulence. More recent research has shown that probiotics can also improve diarrhoea after antibiotic therapy and bacterial gastroenteritis.

You may be familiar with yoghurts and other foods in the supermarket that contain probiotics or friendly bacteria. But be sure to read the labels closely because some of the bacteria in these products aren't the same as those that the research studied. The types of friendly bacteria found in the trials to have a positive effect included *lactobacillus rhamnosus, lactobacillus plantarum* (found in large numbers in unscrubbed and unwashed vegetables),and a concoction of *lactobacill, bifidobacteria,* and *streptococcus* known as VSL#3. Studies of the bacteria *bifidobacterium infantis* also hinted that this bacteria may help by calming down the immune system.

However, there isn't enough research yet to be absolutely sure which types of friendly bacteria you should be looking for. It seems that although the best approach may be to try to swallow a variety of different types of friendly bacteria, even probiotic supplements containing a single species strain may be helpful. One thing that you need to remember is that a single dose isn't enough – probiotics should be taken for several days, possibly weeks, depending on your normal diet and your particular condition, in order to repopulate the gut.

Some experts claim that probiotic bacteria grown in the laboratory lose the ability to stick to the mucosa or lining of the intestines and therefore cannot re-establish a permanent population of friendly bacteria. The experts suggest that only fresh human probiotics (made from friendly bacteria extracted from the faeces of another healthy human being) are able to attach to their new owners and settle down to thrive and repopulate the gut. You may find the idea of being dosed with an extract of someone else's faeces (however hygienically prepared) is a fairly tough concept to swallow! But this concept, called bacterial implantation, does work in some serious bowel infections and is a concept now being tested more extensively by doctors. Fortunately the research is starting to show that probiotic supplements and drinks seem to be adequate for most people.

You don't need a doctor's prescription for a probiotic. If you want to try them you have a variety of choices:

- ✔ Increase the supply from your diet of fruit and vegetables (Chapter 10 explains how).

- ✔ Look out for 'live' yoghurts and probiotic drinks (both dairy-based and non-dairy) in your supermarket chiller cabinet.

- ✔ Ask in your health food shop or pharmacy for probiotic supplements – these come as tablets or capsules.

Codeine

Codeine (and the similar drug dihydrocodeine) is a weak opiate medicine. You can buy formulations that contain codeine combined with paracetamol or ibuprofen in the pharmacy without prescription. People often use codeine as a painkiller, but it has a renowned side effect of causing constipation, as well as drowsiness, nausea, and vomiting.

Some people with IBS come across this constipating effect almost by chance when trying out different painkillers, and then use medicines containing codeine specifically because they may help with diarrhoea. But this isn't a sensible tactic. Loperamide is more effective at treating diarrhoea in IBS and codeine has worrying side effects – for example, you may become addicted to it. If you do use codeine, make sure that you take it only occasionally, in short courses.

Controlling Constipation

The Rome III criteria for IBS, which we describe in Chapter 1, define constipation-predominant IBS solely on stool consistency. Someone with hard stools more than 25 per cent of the time and loose stools less than 25 per cent of the time is said to have IBS with constipation-predominant IBS. So the main aim of treatment is to soften the stools. People often describe infrequent stools as constipation too, but how often we need to visit the toilet varies between individuals and if the stool is soft then infrequency is not usually a significant problem.

Before you start looking at medicines such as laxatives, consider some simple changes to your lifestyle that make a big difference in improving constipation. Constipation in general may be the result of not enough fibre or fluids in the diet and a lack of regular exercise. Constipation can also occur in people in poor health. So basic steps to lead a more healthy life, with at least 20 minutes of brisk exercise every day, a good balanced diet with plenty of fresh fruit and vegetables and at least 6 glasses of water to drink, all help to get your bowel moving.

But many people with constipation-predominant IBS need to take further steps to identify specific triggers that make their symptoms worse, and then try different treatments to find out which ones suit their needs. We look at these options next.

Focusing on triggers first

Most people with constipation just want to have a bowel movement, and they use laxatives to achieve that end. However, if the trigger for constipation is one or more of the things we talk about in Chapter 4 (such as stress or painkilling medications), treating the symptom of constipation instead of the cause can be a losing proposition. It's worth noting that when people need to take constipating medications long term, or when they use large amounts of laxatives, they often find that over time the delicate intestinal muscles become stretched and damaged, preventing them from doing their job. As a result the constipation get harder to treat.

Increasing your intake of dietary fibre is the first approach that doctors recommend for constipation-predominant IBS, and we show you how to do so in Chapter 10. But beware – as we explain in the section 'Bulking agents', earlier in this chapter, research tells us that the benefits of fibre are at best marginal, and at worse overcome by the possible disadvantages. You want to be sure that you mostly increase your soluble fibre intake; insoluble fibre is much tougher on your digestive system. We explain the two types in Chapter 10 and give you a list of soluble fibre foods in Appendix A.

We also recommend that you talk to your doctor about other triggers that may be contributing to your constipation, which we talk about in Chapter 4, before taking over-the-counter or prescription laxatives.

Knowing your options

The list of drug treatments for constipation-predominant IBS isn't long. Constipation treatments are mostly laxatives that can be taken by mouth in various forms – tablet, liquid, granules, gum, and powder. Some of them chemically irritate the intestines to get things moving – *not* what someone with IBS wants to have happen. In fact, dependency on laxatives to get things moving can mean you need greater and greater dosages of the laxative to create a bowel movement, and over time your intestinal muscles stop working on their own.

Keep in mind that most advice about laxatives is based on the clinical experience of doctors and their patients, rather than research evidence or statistics, because researchers conduct few controlled trials on laxatives in patients with IBS. The BSG guidelines are fairly vague about which treatments are really worth trying for constipation-predominant IBS, and come up with very few positive recommendations. This probably reflects the lack of solid research evidence on laxatives.

Read the label on the laxative that you take. The label often says 'for occasional constipation', which means the medication is not meant to treat a chronic condition. A number of doctors, researchers, and people with IBS believe that the use of chemical laxatives for constipation-predominant IBS can actually throw people into diarrhoea-predominant IBS and contribute to the incidence of the alternating diarrhoea and constipation form of IBS.

A number of different types of laxatives and dozens of products are on the market. We describe the main types in the following sections.

Bulk-forming laxatives

Treatment of both diarrhoea and constipation is by using bulk-forming laxatives. This may sound a little odd – how can one treatment have such opposite effects in different people? Bulk-forming laxatives, based on plant fibre, work in constipation by drawing in liquid (like tiny spongy particles that soak up fluid) to help form a bulky stool that's soft enough to pass without effort. In diarrhoea they firm up and slow down the stools.

If you're going to take a laxative, we recommend trying bulk-forming laxatives before osmotic or stimulant laxatives because the latter two have more potential for abuse and dependence and actually hurt the gut over time. (We explain each type in this section.)

Doctors generally consider bulk-forming laxatives to be the safest type of laxative, but they can interfere with absorption of certain medicines. They can also stimulate gas and bloating in the intestines, and may worsen IBS pain in some people. If you don't have excess liquid in your intestines, you must take these laxatives with sufficient water to do the job. Otherwise, they can cause serious gut blockage.

Dietary fibre, from fruit and vegetables, is the most natural form of bulk-forming laxative so you can treat yourself by changing what you eat (we talk about dietary fibre in Chapter 10). However people with constipation-predominant IBS may need to take supplements of fibre, made from natural sources, including:

✔ Bran

✔ Ispaghula husk (also called psyllium)

✔ Methylcellulose

✔ Sterculia

These substances increase the bulk of the faeces and may speed up the passage of intestinal contents through the bowel. But although constipation may improve, and the person often generally feels a little better, these treatments rarely touch the pain of IBS. The bowel continues to twist and churn, albeit with a larger volume of stool that passes by more swiftly.

Overall only 10 per cent of people with IBS get improvements from bulking agents. And you need to keep in mind that randomised placebo-controlled trials show that insoluble fibre such as bran not only has no benefit at all for pain, but may even make the bloating and farting of IBS worse – about one in two people with IBS say that bran aggravates their symptoms. So you may prefer to try the other bulk-forming laxatives such as ispaghula, methylcellulose or sterculia, which are less likely to worsen pain or cause distension.

Sometimes drinking water can relieve mild constipation. Many people live constantly in a mildly dehydrated state without realising it. Be sure that you drink at least one and a half litres of water every day. That means two glasses of water when you wake up (before breakfast), another during the morning, one at lunch, one in the afternoon, one at dinner, and one at bedtime. See, it's not that hard at all! You need more water if you drink dehydrating beverages like coffee or alcohol, or if you sweat a lot with athletic activity. But beware that you don't knock back large amounts of fluids at mealtimes as this can interfere with digestion.

Osmotic laxatives

Osmotic laxatives increase the amount of fluid in the large bowel by drawing more fluid into the bowel from your body, or by retaining fluid you swallow into the gut. Typical osmotic laxatives include:

- **Lactulose:** This is a semi-synthetic disaccharide or sugar that the body doesn't absorb from the gastrointestinal tract. In the large bowel, bacteria break lactulose down into lactic acid and small amounts of other chemicals. This increases the osmotic or 'water-attracting' pressure and slight acidifies the contents of the colon, which in turn causes an increase in stool water content and softens the stool.

- **Macrogols (for example Movicol):** These chemicals don't act on the body itself but stay in the intestines where they hang on tightly to fluid, softening the stool and increasing the number of bowel movements. Research on people with chronic constipation shows that macrogols are more effective and less likely to cause unpleasant reactions than lactulose.

- **Sorbitol:** This is a sugar alcohol made from glucose. Sorbitol works in a similar way to lactulose. You can buy it in some pharmacies as a laxative, but you're more likely to come across it as a sweetener in sugar-free foods, or as a filler in other foods.

  Unfortunately, one of the by-products of the process of breaking down these sugars is gas, and gas and bloating are symptoms you really don't want to add to your repertoire.

Osmotic laxatives may not be the best choice in IBS, and inorganic salts (see the section 'Saline purgatives', later in this chapter) may be preferable to lactulose or sorbitol because they're cheaper and less likely to cause flatulence. However, the research on osmotic laxatives focuses on people with general chronic constipation, rather than those who specifically have IBS, so you may want to try them anyway and see if they suit your particular condition.

 Prunes and figs provide a great tasty and natural way to get a laxative effect. Some experts claim that the high fibre of prunes gives them their zip-along action, but prune juice (which has had all the fibre strained out) is just as effective in getting your transit time going. The real reason why prunes work is that they have a high natural sorbitol content, which gives an osmotic laxative effect.

Saline purgatives

Saline purgatives, which are laxatives based on mineral salts, sound very technical but include a medicine found in many bathroom cabinets – milk of magnesia. These saline purgatives often come in a liquid form that you swallow. As the salts, such as magnesium, pass down through the gut they draw water into the intestine to soften faecal matter. Meanwhile doctors often administer phosphate salts in enemas – at the other end of the gut – to clear the bowel in more extreme cases of constipation or before bowel X-rays or surgery.

One risk from mineral salts, especially if you use them persistently, is that the salt can accumulate and disturb the body's normal salt and water balance. If this happens, you may become overloaded with fluid or salt, which can put excessive strain on your heart. For this reason, doctors do not use laxatives based on sodium salts, because sodium salts are the most important salt in the body and disruption of sodium levels would cause particularly serious problems.

So in general it's best to keep saline purgatives for occasional use only, but as you may be painfully aware, constipation-predominant IBS is not an occasional happening. Unless constipation is a rare event for you, you probably need to make a different choice of treatment and find one that you can use more frequently.

Prokinetic agents

Don't let the term *prokinetic* blind you with science; it simply means 'for movement' – in other words, a drug that speeds up the action of the bowel and the transit time of food. Prokinetic agents are one of the great hopes of scientists working in the work of gastroenterology. However, although some of this type of drug work at the top end of the gut and are used to treat nausea and vomiting, it seems to be more difficult to get the colon working faster. No prokinetic agents have yet been licensed in the UK for the treatment of constipation although several are the focus of research trials.

Earlier in the chapter we talked about how scientists have been looking at drugs that work on the serotonin (5-HT) nerve receptors in the bowel to help diarrhoea-predominant IBS. If serotonin is relevant to diarrhoea, then scientists rightly think that it must be relevant to constipation too. In particular, many researchers are looking at potential prokinetic agents that work at the 5-HT4 sub-group of receptors. One of these *5-HT4-receptor agonist* drugs, called tegaserod, was found to reduce symptoms and improve quality of life in constipation-predominant IBS and entered general use in the USA (but not in the UK). But just as everyone was getting excited about what seemed to be one of the most useful drugs to appear in a long time, worrying reports of side effects meant that it was withdrawn from sale in America (although it is still available in a number of other countries).

However, research into prokinetic 5-HT4-receptor agonists continues and it is likely that in the future you're going to hear a lot more about this group of drugs for the treatment of constipation-predominant IBS.

Stimulant (irritant) laxatives

Stimulant laxatives (also known as irritant laxatives) are chemical laxatives that irritate the bowel lining, which stimulates muscle movement along the length of the intestine, hurrying stool along to its end. Most doctors recommend the drugs in this class of laxatives for short-term use only, because using them can lead to dependency or the need for ever-increasing doses to get the same effect. Therefore, stimulant laxatives don't do much for people who have life-long symptoms of IBS.

Stimulant laxatives include

- ✔ Bisacodyl (and other related chemicals such as cascara – a powerful stimulant whose fearsome reputation your grandmother may be able to tell you about but which is no longer used)
- ✔ Docusate sodium – this probably acts both as a stimulant and as a softening agent (see the section 'Lubricant and softening laxatives', later in this chapter)
- ✔ Dantron (also called danthron)
- ✔ Senna (from natural plant sources)

Always check the ingredients of laxatives that you buy over the counter, or ask your pharmacist to do so. Recent studies indicate that *phenolphthalein,* an ingredient in some stimulant laxatives (such as dantron or danthron) has links with cancer. Although this evidence comes from studies of rodents, not humans, research shows that phenolphthalein may also cause damage to the genes, and manufacturers therefore mostly replace it with safer ingredients. But it's still occasionally used (you may, for example, find it in laxative products if you purchase some abroad) and you may prefer to avoid this possible risk.

Lubricant and softening laxatives

Lubricants lubricate, grease, or oil the stool, enabling it to move through the intestine more easily. Mineral oil used to be the most common lubricant used in laxatives, and is still included in some, but it's not a good choice because it's too heavy for the delicate bowel mucosa. People also used liquid paraffin in the past, but this can cause intense irritation and the formation of lumpy scarred tissue in the mucosa and skin.

Another side effect of mineral oil/paraffin includes malabsorption of vitamins A, D, E, and K. If used in the long term, mineral oil can create severe vitamin deficiency symptoms. In Chapter 9, we discuss vitamins and how important they are to good health and the treatment of IBS.

Despite these negatives, some people with constipation-predominant IBS find that lubricant laxatives suit them well. As we have said several times in this book, IBS is a very individual disease and we advise people with the condition to try a range of approaches in order to find what works best for them.

Stool softeners provide moisture to the stool and prevent it from becoming dry and hard. The main softener is *docusate,* which is basically a detergent that the body doesn't absorb. As you know from washing dishes, a detergent dissolves grease in water. In the body, a stool softener traps dietary fat and then mixes it with the stool, making hard stool much softer. It doesn't attract water like some bulking agents, and it doesn't stimulate the bowel like some laxatives (although a widely used docusate-based laxative known as docusate sodium also has a separate stimulant effect).

Docusate is not very helpful on its own for constipation but can be useful in combination with other laxatives, and during pregnancy and after surgery. It also takes time to work: You usually see the effect one to three days after the initial dose.

The side effects of docusate include nausea, mild abdominal cramps, bloating, diarrhoea, rumbling sounds, severe abdominal pain, and vomiting.

Never take a laxative if you have severe abdominal pains, fever, diarrhoea, nausea, vomiting, or bloody stools. Instead, see your doctor immediately, as these may be symptoms of appendicitis or bowel inflammation.

Laxative mixtures

Many people find that by using a mixture of different types of laxative they get a more reliable result. For example, people often use a bulk-forming laxative to start things moving gently, add in a stool softener to ease things along and, if they still need help, take a stimulant laxative as well, to really get the gut moving.

Go carefully with mixtures like this – the last thing you want is an explosion, especially if you've been blocked up for a long time. You also risk triggering a prolonged bout of diarrhoea-predominant IBS. So start one drug at a time for a few days and then gently build things up. Ideally, get advice from your GP about which laxatives may suit you best.

Suppositories and enemas

Some people, fed up with their constipation-predominant IBS, turn to drastic means. Instead of trying to pour medicines down from the top of the gastrointestinal tract to get things going, they attack the problem from the other end. They use suppositories or enemas to try to clear out their bowel.

The suppositories used to treat IBS are small waxy plugs that you insert into your back passage. The suppository contains a stimulant laxative such as bisacodyl, or a softening agent such as glycerol (or glycerine). These ingredients work in a similar way to the equivalent oral medicine. The lubricant or softener softens hard stools, and the stimulant helps the rectum to push out the soft stools. Direct contact between the stimulant and the delicate mucosal lining of the rectum can bring a very rapid result.

An enema is a liquid treatment containing one of a variety of possible chemicals that's introduced into your bowel via a tube in your back passage. In mild constipation, where only a small amount of liquid needs to be placed just inside the anus, some people feel confident to administer the treatment to themselves (many enemas are provided in a simple self-administration pack) . But you may need help from a partner or the nurse at your doctors surgery. These simple saline enemas (which contain, for example, phosphate salts) are easy to use and don't have to be held in for very long. They're sufficient in most cases to clear the bowel, although you may need to repeat the enema several times.

In severe constipation, when the faeces are very hard, you can use lubricant enemas that contain ingredients such as arachis oil (an oil extracted from peanuts) and leave the enema in overnight to soften the stools. Medical help is vital here because the practitioner must introduce the enema high into the bowel using a long fine tube, so that the enema stays put and works fully.

Only use enemas and suppositories occasionally because they can damage the delicate lining of the gut. If you use them frequently, the gut can forget how to work on its own and may become even less active than ever. After the bowel is cleared, a good diet can help to keep constipation at bay (see Chapter 10 for lots of advice) but many people with constipation-predominant IBS find they also need extra help from oral laxatives.

However, despite this warning you come across people who swear by a daily enema. It may be the only way that they can get relief, but they may then become dependent on enemas as the only way to empty their bowel.

It can be hard to get active when you're not feeling great but don't forget that regular exercise is important for keeping the gut moving. Low levels of physical activity double the risk of constipation for anyone. In the US the Nurses' Health Study, which followed 62,036 women, found that physical activity two to six times per week meant a 35 per cent lower risk of constipation.

Dealing with Pain

Pain is an important defining feature of IBS. If no pain existed in IBS it would be a completely different condition. Most people can put up with diarrhoea and constipation alone. But when you have to deal with gripping, spasming pain, you may not cope so easily.

Pain from spasms can aggravate diarrhoea and ineffectual spasming can result in constipation. A build-up of gas and bloating can also cause pain as sensitive areas stretch and twist. In the following sections, we discuss common medications prescribed to help patients with IBS deal with pain.

Treating spasms

Doctors do not know the exact cause of intestinal twisting and contorting in IBS, but research shows that in people with IBS the muscular walls of the intestines contract and squeeze more, and these contractions reach even more exaggerated heights after eating (especially when diarrhoea is a pre-dominant feature of IBS). So it seems logical for doctors to offer patients anti-spasmodic drugs to try to suppress these contractions and so reduce painful symptoms.

As a result, antispasmodics are the most commonly used medicines for abdominal pain in people with IBS. Although doctors can't agree on exactly how long you can or should go on taking antispasmodics, most suggest that you can safely use antispasmodics when you need them up to three times a day, and that you can take then when you get an attack of pain, or as a pre-ventative measure before meals if food tends to bring on spasms. It is a good idea to review your use of antispasmodics every few months with your GP.

Antispasmodic treatments inhibit contraction of a type of muscle called smooth muscle, which is the muscle found in the walls of the gastrointestinal tract. Two main types of antispasmodics exist: anticholinergics (now more widely known as antimuscarinics) and smooth muscle relaxants. They include (brand names in brackets)

- Alverine (Spasmonal)
- Atropine
- Dicycloverine, also called dicyclomine (Merbentyl)
- Hyoscine (Buscopan)
- Mebeverine (Colofac)
- Propantheline bromide
- Peppermint oil

The research into antispasmodics shows that several drugs have some benefit, improving abdominal pain and generally decreasing symptoms, although
there isn't enough data to tell whether any one antispasmodic is more effective than another. The studies show a 56 per cent improvement with these
drugs compared to 38 per cent with a placebo, and that pain was relieved
in 53 per cent compared to 41 per cent with the placebo.

Two main types of antispasmodic drugs exist, which are divided on the basis
of how they work: Smooth muscle relaxants and antimuscarinic drugs.

Smooth muscle relaxants

Direct-acting smooth muscle relaxants, such as mebeverine and alverine, tend
to specifically affect intestinal smooth muscle rather than smooth muscle
elsewhere in the body. This is important because it means that direct-acting
smooth muscle relaxants are less likely to cause unwanted side effects.

Peppermint oil also works as a direct relaxant of gastrointestinal smooth
muscle and has antispasm properties.

Antimuscarinic (anticholinergic) drugs

Antimuscarinics (previously known as anticholinergics) reduce the contractions and movement of the intestinal muscles but often cause problematic
side effects. These side effects are a particular issue with the commonest
antimuscarinic drug available, atropine, which is not therefore routinely
used in IBS.

Antimuscarinic medication can help to prevent intestinal spasms that occur
with eating when you take the drug 30 minutes before a meal.

Antimuscarinics inhibit smooth muscle contraction, but they can also act at
other places in the intestines and elsewhere in the body where muscarinic
receptors exist. So they dry up secretions in the intestine, and can cause side
effects of dry mouth, blurred vision, drowsiness, nasal stuffiness, rash, itching, decreased sweating, and inability to urinate. This type of medication may
make constipation worse.

Although some people with IBS find antimuscarinic drugs useful, there is limited research evidence to support their use. Scientists do not have clear evidence that alverine is effective, for example, and they link dicycloverine with
significant side effects. However, research shows that people generally tolerate mebeverine well and can use it intermittently as required (before meals,
for example).

Using antidepressants

Antidepressants block the way the brain perceives pain, so doctors sometimes prescribe them in the treatment of IBS. Antidepressants effect neurotransmitters, which play a role in modulating pain. Fortunately, you need lower doses of these drugs to relieve pain than to relieve depression, and lower dosages mean fewer side effects.

Neurotransmitters are chemicals that occur throughout the nervous system and help transmit messages from cell to cell. One cell releases a neurotransmitter, which then passes across to another cell and stimulates it. Each cell has a receptor, usually on the outside membrane, which selectively receives and binds to specific chemicals like neurotransmitters. After transmitting its message, a neurotransmitter goes back into the cell and is recycled and used again and again.

Although dealing with IBS can be tough, the condition itself does not cause depression. But both are common conditions so some people with IBS suffer from depression at the same time. If your doctor offers you antidepressants for your IBS symptoms, the aim of the treatment is to treat your pain not your mental state. It doesn't mean that your doctor thinks that you're depressed, and the dose given isn't high enough to have any effect on your mood if you're depressed.

However, researchers know that around 40 to 60 per cent of people with IBS who seek out medical intervention also have symptoms of anxiety, panic attacks, and depression. (Among people who don't have IBS, 25 per cent have these symptoms.) So if you do feel down, make sure your doctor knows this so that he can consider it separately.

Antidepressant drugs do not have a licence from the governmental regulatory body in the UK for use in pain or IBS-related pain. But doctors have used them for this reason for years and their effects are fairly well known. Doctors can use drugs 'off-licence' like this when they think that it's appropriate (and many drugs are used off-licence in different conditions) but the drug manufactures can't promote them for unlicensed uses.

Blocking the perception of pain

Antidepressants come in a variety of types, and your doctor chooses which one to use depending on your symptoms.

Doctors have used a group of medicines known as tricyclic antidepressants (TCAs) for decades in many different conditions for their ability to alter pain perception, especially during acute stress. This alteration of pain perception is separate to the drugs' anti-depressant or anti-anxiety effect.

TCAs also act directly on the smooth muscle in the gut to reduce intestinal spasms, and so reduce pain in a different way too. In addition TCAs affect the serotonin system, boosting levels of the neurotransmitter, which may also decrease activity in the enteric nervous system and reduce gut motility.

However, one recent report found only a minimal improvement in IBS pain with tricyclic antidepressants. Even so, experts are adamant that they do provide some relief among people with predominant symptoms of diarrhoea and pain, particularly in severe or difficult-to-treat cases. As a result, TCAs are offered to about 10 per cent of IBS patients, usually those whose symptoms don't respond to other treatments.

Researchers using sophisticated imaging techniques such as MRI have found that when a toxic stimulus irritates the intestines, there is a particular response in the brain. The body activates the part of the brain that perceives this stimulation, and amplifies the perception of pain. Antidepressants can act to decrease pain perception. The antidepressant doesn't cure the pain, just depresses your perception of the pain.

Reviewing research on antidepressants

The BSG guidelines refer to several randomised placebo-controlled studies that show that low-dose TCAs effectively decrease symptoms. Researcher studied five TCAs thoroughly (amitriptyline, trimipramine, desipramine, clomipramine, and doxepin). It seems that patients with diarrhoea-predominant IBS get the greatest benefit from the drugs. Unfortunately, even though the patients take low doses of TCAs, side-effects such as constipation, dry mouth, drowsiness, and fatigue occur in over one-third of patients. These side effects can put patients off taking the drugs regularly or for as long as they need to in order to get relief. Although a patient may see an effect as soon as one week after starting a TCA, they must take the drug for several weeks to see the full benefit.

Doctors also try a more modern group of antidepressants, the selective serotonin reuptake inhibitors (SSRIs), to treat IBS. Doctors widely prescribe these antidepressants, which people tolerate well, in the treatment of anxiety, depression, and disorders where people express their psychological distress through physical symptoms (known as somatisation disorders). But do SSRIs work in IBS? Four randomised placebo-controlled studies of SSRIs in IBS show general improvements in wellbeing without significant change in bowel symptoms or pain. However, all but one of the trials only involved small numbers of patients. A large cost-effectiveness trial showed that a standard dose of an SSRI antidepressant produces a significant improvement in health-related quality of life at no extra cost in patients with chronic or treatment-resistant IBS. After the trial, patients on SSRIs were more likely to want to continue with the drug (84 per cent versus 37 per cent on a placebo), so it seems clear that these medicines provide a benefit even if they don't change bowel symptoms.

Antidepressants alter intestinal transit time whether or not they alter mood. Certain drugs, like the TCA imipramine, can slow down the bowel, which can lead to constipation. This is due to antidepressants' anticholinergic activity, which can also cause symptoms of dry mouth and impotence. On the other hand, SSRIs appear to cause more diarrhoea, as well as side effects such as nausea, headaches, insomnia, and sexual dysfunction.

Working with Wind

Along with pain and altered bowel habit (diarrhoea or constipation), excessive gas production in the gut is one of the commonest problems in IBS. And like the other symptoms, treating it isn't easy.

Many people find that they can reduce their gas problem by carefully tweaking what they eat – Chapter 10 has lots of useful advice on how to weed gas producers (such as difficult-to-digest sugars, or gassy vegetables like beans or Brussel sprouts) out of your diet.

But it can be difficult to eliminate all gas-related food without severely restricting your diet. One type of treatment that may help (but which seems to be increasingly difficult to source) is a natural enzyme, alpha galactosidase, that's made by a mould. Taken as a liquid or tablet with meals, this enzyme breaks down some of the difficult-to-digest complex sugars in vegetables so that your body can absorb them in the small bowel, rather than letting them pass into the large bowel where bacteria ferment them and produce gas.

Alpha galactosidase is effective in decreasing the incidence of intestinal gas. The enzyme is known as Beano in the US, where it's widely available. In the UK, you usually find it in health food stores, often on the shelf marked 'Enzymes for Vegans'.

Other treatments for gas include simethicone and activated charcoal. You may have seen simethicone promoted as a treatment for colic in small babies. In this instance the chemical helps the baby to burp up wind from their stomachs and so (theoretically at least) prevent the gas from passing down into the intestines and causing problems with colic. But simethicone has no effect on the formation of gas lower down in the colon and so is unlikely to help IBS bloating. If you want to give it a try anyway, you can buy simethicone in pharmacies, in a chewable tablet form. Activated charcoal does reduce the formation of gas in the colon, though the way in which it does so is unknown. Although it's odourless and tasteless, it may be hard to swallow.

Part III
Healing and Dealing with IBS

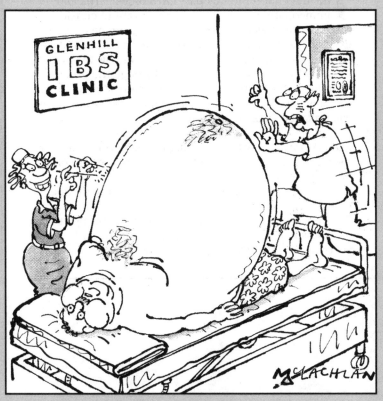

'No, no, no!! — <u>not</u> the acupuncture!!!
— not on this patient!!'

In this part . . .

The first chapter in this part introduces herbs and homeopathic medicines you may want to consider when putting together a treatment programme for your IBS. We also recommend that you place a lot of emphasis on your diet, so in this part we show you how to eat an IBS-friendly diet. We also walk you through the process of avoiding potential triggers and then reintroducing them to see how your body reacts – the simplest way to determine what may be causing you pain.

Exercise is also key to alleviating IBS pain, especially for people who suffer from wind and constipation. We offer lots of suggestions for great exercises to try, as well as motivation to make exercise part of your daily routine.

Finally, we introduce a wealth of other therapies you may not know much about, such as hypnotherapy and acupuncture, that can help you reduce stress.

Chapter 9

Controlling Your IBS

· ·

In This Chapter

▶ Taking charge of your condition

▶ Keeping an eye on your bowel

▶ Being your own doctor

▶ Developing good habits

· ·

*O*ne person can do huge amounts to help with your IBS – you! Of course, GPs, gastroenterologists, nurses, dieticians, complementary therapists, and many other health professionals provide invaluable sources of advice and can help establish the diagnosis, arrange tests, and prescribe treatments. But you are at the centre of all this, at the controls of every aspect of your life and how it plays a part in your condition. Think of the health professionals as your orchestra and you as the conductor, leading the music in the way that feels right for you.

Self-Managing Your Symptoms

Doctors these days appreciate that effective self-management is the key to many chronic conditions. The person with the symptoms needs to under-stand their disease and how they can re-organise their lifestyle to cope with and control it.

The UK government funds a nationwide programme called the Expert Patients Programme that supports people in managing their own long-term conditions, from heart disease and diabetes to asthma and – yes – IBS. The programme aims to enable people to develop skills that increase their confidence, improve their quality of life, and help them better manage their condition.

A network of trainers and around 1,400 volunteer tutors who also have long-term medical conditions run the courses around the country. You only need to commit to two or three hours a week for six weeks.

The programme focuses on five core self-management skills:

- ✔ Developing effective partnerships with healthcare providers
- ✔ Making decisions
- ✔ Solving problems
- ✔ Taking action
- ✔ Using resources

The course helps you to develop your communication skills so you can ask for what you need, manage your emotions, enjoy daily activities, interact with the healthcare system, find health resources, plan for the future, understand exercising and healthy eating, and deal with fatigue, sleep, pain, anger, and depression.

Ask at your local surgery about how you can sign up for a course on the Expert Patients Programme or check out the Web site at www.expertpatients.co. uk. Meanwhile, we look at developing a lot of those important skills in this chapter.

Relying on the Doctor Within

The most important aspect of managing your IBS is to take charge of your condition. IBS has a lot of symptoms, with plenty of ups and downs, and you need to be on top of what's going on. You probably don't have the time, money, or energy to go to your doctor every time you have a symptom. But we guess you probably do have the time to read this book and be clear about what IBS is, and what you can do for yourself.

Assuming power

Being in charge of your IBS is much more empowering than thinking that your doctor knows more about your body than you do. In fact, the attitude of being empowered may help turn off the stress trigger of IBS. You may be tempted to just hand over the responsibility for your health to someone else; with some conditions, especially if you need surgery, this makes sense, but with a functional condition such as IBS, where changes in lifestyle are so important in managing the condition, being in charge of yourself is best. If it is you that is making most of the decisions about very personal choices such as adapting your diet or how you deal with stress, you are more likely to find ways that work for you.

Dealing with your IBS

With the NHS straining under financial pressures and GPs burdened with huge lists and able to allocate only a few minutes for each consultation, many doctors don't have the time to sort out your diet, lifestyle, and stress in relation to IBS. Therefore, reading this book to understand the ins and outs of IBS and how to manage your condition on a day-to-day basis is a great step.

Looking after your IBS may be something you can do on your own, as long as you know the rules. The rule with gastrointestinal symptoms is to watch for alarm symptoms (which we list in Chapter 6) and see your doctor if you have them. The self-care approach comes after your doctor diagnoses IBS – not before. If you are in denial about severe gastrointestinal symptoms and keep telling yourself you don't have IBS, you may be missing a more severe condition.

The doctor within you probably knows that you need to eat a healthy diet and exercise regularly – you don't need a GP's prescription for these. We look at organising your diet and exercise later in this chapter.

Taking steps to improve your eating and exercising habits is up to you. Nobody else can make diet changes for you. But change is a hard thing to do. Sometimes we are more comfortable in a bad place that's familiar than a new place that seems scary. If you find yourself feeling overwhelmed by what you think that you should do, try some of the stress-busting techniques we talk about in Chapter 12.

Developing a healthy scepticism

As you make strides toward taking control of your IBS, you may hear about miracle 'cures' that other people with similar symptoms swear by. We encourage you to read as much as you can about IBS and to talk, whether in person or online, with others who share your situation, but we do urge you to be cautious. Sometimes even people with the best intentions give suggestions that just don't help.

Consider this situation: You take a new vitamin or mineral supplement, or you try a new diet, and the results are amazing. Your IBS symptoms disappear and you want to tell everyone. A dozen or so people are so inspired by your story that they try your miraculous cure. A third of them also get good results, but the others experience no change. The people who are cured keep spreading the word – and a health fad starts.

Or what if you thought for years that you had IBS but find out you actually have gluten intolerance (coeliac disease)? You may tell everyone you know that all the symptoms you suffered for years were due to eating gluten foods, and you warn everyone about the dangers of eating toast. But someone else's IBS symptoms may be caused by fruit, or antibiotics, or stress – eliminating gluten won't do that person any good at all.

One person's food is another's poison. In Chapters 8 and 10, we talk about the medications and dietary supplements used to treat IBS. Each drug works well for some people but not others – and each causes side effects in some people that far outweigh any benefits. The same is true for diets: What works wonderfully for one person may cause another person even more problems.

The way to deal with IBS is to follow a systematic approach, methodically checking through every condition that you may mistake for IBS (with the help of a doctor) and every trigger for IBS (perhaps with the help of this book). Only by doing so are you likely to determine the source of your symptoms.

Because many people with IBS symptoms don't get the help they need from conventional medicine, hundreds of chat groups and online resources exist for the condition. Some of these are very useful, but buyer beware! You may get advice from someone who knows less than you do. The Internet is littered with misinformation, half-truths, and anecdotes dressed up as facts. Reading this book is the first step to getting the full scoop on IBS and sorting out the realities from the myths. And in Chapter 20, we offer suggestions for other reliable sources of information on IBS.

Keeping a Diary of Symptoms and Life Events

When doctors look for a diagnosis, they know that what matters aren't symptoms alone but *patterns* of symptoms. How problems play out over time and in response to other factors in your life gives a much more detailed picture of disease. For example, does exercise make your pain worse? How does your bowel frequency change when you are on holiday? Is bloating a particular problem after a trip to your local Indian restaurant? Do you notice a change in your condition when you start a new job? These sorts of questions help to explain the systems involved in a symptom and pinpoint causes, perhaps showing whether pain is due to exercising or indigestion after a spicy meal.

By keeping a diary of everything going on in your life, from your health and IBS symptoms to your emotions and physical activity, you can understand your IBS better and get to know the events that aggravate your symptoms, and the factors that soothe them.

Recording each day

If you like the idea of keeping a symptoms and life-events diary, find a notepad or invest in a diary that gives a reasonably large space for each day. Try to pick a fairly typical month in your life to record, and then each day note the following in your diary:

- ✔ **Bathroom habits:** Make a note of when you use the toilet and whether the motions are explosive, loose, normal, or constipated.

- ✔ **Emotions:** Try to attribute a general feeling to each day, such as 'busy', 'dreary', 'fun', or 'miserable'. You may even want to devise your own scoring system. Then add particular emotions, for example note down if something made you feel very happy or very low.

- ✔ **Exercise:** List your trips to the gym, the distance you walked to get to work, and any other exercise.

- ✔ **Meals:** Note when, what, and how much you ate. Try to list the basic ingredients of each meal, and the brands of pre-prepared foods.

- ✔ **Sleep:** Note your sleeping and waking times, and mention the quality of your sleep.

- ✔ **Stress:** Note all stressful events and feelings of anxiety, and what they relate to.

- ✔ **Symptoms:** Write down all your symptoms as they develop, including pain, bloating, nausea, and fatigue. Describe the symptoms as well as you can.

- ✔ **Treatments:** Record all medications, complementary therapies, and treatments you have.

At the end of the month, read through the diary and look for links between your IBS and the events marked each day. You may find that simply filling in the diary each day has already helped you to see the way your IBS fluctuates or reacts to different aspects of your lifestyle. See if you can find a pattern to your condition. Mark the days when your IBS is particularly bad with a red cross, then look for other diary entries that seem to crop up frequently on those bad days or the preceding days. Can you link triggers with symptoms?

If you can't see any particular patterns to your symptoms, you may want to go through the diary with your GP – perhaps ask the receptionist to book you a double appointment to do this.

Paying attention to your body

To successfully manage your IBS, you have to see your IBS symptoms as signs of things that have to change. You got the IBS symptoms for a reason, whether it be infection, food, or stress. The first step in getting rid of your symptoms is to acknowledge why you got them in the first place. Sticking your head under the sand like the ostrich is not going to help.

You're better off identifying what triggers your symptoms than just going to a doctor and saying, 'I have no idea why my bowels are acting up. Can you give me a pill?' (As we explain in Chapter 8, pills are another thing that your bowels may react against.)

It's your body, and you're in charge. You know what you like, what you don't like, what symptoms you're prepared to put up with and what you won't tolerate on any terms. For example, maybe you enjoy eating curries so much that you're prepared to suffer, now and then, the turmoil that spicy foods generate. IBS is very much a condition that people experiment with. After all, you feel awful, nobody seems to have the one answer to how to feel better, and you have to experiment to find out what works for you. Just be sure that you experiment with the right information and tools so that you can come out on the other end winning the battle against IBS.

After you've completed the diary and identified relevant aspects of your life that affect your IBS, the next stage is to address those factors. After this is in hand – perhaps a couple of months later, you can start the diary all over again. You can gauge whether the changes to your lifestyle that you've put into place have had any effect on your condition.

Reducing the stress in your life

No one lives a stress-free life. Stress drives and motivates us, but it shouldn't overwhelm us. Stress is a well-known trigger that causes havoc for many people with IBS. But how clearly have you identified the stresses in your life and worked out how to deal with them?

Stress has a nasty habit of flitting in and out of your mind without getting the attention it needs. You can use the symptoms diary idea to keep a record of your stress and focus on some of the causes, develop an insight into how you react to stress and if your reactions are appropriate, and identify what level of stress you can cope with.

If you think that you have a lot of stress, when you fill in your symptoms diary record any incident stressful enough for you to feel that it's significant. Then note the following information about the incident:

✓ **Date and time:** Note when the stress occurred.

✓ **Level of stress:** Record how stressed you felt, using a scale of 0 to 10, where 0 is the most relaxed you've ever been and 10 is the most stress you've ever experienced.

✓ **Symptoms:** Note whether you felt, for example, cramps, 'butterflies', anger, headache, or a raised pulse rate.

✓ **Cause:** Try to be as honest and objective as possible and note the fundamental cause of the stress.

✓ **Alleviation:** Note what action you took to reduce the stress and how well this worked.

✓ **Afterwards:** Note your mood and how effectively you got on with things after the stress. Try using a scale of 0 to 10, where 0 is falling to pieces and 10 is feeling calm and in control.

Keep a stress diary for a month, then try looking back at the different stresses you experienced over the month. List the types of stress and how often they occurred. Put the most frequent stresses at the top of the list – these common stresses are probably areas of your life that you need to deal with. Prepare a second list, putting the most unpleasant stresses at the top of the list and the least unpleasant at the bottom. Then try to eliminate or work out how to control the stresses at the top of the list – this may require a lot of brainwork.

Going through the list of stresses, look at your assessments of their underlying causes and how well you dealt with them. You may see which stress management skills seem to work for you by doing this.

Finally, look at how you felt when you were under stress and how this related to your symptoms of IBS. In this way you can identify what the most important and frequent sources of stress are in your life, and how far these aggravate your IBS. You can then address these stresses or, if you can't escape them, find ways to anticipate and prepare for them.

You can find out more about techniques for dealing with stress and difficult emotions in Chapter 12.

Eating for Health

The first step in managing bowel symptoms is to watch what you eat. If you keep a symptoms and life-events diary, as we describe earlier in this chapter, the diary may help you to identify food or drink that makes your symptoms worse. Then you only need make a small step to draw the conclusion that is the food or drink is bad for you. You don't need to pay a doctor or a dietician to tell you what you already know.

You probably also know quite a lot about general principles of healthy eating, even if you don't take too much notice of it. From a very young age, parents, schools, TV, and magazines bombard us with messages about healthy foods. We find it hard to imagine that none of this has ever got through to your brain. Most people know that a balanced diet with plenty of fresh fruit and vegetables helps to keep them healthy, although someone with IBS may have to pick and choose a little more carefully. And being generally healthy plays a part in keeping IBS and its triggers under control.

So have faith in your ability to manage your diet. We devote Chapter 10 to information that can help you to become wiser about what and how you eat.

Encouraging Good Bowel Habits

Most parents spend some time and effort when toilet training their children, emphasising the benefits of a regular habit. A mum may give her child frequent opportunities to sit down peacefully on the toilet or potty, in a quiet spot undisturbed by others, often with a story book or some sort of entertainment, and then let the child get on with it. As soon as a pattern emerges, the mum encourages the child by taking her to the toilet at the same time each day, or allowing her to visit the toilet whenever the child recognises that their bowel needs to empty.

But then look at the adults' own habits – we rush here and there, dashing into the loo for a hurried effort while phones ring, or holding it all in because we have other things to get on with. You need to get back to your childhood and give your bowels a chance to do what they have to do, when they have to do it.

Make your toilet a haven and pay it a regular visit. Some people (mostly those who tend to constipation) find it takes a period of relaxation before their bowel opens – so let it have the time it needs. The body does adapt to a particular rhythm, so encourage your bowel by setting a regular timetable every day for 15 minutes uninterrupted in the loo. Don't worry if at first nothing happens (and certainly don't strain to pass a motion). Eventually, you can find that your body anticipates the opportunity and makes the most of it.

A bit of thought about what you eat also helps to keep you regular – Chapter 10 talks about the foods you need to consider if you want to deal with diarrhoea or constipation. Good bowel habits may also be helped by the careful use of medicines such as laxatives – but you may risk becoming dependent on these. You can find out more in Chapter 8.

Taking Regular Exercise

We all know that our bodies need regular exercise. But plenty of people pretend not to know!

If you want to be in charge of your IBS then you have to boss your body into action even on those days when it tells you that it really doesn't feel like it. Your doctor can remind you that regular exercise improves bowel habit, helps pain management, lifts mood, and generally improves wellbeing until she's blue in the face, but only your inner doctor can actually boot those muscles into action.

Only you know which exercises you enjoy and are more likely to stick at. A health professional can't choose your exercise programme for you, and if she did she'd probably pick what she herself likes to do. You set the programme and decide on what fun you want and who you want to exercise with. And if you're not sure what sort of exercise to do, don't ask your doctor but find a sports coach or gym trainer to explain pros and cons of different forms of exercise. Or just have a go at something new and see how you get on.

In Chapter 11 we look at the basic principles that you need to consider when working out an exercise programme.

Relaxing – Your Way

The connection between stress and IBS is fascinating, unless you're the person trying to sort it out. Then it can be downright frustrating, which doesn't help your case one bit. And what's stress for one person is excitement for another. Relaxation is a basic health need that we use to defuse stress and recharge our energy levels, but we all see the world differently: Although one individual may suggest snuggling quietly on a big sofa and watching a good movie, another may feel cooped up and prefer relaxing by dangling on a rope from a hang-glider.

Relaxation – whatever that means to you – is a vital technique, which we look at in Chapter 13. It has two important components that relate to whether we're awake or trying to get to sleep, which we discuss in the following sections.

 Right this minute, take a deep breath. Fill your lungs deeply, and make your abdomen expand. If you can't do that, or if it feels tight and uncomfortable, you have abdominal tension that translates into intestinal tension. And it only makes sense that if you try to hold in gas and diarrhoea, you have a tense abdomen as well.

Making time for you

Most of us benefit from at least a couple of periods in the day when we're under no pressure to perform or produce results, where we can do exactly what we want to do, kick off our shoes, daydream, or idle away time. Think about those instances or situations when you feel happy or mellow – perhaps listening to music or doing a crossword.

Try to find something that relaxes you and make a place for it in your schedule. Put yourself first for at least a few minutes and tell yourself that others may reap the benefits of your reduced stress levels. If you find it hard to relax, try yoga, visualisation techniques, a gentle stroll in a nearby park, or an aromatherapy session. And if these all sound so boring that you may go crazy, accept that relaxation for you may simply mean doing something that breaks you out of your normal daily humdrum routine.

Sleeping for health

The other aspect of relaxation that you need to practise until you get it right is sleep. Good deep sleep is a priceless restorative that improves wellbeing and raises pain thresholds. But people with IBS are more likely to suffer from insomnia and may have significant problems getting off to sleep. Self-reported sleep disturbance is one of the non-intestinal symptoms of IBS that markedly affects quality of life.

You can do plenty of things to improve your chances of a good night's sleep. The key is something called sleep hygiene – a set of rules and recommendations just as critical to your health as kitchen hygiene:

- ✔ **Avoid late night stimulants:** Coffee (even decaffeinated), tea, hot chocolate, and alcohol can all disrupt normal sleep as they contain chemicals that stimulate the brain or upset its normal activities. Try herbal teas (especially camomile) or milk instead.

- ✔ **Don't work yourself up trying to sleep:** If you can't get to sleep in 20 minutes, get up and sit quietly somewhere for a while before trying again. Don't put on bright lights as this tells your brain it's time to wake up. Don't lie in bed watching TV either.

- ✔ **Exercise during the day:** Getting active during the day, and tiring yourself out physically, is a great way to promote good sleep, but try not to exercise late in the evening. A gentle walk in the cool night air is fine but intense activity raises your body temperature and gets your brain buzzing, both of which interfere with the wind-down towards sleep.

- ✔ **Keep the TV out of the bedroom:** Reserve your bedrooms for sleep and sex – another good sleep-inducing activity.

✔ **Make your bedroom the perfect environment for sleep:** It needs to be comfortable, not too hot or cold (experts recommend 16–18°C), and not noisy, smoky, or poorly ventilated. Decorate the room in relaxed colours – green is very soothing.

✔ **Steer clear of large amounts of food late at night:** However, a light snack about an hour before bed may help to induce sleep.

✔ **Stick to a regular routine:** Go to bed at the same time (or as close as possible) and get out of bed at the same time.

✔ **Try to avoid sedatives:** They may help in the short term during very stressful times but sedatives induce an abnormal type and pattern of sleep, and can cause daytime drowsiness.

✔ **Think about nap times:** Daytime naps are the subject of great debate. Some believe that a short snooze can help you to feel better during the day, but a big nap can disrupt your daily sleep pattern.

✔ **Wind down in the evening:** Prepare yourself for sleep each night with a regular relaxing routine. A hot bath can help but don't make it too hot as this can leave you feeling uncomfortable. The drop in body temperature afterwards induces sleep.

Talking to Others

IBS is a common condition – it affects as many as 1 in 10 people. So out there, all around you, are hordes of people who have become experts in IBS simply through the need to manage their own condition. They've been through a lot of what you've been through, and trawled their own information sources, finding things that help and other things that don't. A huge range of professionals also have useful advice to offer, and you can turn to family or friends who care about you and are good listeners, ready to help you let off a little steam about your troubles.

Talking to others can be fantastically therapeutic and is often a great stress reliever that may help you to accept your symptoms. But despite the fact that the British are renowned for their ability to talk about their bowels, many people still find it hard to talk about the sort of problems that IBS can cause. However, if you truly want to be in control of your IBS this may be a barrier worth breaking down. If talking seems too difficult, start with the professionals. Talk to your GP about your symptoms – you can't say anything that shocks her or that she hasn't heard many times before. Then move on to practise with the surgery nurse, the dietician, the pharmacist, the woman at the desk in the local library, a kindly work colleague . . . The more you talk, the easier it gets, and soon you'll be sharing tips with the cashier at the supermarket till as you discuss the varied contents of your IBS-friendly shopping basket.

Gill struggled to cope with her IBS symptoms for more than two years. She was far too embarrassed to tell anyone at work, but often wondered if her colleagues thought she was skiving when she disappeared to the toilet several times every hour. This made her feel so worried and stressed that her IBS seemed to get even worse. It was a vicious circle. One day a woman came into the shop and asked if she could use the toilet urgently because she had problems with IBS. Gill listened in astonishment as another of the shop assistants sympathised with the woman and explained that she too sometimes had to rush to the toilet for the same reason. As they discussed some of the triggers they'd experienced, Gill found herself joining in the conversation – and finding out some helpful facts. The next time she needed the loo (which oddly enough, wasn't for some hours) she quietly mentioned why to the other assistant and was relieved to get a very sympathetic response.

Chapter 10

Eating an IBS-Friendly Diet

• •

In This Chapter

▶ Removing possible offenders from your diet

▶ Letting your body go through detox

▶ Taking additional foodie steps to combat your symptoms

• •

*Y*ou probably know the saying 'You are what you eat'. For people with IBS, another truism is 'You suffer from what you eat'.

Many foods – and even the act of eating itself – can trigger an attack of IBS, as we mention in Chapter 4. Through a combination of diet, which we address in this chapter, and stress reduction, which we tackle in Chapter 12, we hope to help you put an end to your food–IBS connection.

The goal is to identify the food factors that may trigger your symptoms, eliminate those foods, and reduce your symptoms. When your symptoms are under control, you – not your food – are in charge.

Most diets start out by eliminating some foods – and our diet for IBS is no different. In fact, most doctors, dieticians, and nutritionists who treat IBS successfully start their patients with an elimination and challenge programme. And remember: Cutting out foods doesn't have to be bad news – great-tasting substitutes for some of the foods that trigger IBS can make the food elimination process much easier to handle.

We don't tout a specific IBS-diet. Everyone with IBS has different food triggers and preferences, and so we don't tell you what to eat. Instead, we suggest lots of options and help you to determine what's best for you.

We know that changing the way you eat isn't easy. But we also know it's possible, and the result may be freedom from your IBS symptoms.

Keeping a Diet Diary

Most of us are surprisingly forgetful when it comes to analysing what we eat. Out of sight after it's down the hatch, the exact contents of a meal soon slips out of our mind. So the best way to be certain about what you eat and how it relates to your symptoms is to keep a diary of what you eat and drink.

A diet diary helps you to see how certain foods match the appearance of symptoms, and which foods may cause your IBS problems. This is especially important during an elimination diet as you reintroduce foods that you have been avoiding (more on this in the later section 'Eliminating Possible Food Triggers'). Diet diaries also help you to understand your pattern of eating, when you tend to get hungry, how you snack, and the times you tend to sit down to a meal. This can help you to work out healthier habits, or change your schedule to cut down on the need for instant grub to keep your energy going (the sort of snack foods that most people reach for, such as a sandwich, crisps, cake, or chocolate, are more likely than planned meals to contain foods that trigger IBS). A diet diary is also a great motivator – if you set aside a set period such as four weeks to get your diet right, you're more likely to stay the course.

Try to be as honest as you can. Don't rely on your memory at the end of the day. Record your diet as you go.

We talk about making a symptom and life-events diary in Chapter 9. Use our suggestions in that chapter as a basis for keeping a diet diary, making sure you note the following important points:

- ✔ **What you eat and drink:** Record every single thing that passes your lips, including meals, snacks, drinks (even water), and those stolen morsels such as chewing gum in the car and the remains of your child's fish fingers. Be as specific as you can, including noting brands for packaged foods, as you may want to go back and scrutinise ingredients on the labels. Don't forget extras like sauces, gravies, mayonnaise, and salad dressings.

- ✔ **When you eat and drink:** Give specific dates and times. This may seem like a long and tedious chore, but it's worth it when you finally pinpoint your IBS triggers.

- ✔ **How much you eat and drink:** You don't have to weigh each ingredient, but at least estimate portion sizes. Some people find that they can tolerate small amounts of a certain food (or put up with a small amount of symptoms) but large portions spell trouble.

- ✔ **Spicy details:** Note when you eat something very spicy as this can contribute to IBS, particularly to diarrhoea.

- ✔ **Social drinks:** Write down all the alcohol and other drinks you consume when socialising – alcohol is an important trigger of IBS for some people.

✔ **Your symptoms:** Note all the times you experience IBS symptoms, as this may be important in relating problems such as diarrhoea or bloating to specific meals. (If you write out your diary as a day to a page with events noted in chronological order, it may be easier to spot what follows and how triggers for IBS may lead to trouble.)

✔ **Your feelings related to eating and specific foods:** Was it tasty, satisfying, or disappointing? Charting your feelings may be useful when changing your diet and looking for foods to substitute for those causing problems.

✔ **Other thoughts:** Include any other notes relating to each meal that may be relevant as a trigger, such as 'Ate in a hurry as late for work – feeling stressed'.

Watching what you eat

After you complete a food diary for a couple of weeks, sit down and take a cold steady look at the sorts of food that you eat, and ask yourself the following questions:

✔ **Do you eat a healthy balanced diet?** IBS or no IBS, you need to be aiming for foods that maximise your general health. The healthier you are, the better you cope with the pain and misery of IBS. To ensure that you're munching a healthy diet:

- Eat plenty of carbohydrate-rich foods such as breads, potatoes, pasta, and other cereals.

- Fill up on fruits and vegetables.

- Have moderate amounts of milk and dairy products, meat, fish, or meat/milk alternatives.

- Limit amounts of foods containing fat or sugar.

Because no single food can provide all the essential nutrients that the body needs, eat a wide variety of foods to provide adequate intakes of vitamins, minerals, and dietary fibre.

✔ **Can you see any obvious patterns in your diary?** Look for links between particular foods, the time of meals, size of meals, the way you prepare foods, and the appearance or worsening of IBS symptoms.

You may find it difficult to see a pattern, especially as some people find that it can take several hours before a reaction to a food develops. As we explain in Chapter 2, the time it takes for food to travel through the gastrointestinal tract from mouth to colon is very variable and can be many hours. It may also take a while for the immune system to trundle into action.

Dodging disastrous diets

We can't recommend a single diet for IBS because triggers vary from person to person. A wheat-free diet helps some people but means unnecessarily missing out on some very tasty and nutritionally useful foods for many others. The only way we can cover all suspects in a diet that won't trigger IBS symptoms is to tell you just to drink water – not exactly a balanced diet!

But we can give you some guidance about the sort of food groups that are frequently to blame in IBS, which you can pay extra attention to. We discuss lots of trigger foods in detail in Chapter 4, but as a quick guide you may want watch out for the effects of the following:

- **Cowboy diet:** Beans, beans the musical fruit, the more you eat the more you toot . . . So goes the popular saying, and no wonder because it's true. High in fibre and a natural sugar called raffinose that some people can't tolerate, beans, lentils, and other legumes are top fodder for your colonic bacteria. See Chapter 4 for more on the effects of beans.

- **Dairy diet:** Although they have lots to offer within a healthy balanced diet, dairy foods can also upset the gut. Check out Chapter 4 for the low-down on lactose intolerance.

- **Drinker's diet:** Coffee is a villain in IBS for many reasons. Coffee is highly acidic and irritates the stomach, and stimulates motor nerve activity in the colon, producing a laxative effect. Even decaffeinated coffee has a similar stimulant action on the intestines. But decaff may stop your body's stress hormones levels rising due to caffeine as well as coffee's dehydrating effects. Coffee can also decrease magnesium absorption from food (magnesium plays a part in keeping the gut moving).

- **Fibre diet:** Fibre is a notorious character in the IBS world – both fiend and friend. We can't generalise much because people with IBS seem to react so differently to fibre. Chapter 4 tells you more about this slippery character.

- **Fruity diet:** Watch out for fruit and foods containing the fruit sugar fructose, such as snacks, manufactured foods and pre-prepared meals, and sweeteners. Chapter 4 has more on fructose intolerance.

- **Sandwich diet:** Gluten is a natural plant protein found in wheat, barley, rye, and possibly oats, and therefore in most bread. Gluten can cause an immune reaction in vulnerable people which damages the lining of the small intestine, disrupts the absorption of food and leads to symptoms that doctors may mistake for IBS. Wheat allergy is another possibility to consider (see Chapter 4).

- **Weight-loss diet:** Artificial sweeteners such as sorbitol zip straight through the intestines, dragging fluid with them. So diet foods can aggravate IBS symptoms such as diarrhoea and bloating (You can find out more about sorbitol in Chapter 4).

Making Smart Food Choices

In this section we offer some general suggestions on how you can be a smarter eater. You may be surprised at how making small changes to the way you eat can improve the way you feel. Avoiding certain combinations of food, cutting out fatty foods, and simply knowing what's right for you can all help your IBS symptoms.

Combining food wisely

Food combining was all the rage a few years ago, and the theory behind it may be relevant to IBS. Food is split into three main types:

- **Carbohydrates:** Carbs fall into two categories: simple sugar carbs (think white bread, cookies, and crackers) and complex carbs (such as vegetables, grains, and beans). Your body breaks down all carbohydrates into sugars, which provide the energy you need to operate.

- **Fats:** Fat is an important source of energy but some dietary fats are much healthier than others. The main types are saturated fats (from animals and some plants, such as butter, milk and palm oil), and mono- and poly-unsaturated fats (sometimes called MUFAs and PUFAs, these are found mainly in fish, nuts, seeds and olive or sunflower oil and are the healthiest type of fat).

- **Proteins:** Proteins are essential for growth and repair. Common sources of protein include fish, poultry and red meat, dairy products, eggs, beans and nuts.

You digest each type of food at very different rates. Proteins stay in your stomach for about three hours, and fats can hang out in the stomach for about six hours. But the simple sugars in carbohydrates need to get out of the stomach as soon as possible, and through to your small intestine where enzymes break them down.

If you eat a mixture of these food types, the simple carbs (especially refined sugar), may get trapped with the protein or fat in your stomach. When sugars hang around in your stomach, they can ferment and create gas. Younger people usually have enough stomach acid to digest the fermentation, but as you get older, the burps and belches can develop into a chorus of indigestion. So what do you do? If you're like many people, you take antacids. But in Chapter 3 we explain that antacids aren't the answer because they further deplete your stomach acid, which means food may not get completely digested.

If you have IBS, we recommend cutting out simple sugars, such as the sugar in your tea. (In Chapter 4, we explain why refined sugar and even the sugars in fruit may trigger IBS symptoms.) But if you can't completely eliminate sugar from your diet, you may want to try eating it separately from protein and fat. In other words, don't eat meat, fish, poultry, eggs, cheese, milk, or butter at the same time you eat concentrated sugars like fruit, fruit juice, or refined sugars in pastries, cakes, fizzy drinks, or sweets. As long as fruit isn't a trigger for your IBS symptoms, try to eat fruit about 30 minutes before a meal.

Because it takes three or four hours to move a protein meal out of the stomach, eating dessert right after a heavy meal can also lead to fermentation and indigestion. If you have tummy troubles, we recommend skipping dessert with a meal and occasionally indulging your sweet tooth three hours before or after a meal.

Reducing fats

A universal piece of advice we can offer for anyone with IBS symptoms is to reduce the amount of fat you consume. Most people in the Western world eat far too much fat – the standard recommendation is that no more than 30 per cent of your daily calories should come from fat.(currently about 35% of calories in the average UK diet are from fat).

Fat in the diet causes lots of bells and whistles to go off in your body. Enzymes from the pancreas and bile from the liver both digest fat, and large amounts of bile in the intestine can be irritating and cause cramping pain. Fatty foods include full-fat dairy products, certain cuts of meat, fried foods, and chocolate.

To reduce your fat intake, remove the skin and fat from your meat, choose reduced-fat or low-fat foods, and microwave, bake, or steam instead of frying or roasting.

Take care when selecting processed foods as labels can be confusing or misleading. 'Healthy' foods aren't necessarily 'friendly to IBS' foods. Low calorie foods, for example, may be low on fat and sugar but contain artificial sweeteners such as sorbitol which can aggravate symptoms. Always check the list of ingredients.

Use monounsaturated or polyunsaturated fats and oils such as those that come from olives, rapeseed, sunflowers, or corn, rather than saturated animal fats such as butter and lard. You also need small amounts of two types of essential fats: omega-3 fatty acids (found in oily fish, walnuts, omega-3 enriched eggs, and rapeseed and soya oil) and omega-6 fatty acids (found in vegetable oils such as sunflower, corn, and soya oil).

Not all oils are created equal. Some healthy fats harm can hurt IBS and some unhealthy ones may help. In general, we advise you to avoid saturated fats, but some saturated fatty acids are less harmful than others. Research suggests that coconut oil may have particular benefits in IBS, as the digestive tract absorbs the fatty acids found in coconut oil more efficiently than the fatty acids found in some vegetable oils. You can use coconut oil for cooking, and some people mix it into protein drinks. And while we also generally recommended that you use mono- and polyunsaturated fats, research suggests that the fatty acids found in some polyunsaturated oils – such as soy, corn, and other vegetable oils – may cause inflammation and irritation in people with intestinal problems.

Knowing what's healthy for you

People sometimes tell us that after they began eating 'health foods' they developed symptoms of IBS. They thought they were doing something good for their health but got blindsided by their digestive tract. The foods that many people move to when they make a bid to change their lifestyles include wholemeal or wholegrain bread, soy products, and fruit. But – as we explain in Chapters 4 and 7 – these foods can cause IBS symptoms in some people.

Here are some ways that healthy foods can cause problems in certain people:

- ✔ Gas and bloating are common symptoms when people start eating more roughage or fibre.
- ✔ The extra roughage from wholemeal products can kick-start diarrhoea in susceptible people.
- ✔ Eating more wheat can uncover underlying gluten intolerance (also called coeliac disease, which we explain in Chapter 4), causing constipation or diarrhoea.
- ✔ Soy milk, soy cheese, soy protein powders, and soy products, such as 'vegetarian meat', can cause susceptible people to develop gas and bloating. (As we note in Chapter 4, soy is very difficult to digest, especially if your body doesn't ferment it.)
- ✔ As we explain in Chapter 4, if you don't have the enzymes to digest fruit, you suffer the intestinal consequences.

If you want some good general advice about the basics of healthy eating, try www.nutrition.org.uk, the website of the British Nutrition Foundation.

As you read this book, and any other resources that recommend dietary changes to address your IBS, bear in mind that your body is different from any other body. A health food for one person may be an IBS trigger for you. Pay attention to your body's signals as you eat different foods, even healthy ones, and at the first sign that a particular food offends your system, cut it out of your diet. For more on cutting out certain foods, have a look at the next section in this chapter.

Eliminating Possible Food Triggers

In this book we place a lot of emphasis on food triggers for IBS and conditions such as food allergies and intolerances that people sometimes mistake for IBS. You probably use the process of elimination (where you cut out foods to see if symptoms settle) and challenge (where you then bring the same food back into your diet to see if it stirs up trouble again) constantly without knowing the name for it. You eat something that you realise (too late) triggers a reaction, so you eliminate that food for a while, out of fear for your gut. The next time you face that food, you may try it just to see what happens.

An elimination and challenge diet to find the food triggers of your IBS doesn't need a doctor's prescription. You can take this step on your own, but you have to use your common sense and intuition and look upon it as a clinical trial of one person.

The memory of pain is often short-lived, and you may forget that after eating a certain food two months ago you spent three hours keeping family and friends away from the toilet. We recommend using a structured elimination and challenge experiment, so you can prove to yourself which foods bother you. Plus, people with IBS rarely have just one trigger food, so eliminating just one food at a time may not help much at all. You need a plan that helps you eliminate as many triggers as possible.

You'll probably waver on your elimination diet now and again. A birthday party, a holiday, a friend waving a cake under your nose – any number of temptations can cause you to stray. But you can still develop from the experience and be stronger with the next effort.

If you follow an elimination diet and choose to sample a forbidden food in the midst of it, we suggest you do so close to home – and close to the toilet. When you take trigger foods out of your diet, even for just a few days, sometimes a mere taste can send your bowels into spasm.

Taking two weeks towards better health

Before you even start eliminating foods, make notes about your IBS and how you feel. How many bowel movements do you have a day (or a week if you suffer from constipation)? When do you have most of your pain, gas, and bloating? What foods do you think aren't your friends? Write it all down, and then make daily entries during your elimination adventure. Keeping a diary of your journey is very useful because often you don't remember how bad you felt before you made a big lifestyle change.

In Chapter 4 we offer a detailed account of some of the common triggers of IBS and other conditions mistaken for IBS. We suggest that you avoid the following potential triggers completely during your elimination diet:

- Alcohol
- Coffee and tea
- Dairy
- Food additives and 'diet' products
- Fried foods
- Fruit
- High-fructose corn syrup
- Processed foods
- Spicy foods
- Sugar
- Wheat

Try eliminating these foods for at least two weeks to get them totally out of your system. Your immune system may react to these foods, so avoiding them for two weeks allows your system to settle down and the irritation to subside.

Yes, we can hear the storm of protest. Life as you know it is now over! You have nothing left to eat! How can you possibly survive? If that's your reaction, though, that means you've been surviving on bread, doughnuts, and coffee (with cream and two sugars) for far too long. Maybe now is the time to change – for the good.

Dairy can be hard to digest, and simple sugars can spell fermentation in the gut. Additives, fried food, alcohol, and coffee can all trigger symptoms of IBS, so you really are better off without them.

You may be pleased to hear that you can happily munch away on the following foods:

- Fresh meats, poultry, and fish
- Nuts and seeds
- Unprocessed oils containing the right sorts of fat – flax, olive, sunflower, and coconut

✔ Vegetables

✔ Whole grains, such as rice, millet, quinoa, amaranth, and kasha

✔ Water, home-made lemonade, and herbal teas

In the section 'Translating Your Results into Better Habits', later in this chapter, we offer a suggested shopping list and some tasty recipes to try while you're on the elimination diet – and afterwards too, we hope, when you realise how beneficial healthy eating can be.

Doing the detox

Detoxing is an aspect to all elimination diets. For example, you may know that if you're a regular coffee drinker and decide to eliminate coffee, you can get headaches from the caffeine withdrawal, which are a result of detoxing. In this section, we give you some tips on how to make the detoxing process (whether from caffeine, sugar, or other addictive foodstuffs) less painful.

If your diet consists mostly of bread, dairy, sugar, and coffee with some protein and a vegetable or two thrown in as an afterthought, your body may react when you eliminate bread, dairy, sugar, and coffee. But if you understand what's really happening, you can do something about the detoxing symptoms that you experience.

Here's what happens in your body when you eliminate simple sugars and other addictive foods and drinks: Your blood levels of sugar or caffeine, for example, may dip and your body, which adjusted over the years to being bombarded with the chemical, may take time to readjust. Meanwhile you feel jittery and irritable, and have a throbbing headache. Comforting habits such as the ritual of coffee-making, clutching a cigarette or the shared joy of cakes with tea disappear, leaving large voids in your routine, and you have to find other things to do which may help you cope with the physical and psychological demands of your addiction. You feel so yucky that you just don't want to continue and returning to your habit seems your only way out.

Here are some suggestions to help you deal with detoxing during the first two weeks of changing your diet:

✔ **Drink water:** Drink eight glasses of filtered or bottled water every day to flush out your system. Using the morning elixir that we describe in the previous section is even better. If you enjoy the comfort of a hot-drink-in-a-mug sensation then herbal teas or just plain boiler water may be an option.

✔ **Eat good food:** In the section 'Translating Your Results into Better Habits', later in this chapter, we offer you a shopping list and some recipes to help you improve what you eat both during and after your elimination diet. Try them!

✔ **Give psyllium a chance:** If you have constipation-predominant IBS, take psyllium husk capsules or powder to maintain two bowel movements a day and sweep out the debris.

✔ **Keep a diary:** Write down how you feel when you find yourself reaching for something that you know you should eliminate from your diet.

✔ **Swallow probiotics:** Try taking probiotics (we talk about these in the section 'Probing probiotics', later in this chapter) from the first day of your elimination diet.

✔ **Try magnesium:** Consider taking magnesium citrate powder or magnesium citrate capsules. Magnesium is necessary for energy, muscle relaxation, keeping the gut moving, and sound sleep. It also protects the heart and helps to prevent diabetes. But be careful – Magnesium salts can have a powerful laxative effect and aggravate diarrhoea-predominant IBS.

Challenging individual foods

After you successfully follow the elimination diet for at least two weeks and your IBS symptoms seem to be under some control, you can move on to the next part of the experiment – figuring out what you can add back. Here are the basic steps you take:

✔ Continue following the elimination diet.

✔ Add back one portion of one new food each day.

✔ Keep a journal of your reactions to the food.

Gas and bloating are big clues that a food is not your friend. These symptoms usually come quite quickly after eating an offending food. If your IBS symptom is predominantly diarrhoea, you may have that reaction within just a few hours. But constipation-predominant IBS takes a lot longer to appear, so the gas and bloating are your first clues. If you actually have an allergy to a food that you add back, you either experience very sudden symptoms such as cramps and/or facial flushing, or a more gradual appearance of a rash, stuffy sinuses, and/or headaches.

It's important to follow our recommendation to add only one portion of a new food per day. If that food gives you a reaction, then you can mark it down as something that triggers your IBS and you can avoid it in future. If you don't have a reaction, you are then able to eat this food freely. However, we recommend that you don't bombard your gut with too much of any one food, especially during this delicate stage of testing because it may disrupt your analysis of the effects of other foods that you try. Some people find that they can tolerate a food (such as a spicy food) in moderation but that they need to gradually build up to eating it regularly, or that their gut just can't cope with it on a daily basis. Just how much of a food you can take is something that you will need to work out a little later on, after the basic elimination/challenge diet.

If you did get a reaction to the food, you may have to wait for another day or two for your gut to calm down again and get back to its usual state before testing another food.

Pay careful attention to your reactions to foods that you reintroduce. If you try some wheat and just feel a little gassy afterwards, heed this warning sign. Some gassy grumbles following a bit of wheat today can turn into an hour on the toilet tomorrow. Any reaction in your digestive tract is reason enough to take care with a particular food, and maybe wait a day or two to see if further troubles appear. You might want to try the food again once your gut has settled to see if it gives the same effect. You can also experiment with different quantities of the food to see if there is a limit that your gut can tolerate (this is often the case with lactose intolerance where people can often manage small amounts of milk in a cup of tea but not a whole glass of milk).

If you test wheat, dairy products, and sugar, be sure to experiment with foods containing only one ingredient. For example, bread contains wheat, yeast, and other ingredients, so don't test your reaction wheat by eating bread: Instead, eat plain shredded wheat covered with a bit of boiling water.

If you have a negative reaction to wheat, you have a choice to make. It's actually much easier to live without wheat today than it was 15 or 20 years ago. We now use plenty of other grains to make breads, cereals, or side dishes – millet, quinoa, buckwheat, and amaranth are the ones with the least gluten. But watch out for other foods too: Wheat flour is an ingredient in many cakes and pastries, for example, as well as a thickener in lots of sauces.

Don't challenge wheat, dairy, or any other food if you already know or suspect that you're allergic to it. Even after just two weeks of avoiding allergenic foods, you may become more sensitive to them.

Translating Your Results into Better Habits

Whether the elimination and challenge process indicates that one food offends you or a dozen are to blame for your IBS symptoms, we hope you use the opportunity (and your heightened willpower after two weeks of sacrifice) to make some lasting changes to your diet. In the following sections we help you choose healthy substitutes if you find that your favourite foods trigger IBS, and suggest some great gut-friendly recipes to get your taste buds tingling.

Substituting good foods

If you discover that one of the staples of your diet is the cause of your IBS misery, you may decide to cut out the offending food. But doing so can leave a gaping hole in your eating habits. So you need to substitute this food with another food that you can use in a similar way. This can be a great opportunity to explore the aisle of the supermarket that you never venture into and discover the joys of food that you haven't tried before.

Many of the foods that turn out not suit your body when you reintroduce them after elimination made an important nutritional contribution to your wellbeing, even if they did stir up IBS. So after you identify problem foods, you must make substitutes that are equally nutritionally valid. For example, if wheat is a problem, aim to replace it with another complex carbohydrate and a source of fibre (if fibre suits you). You also need to ensure that other foods in your diet now supply the vitamins and minerals you got from wholemeal bread (such as calcium, iron, B vitamins, folic acid, and selenium).

In Table 10-1, we suggests lots of alternatives for common trigger foods.

Table 10-1	Substitutes for Common IBS Trigger Foods
Trigger Food	*Foods to Substitute*
Wheat	Breads, cakes, cereals and snacks made from rice flour, potato starch, rye, quinoa, amaranth, and oats
	(If you have coeliac disease, make sure you choose gluten-free products)
Dairy	Rice milk, almond milk, soy milk
	(If you have lactose intolerance, try lactose-free milk or use lactase drops)
High fructose fruit (especially in apples, pears, prunes, plums, grapes, and dates)	Low fructose fruit (strawberries, raspberries, oranges, pineapples, and bananas)
	Extra vegetables (but be careful with sweetcorn, tomatoes, and carrots)
Beans, lentils, and other legumes	Try different types as some people cope with some varieties
Saturated fats (such as butter)	Olive, sunflower, flax and coconut oil, and spreads based on these

(continued)

Table 10-1 *(continued)*

Trigger Food	Foods to Substitute
Fatty meats	Leaner and skinless cuts (fat lies beneath the skin)
Fried foods	Steamed, microwaved, or baked foods
'Diet' foods and drinks (through sensitivity to sweeteners such as sorbitol)	Foods that are naturally low in calories, such as vegetables Bottled or filtered water
Coffee and tea	Herbal teas
Food sweeteners	Natural sweeteners, such as honey and maple syrup

You may well read the labels of a few of your favourite packaged foods and think that most things contain at least something on the above list in Table 10-1. It can take quite a lot of detective work to check the ingredients in processed foods, and look for substitutes. Fortunately supermarkets have become much better at labelling their foods and are developing growing ranges of foods free from the sorts of ingredients that are common triggers of IBS. For example, many large supermarkets carry a range of wheat-free foods, while others will consider stocking these sorts of goods if you ask them to. Health food stores are another good source, and often have several of these sorts of alternative versions of common processed foods such as biscuits and cakes, or chilled meals such as shepherds pie.

Planning and shopping for health

Your daily menu needs to include the main food groups to ensure you get complete nutrition. Try to eat the following at least once a day:

- ✔ A whole grain dish (made of a grain you can tolerate after the elimination diet).

- ✔ A source of protein, such as fish, chicken, or eggs (or a vegetarian option such as nuts).

- ✔ Five or more portions of fruit and vegetables, including at least one of green vegetable (such as broccoli, runner beans, cabbage), one serving of red, orange or yellow vegetable (such as tomatoes, peppers and carrots) and one of fresh fruit (e.g. apples, oranges, pineapple, banana, cherries). Aim for variety.

- ✔ A source of high-quality fats, such as flax oil, coconut oil, avocado, nuts, or seeds.

✔ Complex carbohydrates to provide some slow-burn energy – the whole grain dish we recommend above will provide carbohydrates but this type of food should be a central part of a healthy diet so you may want to also have a starchy food such as rice or potatoes at least once a day.

Following is a shopping list that can help you find foods that will, we hope, become your new best friends.

✔ **Grains:** Rice (ideally brown or basmati rice), barley, quinoa, millet, kamut, spelt, buckwheat, amaranth, oatmeal, cream of buckwheat.

✔ **Non-dairy milks:** Rice milk, almond milk, oat milk, hazelnut milk, soy milk.

✔ **Nuts and seeds:** Almonds, walnuts, brazil nuts, sesame seeds, pumpkin seeds, sunflower seeds, cashews, pecans, pine nuts, pistachios, coconut, chestnuts, macadamia, hemp seeds, flax seeds.

Many commercial combinations of nuts and seeds are available for you to try and enjoy. But keep in mind that it may be difficult to work out which one is the problem if the mixture aggravates your IBS.

✔ **Oils:** Extra virgin olive oil, flax seed oil, sesame oil, coconut oil, sunflower oil, flax oil.

✔ **Snacks:** Corn chips, popcorn, vegetable chips (containing beetroot, carrot, and parsnip, for example), granola (check the ingredients), rice cakes, banana chips, yoghurt-coated berries, dried pineapple.

✔ **Soy protein:** Tempeh, tofu, textured soy protein, soy yogurt.

Fermented soy products are easier to digest, although some people can tolerate unfermented soy.

✔ **Sweeteners:** Maple syrup, raw unrefined honey.

Choosing healthier ways of cooking

In addition to different foods and how they can help or harm in IBS, how you prepare and cook those foods also matters. We all have our own preferred ways to cook, but bear in mind that your carefully selected menu of IBS-friendly food is no good if the food is badly cooked, indigestible, or doused in IBS-inducing fat.

Here are some of the pros and cons of different types of cooking:

✔ **Raw foods:** Uncooked fruit and veg often contain more nutrients than cooked, because heating destroys some nutrients. Raw food may also be covered in friendly bacteria, helping you to top up levels in your gut. The downside is that skins of fruit and veg may be tough and hard to digest, aggravating diarrhoea-predominant IBS.

✔ **Frying:** The fat used in frying can be a trigger for IBS and it contains a lot of calories. If you must fry, try to use monounsaturated or polyunsaturated fats such as olive oil and sunflower oil.

✔ **Roasting:** This tends to have high fat levels. If you enjoy roasts then try to use minimal amounts of added fat. Look out for 'healthy roasting' kitchenware designed to cook a meat joint in its own juices, and drain meat or roast vegetables well (or pat dry) to remove as much fat as possible before serving.

✔ **Baking:** This is often a very healthy way to cook foods because it uses less fat and can preserve juices and vital nutrients. Just wrap up your fish in tinfoil, run a skewer through a potato or throw a few chopped veg into a tray and drizzle with olive oil, stick it in the oven and enjoy reading a good book while things cook up. Bear in mind that baked potatoes are a good source of fibre too.

✔ **Boiling:** The hot water can leach away vital nutrients such as vitamins, and there is a risk of soggy veg. But if you use the boiled veg water to make gravy you may be able to rescue some of those nutrients.

✔ **Steaming:** This is one of the healthiest ways to cook, because it is least likely to destroy nutrients such as vitamins and minerals. Try using the steaming water to make a sauce or gravy, so ensuring that you get as many of the nutrients as possible.

✔ **Microwaving:** Zapping your food in a microwave is an easy, quick way to cook. It's a healthy way to cook vegetables too because very little liquid is needed and the vital nutrients don't tend to leach out or be destroyed.

Treating Symptoms with Supplements

The best approach to treating IBS symptoms involves making positive lifestyle changes rather than using medications to mask the problem. These lifestyle changes include eating healthy foods (we hope we give you lots of ideas here in this chapter), exercising (which we talk about in Chapter 11), not smoking, reducing alcohol consumption, and dealing with stress (we offer lots of anti-stress tips in Chapter 12).

Dietary supplements are an additional tool. These supplements include digestive aids and probiotics. As with the medications we discuss in Chapter 8, not everyone with IBS symptoms benefits equally from using dietary supplements. You may find that a certain supplement makes a world of difference for you, but that doesn't mean it has the same profound effect on your friend.

Unlike the medications we discuss in Chapter 8, most of the supplements we talk about in this chapter have few side effects. Most people can try these supplements, in the dosages recommended on the packaging or by a doctor, without having to fear serious repercussions. You can buy these products without a prescription in most health stores and pharmacies, but we advise that you discuss them first with a health professional such as your GP, a nutritional therapist, a naturopath, or a herbalist, who will help you work out what is suitable for your needs.

Healing with herbs

People have used herbs for centuries to treat digestive complaints. In this section we mention some of the most common herbs used to treat IBS – but remember that, as with any treatment for IBS, some herbs may help you greatly and some may not.

Its possible to use many of these herbs as a therapy simply by adding them to your cooking (caraway seeds, for example, are a great digestive aid). However if you use them this way the amount of active ingredients in some herbs may be small. A more reliable way to get a good dose of the herb is to take it in the form of a pre-prepared formula (as a pill or capsule for example).

If you decide to try a herbal formula for IBS, bear in mind the following:

- ✔ **Study the ingredients:** Make sure you don't take a laxative herb if you have diarrhoea-predominant IBS.

- ✔ **Choose liquid and capsule preparations:** The body finds it easier to digest and assimilate liquids and capsules than tablets.

If you don't experience relief from your IBS symptoms after trying a pre-packaged herbal formula, don't give up on herbs yet. Consider making an appointment with a master herbalist who practises herbalism or traditional Chinese medicine (TCM). After a detailed discussion, a master herbalist customises a one-of-a-kind herbal remedy for you. To find a good herbalist or TCM doctor, ask at your doctor's surgery or local health food store, or ask for recommendations from friends.

Throughout this book, we stress the importance of recognising that your IBS symptoms and triggers are unique to you, and a unique herbal formula may just be what the TCM doctor ordered.

The smooth muscle relaxation that most of the following herbs are capable of also makes them very beneficial for preventing and treating PMS and painful periods.

Never use herbal treatments if you could be pregnant, without the advice of an experienced health professional. Some herbal remedies can stimulate the womb and increase the risk of miscarriage or premature delivery, while others may damage the unborn baby. Rosemary for example, is thought to be generally safe at the level found in most foods but may be unsafe in pregnancy when used in the medicinal amounts found in supplements. Angelia root may stimulate the uterus and induce labour while Goldenseal can cross the placenta to the baby.

There are many different herbs to chose from, each with different effects, so try to select those which match your particular condition. Here are some suggestions:

- **Angelica root:** Angelica root is also known as dong quai. The Chinese cook angelica and eat it as a vegetable. Angelica is sometimes called a 'female herb' because it has such a beneficial antispasmodic effect on menstrual cramps. The same can be said for intestinal cramps, gas, and bloating. Women with IBS often have symptoms of PMS too: By working in both areas, angelica may be very beneficial for women.

- **Anise:** This has a sweet liquorice taste. An oil in anise seeds helps aid gastric juice production. Anise relieves gas and bloating, prevents vomiting, and settles colic. It's also an antispasmodic used to prevent and treat gastrointestinal cramping. Anise is appropriate for use in both constipation and diarrhoea because it normalises bowel activity, making it very useful in IBS. The herb is also a mild sedative and calms irritability and nervousness.

- **Bitter herbs:** Bitter orange peel, gentian root, artichoke leaf, areca seed, and dandelion root all have a role in intestinal health. These herbs are bitter, stimulating gastric juices, and they also increase bile production, which helps digest fats. Areca seed comes from the dried ripe fruit of *Areca catechu*, a tree that belongs to the palm family found in the tropics. Practitioners use areca seeds to treat parasites, abdominal distension, and constipation.

- **Caraway:** This ancient herb is safe for squirmy children and colicky infants. Caraway seeds are an aid to digestion: They treat indigestion, colic, and nervous tension. Chefs add this herb to heavy foods to prevent indigestion. Caraway increases production of gastric juices, prevents intestinal spasm, and is a natural antibiotic. Research shows that several chemicals in caraway relax smooth muscle tissue in the intestines and either prevent or help eliminate gas.

- **Chamomile:** People use chamomile for gastrointestinal spasms and as an anti-inflammatory. Chamomile is a very relaxing herb and may help anxiety and nervousness. It relieves gastrointestinal tension by calming smooth muscle tissue, therefore relieving indigestion, gas, and bloating.

Chamomile is a member of the daisy family, which also houses ragweed, a well-known allergen. A potential side effect of chamomile is an allergy to it.

✔ **Fennel:** This is a common ingredient of Indian cuisine. It has a mild licorice taste. Fennel soothes the bowel by eliminating gas and bloating. An antispasmodic herb, it increases the production of gastric juices, which aids digestion. Research shows that fennel is safe for daily use and effective for use in gas, bloating, and abdominal pain. Studies on fennel show that it normalises the contractions in the intestines and relieves colic, heartburn, abdominal pain, and indigestion. Fennel also has antibacterial properties, which may make it useful in post-infectious IBS (Chapter 4 talks about this type of IBS).

✔ **Ginger:** Ginger can prevent pregnancy-related nausea and vomiting and seasickness. Ginger is also useful for indigestion, acting as a strong digestive enzyme, and people also use it to treat and prevent gastrointestinal cramps. Ginger is an antispasmodic that normalises the tone of the gastrointestinal muscles.

✔ **Oregano:** Italians often cook with this strong-smelling herb. Oregano relieves nausea, vomiting, diarrhoea, and muscle spasms. The oils in oregano act as antispasmodics and anti-inflammatory analgesics. They increase gastric juice production and eliminate gas and bloating. The calming effect of oregano works on the whole body.

✔ **Peppermint oil:** This relaxes the intestine, relieves bloating, calms intestinal spasms, and acts as an intestinal painkiller. Doctors believe peppermint oil is safe enough to give to children with IBS.

Dosing on digestive enzymes

Complementary therapists often recommend supplementing your diet with digestive enzymes, especially to reduce belching and flatulence, although no good evidence exists to show that these enzymes improve IBS symptoms. You can get your digestion going yourself simply by chewing properly (at least 40 times per bite of food), but taking supplemental enzymes may improve the efficiency of your body's own efforts – especially if, due to illness or older age, your gut doesn't produce its own enzymes very well. The aim of taking supplemental enzymes is to ensure that no incompletely digested food reaches your large intestine, creating fodder for bacteria that results in irritating toxic molecules (check out Chapter 3 for the low-down on these lowlifes).

Digestive enzymes and digestive supplements may contain various combinations of the following ingredients:

✔ **Amylase:** Naturally produced in the mouth and by the pancreas, this enzyme digests carbohydrates.

✔ **Betaine hydrochloride:** Provides a source of hydrochloric acid that enhances digestion in the stomach.

✔ **Bromelaine:** Helps to break down proteins.

✔ **Lipase:** Helps to digest fat.

✔ **Papaya:** A fruit source of protein-digesting enzymes.

✔ **Pepsin:** For protein digestion in the stomach.

✔ **Peptidase:** For protein digestion in the small intestine.

Digestive enzymes are best taken in the middle or towards the end of a meal. With these supplements, the proof is in the pudding. You should notice a difference in bloating, belching, and flatulence when you use these supplements. But if these symptoms don't improve you are better off saving your money and trying other tactics we suggest in this book, such as changing your chewing habits or using medication.

Probing probiotics

Probiotics are supplements of live good or 'friendly' bacteria that improve the balance of different organisms living in the gut and suppress inflammation in the intestinal wall. Scientists don't yet fully understand how they chase off the more harmful bacteria.

Researchers say up to 400 different kinds of good bacteria live in the gut, and (not surprisingly) many different types of probiotic supplements are available. But the commonest probiotics are species of bifidobacteria and lactobacilli. Lactobacilli have a long history of use in the dairy industry and are naturally present in the intestines. Manufacturers now add bifidobacteria to some foods.

Probiotics supplements are usually in the form of a powder for reconstitution with fluid, or as an oil or capsule containing the bacteria. You can also try probiotic yoghurts and non-dairy drinks but the dose of bacteria in these is usually much less than in the supplements.

The best source of probiotics is probably natural foods, especially vegetables and fruit that haven't been too enthusiastically scrubbed clean as the bacteria live mostly on the surface. So several portions of rinsed (but not scrubbed) fresh, raw vegetables a day may keep your good bacteria levels topped up.

People with IBS may have lower amounts of bifidobacteria and lactobacilli in their gut, and it may be difficult to take in enough probiotic bacteria through food sources alone, so supplements may be a reasonable choice. Recent research shows that probiotic supplements may help to regulate the motility or movement of the intestines, improving pain and flatulence in IBS.

It's only early days in research in this area, and researchers need to conduct much bigger studies of thousands of people with IBS to establish which strains of bacteria are best and what dose people need. But headlines are starting to appear in the medical journals that talk about the great potential for probiotic treatments. It's looking very exciting, so watch this space!

Seeing How Diet and Stress Interact

What do you do when you were feel particularly stressed? The chances are that you turn to one of your favourite comfort foods – maybe chocolate or a big sticky bun – or even coffee or alcohol. Maybe when things are really bad you get so agitated that you feel nauseous and simply can't eat anything for quite a while. When stressed, not many people find themselves reaching for some vegetables or carefully cooking up a nutritious meal.

The links between stress levels and the sort of food we eat are powerful. How we feel directly influences our diet. Many of the foods that make us feel better in our emotions (temporarily, anyway) aren't the most healthy, and may even be infamous villains in the world of IBS. Chocolate – full of refined sugar and fat – can easily stir up the gut, triggering a spasm of diarrhoea, and cakes contain wheat proteins that can aggravate bloating and wind.

Stress also directly affects the gastrointestinal tract, as we explain in Chapter 4. The emotions of stress that we experience in our brain impinge on the enteric nervous system (the 'brain' of the gut) because both 'brains' work in close harmony. The two brains also encourage the autonomic nervous system to join in with their fun and games. So stress and anxiety can stir up the nerves to the gut, causing nausea or diarrhoea, both of which may influence what we feel like eating.

One thing is certain – if you feel stressed you're unlikely to eat the most healthy, IBS-friendly foods. The idea of calmly prepared meals may be abandoned as instead you grab for anything that sustains your flagging energy and sinking mood. Stress is bad for nutrition. To deal with stress, so that you eat better, head to Chapter 12, where we offer lots of stress-busting suggestions.

Chapter 11

Alleviating IBS with Exercise

. . . .

In This Chapter

▶ Considering the types and benefits of exercise

▶ Starting an exercise programme

▶ Finding the right exercise for you

. . . .

*I*f scientists were to put all the benefits of exercise in a pill, it would probably be a multi-million-pound seller. Study after study shows that exercise
can affect every part of the body in a positive way. The trouble is, exercise is
something you – and you alone – have to take the time to do.

Exercise is certainly very beneficial in IBS. But don't worry: Exercising doesn't
have to mean 'going for the burn'. Even just the regular swaying or rocking
sort of movement you may experience on a boat, for example, can be enough
to strengthen the muscles of the abdominal girdle and create a positive change
in constipation-predominant IBS. But buying a yacht is probably the most
expensive remedy for constipation that you can ever find. Much simpler –
and cheaper – forms of exercise are walking, swimming, cycling, dancing, yoga,
or pilates (a system of practising small, precise, and purposeful movements
to strengthen and balance the muscles).

IBS is a younger person's condition, and inactivity can be a contributing factor.
Studies have found that:

✔ More than 60 per cent of adults don't move as much as they should to
keep fit and healthy.

✔ Over one-third of English adults are officially inactive, participating in
less than one 30-minute session of exercise each week.

✔ Only 37 per cent of men and 24 per cent of women meet the UK government's current recommendations for the amount of physical activity
that we need to stay healthy.

✔ An alarming 50 per cent of young people (aged between 12 and 21) aren't
vigorously active on a regular basis – the simple exercise formula needed
for good health.

In this chapter, our aim is to motivate you to start – and stick to – an exercise routine that can improve every part of your body, including those parts most affected by IBS.

Defining Exercise

We mostly hear about two types of exercise. The first is *aerobic,* which causes a lot of air to move through your lungs because you're huffing and puffing while running or playing tennis. The second is *strength training,* which builds muscles. This may conjure up images of big, sweaty men lifting weights heavier than you, but actually strength training is something we can all do in simple ways every day.

Aerobic exercise and strength training are great for your health. But people often overlook a third type of exercise: stretching, or flexibility exercise. Many people think of stretching as a warm-up or cool-down for aerobics or weight training, but stretching is a form of exercise all by itself. In the following sections, we address the benefits of all three types of exercise.

Allowing air in

When you think of exercise, you probably picture aerobic exercises such as running, swimming, and cycling. Perhaps that's why you find it so hard to get started on an exercise programme: Maybe you just can't imagine yourself in a pair of tight shorts with a number on your back doing a marathon.

Aerobic exercise focuses on your heart, lungs, and muscles. Working your muscles and speeding up your heart makes your body demand more oxygen. Your breathing rate increases in order to draw in more oxygen, and as your circulation increases it drives more and more oxygen to every part of your body. You sweat and glow with the effort. This type of exercise gives you an endorphin high and increases your stamina, as well as putting your cardio-vascular system through a good workout.

Don't think that you have to do a 10-kilometre run to receive the benefits of aerobic exercise. A brisk 20-minute walk, at a speed just fast enough to leave you slightly out of puff, is all you need to get your endorphins primed and pumped. The same is true for cycling or swimming – in fact, any brisk activity works, as long as you put some welly into it.

Building strength

Muscle burns calories. The more muscle mass you have, the more calories you burn and the more weight you can lose if you're on a weight-loss diet. Therefore, strength training (which builds muscles) is now very popular. Having stronger muscles is not just about losing weight though – it also reduces fatigue from daily activities and chores.

You don't have to lift weights to do strengthening exercises. Although this is the most effective way to build muscles, many sports (especially those where you work against resistance, such as rowing and walking uphill) can help achieve more muscle mass. But be sure to balance your activities to build up different groups of muscles around the body – get expert advice from the trainers in your local gym or sports centre.

Finding flexibility

Stretching exercises put special emphasis on your joints. During stretching exercises, you take joints in the body through a full range of motion. Stretching helps to keep your joints moving freely and strengthens the muscles and ligaments around the joints to make them more stable, balanced, and able to resist stresses and strains of daily life.

If you don't give your joints a regular workout (other than getting in and out of chairs), you can see what may happen by looking at people with disease or damage to the joints such as arthritis. The joints become stiff and painful, and the muscles around the joints grow weaker or waste away, leaving you more vulnerable to other illness. The immobility gets worse – the more you can't walk, the harder it gets to break the vicious cycle and get back to exercise.

Yoga is the main stretching and flexibility exercise that we talk about in this book. That's because yoga is one of the most beneficial exercises for IBS. You can find examples of helpful yoga exercises in the section 'Loving Yoga', later in this chapter

Benefiting from Exercise

We've compiled one of the most comprehensive lists you can find of the benefits of exercise. Regular exercise can:

✔ Balance serotonin (the neurotransmitter that controls the movement and sensitivity of the bowel) in the gut

✔ Improve digestion

✔ Improve mineral uptake in the skeleton

✔ Improve posture

✔ Improve self-confidence and self-esteem

✔ Improve the flow of fluid through the lymphatic vessels that drain the tissues

✔ Increase circulation, which increases delivery of oxygen to the tissues, giving your face and skin a healthy glow

✔ Increase core body temperature, which improves enzyme function for digestion and metabolism

✔ Increase endorphins (the feel-good neurotransmitters in the brain)

✔ Increase immune system resistance

✔ Increase mental acuity and the ability to concentrate

✔ Increase metabolism, burn calories more efficiently, and improve the appetite

✔ Increase sexual drive due to the extra energy and increased hormone output

✔ Increase the production of oestrogen, progesterone, and testosterone

✔ Lower cholesterol and fat levels in the blood levels

✔ Move gas through the intestines and reduce symptoms of abdominal bloating

✔ Reduce anxiety, depression, irritability, and mood swings (as a result of endorphins, serotonin, deeper breathing, and improved posture)

✔ Reduce stress, both mental and physical

✔ Stabilise the heart rate and strengthen the heart

✔ Stimulate and condition the muscles

✔ Stimulate the nervous system

As if these reasons to exercise weren't enough, a 2004 study at the Harvard School of Public Health found that physical activity seems to have a direct effect on the brain itself. This survey of more than 18,000 women showed that exercise promotes the production of chemicals in the brain, called *nerve growth factors,* that improve the brain cells' survival and growth.

The majority of women with IBS also have symptoms of PMS. Research shows that exercise is helpful to reduce or eliminate the symptoms of PMS because exercise reduces stress and tension, acts as a mood elevator, provides a sense of wellbeing, and improves blood circulation by increasing the natural production of endorphins.

Reducing health risks

It's never too late to start exercising. Studies show that just small improvements in physical fitness can significantly improve your health and even lower your risk of death.

The exercise programme you follow for IBS not only helps to control your symptoms, and increase your wellbeing and productivity, but also gives you an edge on many other diseases. And if your friends worry about developing IBS, you may mention to them that exercise decreases the risk of getting IBS.

The net result for people with IBS who take the time to exercise is an overall improvement in physical strength, energy, and endurance, which banishes fatigue and muscle tension. The Seattle Pacific University – which found that women who have IBS less likely to leap about – also found that when women are very active, they report less severe symptoms, especially less fatigue. The stress-reducing effects of exercise alone are enough to calm anxiety, irritability, and depression. Meanwhile, boosting the immune system results in greater resistance to disease.

Maintaining your muscles

Your body is incredibly adaptable, but if you don't move your muscles for about three weeks, you start to lose them. Have you ever injured one of your limbs? If so, you probably remember that your muscles don't take long to turn to flab. Unless you exercise, your muscles think that you don't care, and they go on strike.

The good news is that when you start to exercise, it takes only about three weeks to see a noticeable increase in strength, muscle bulk, and stamina. A moderate exercise programme involves spending 30 minutes a day or an hour four times a week walking, swimming, running, or trampolining.

Focusing on psychological fitness

Having IBS is stressful. If we can't convince you to exercise for any other reason, try making exercise an important part of your overall wellness programme in order to reduce stress. Taking a brisk walk with a positive attitude lifts your endorphins and your mood. A morning walk can improve your mental concentration and creativity and make your work easier.

Any type of exercise can reduce anxiety and depression. The calming, meditative postures of yoga, where you take deep refreshing breaths and become centred and grounded, are a balm to IBS. In some studies, exercise outshines psychotherapy and antidepressive medication for relieving mild to moderate depression.

Another psychological benefit to exercise is that it may help to relieve insomnia and sleep disturbance. However, we recommend not doing heavy exercise at night. Instead, try saving a few yoga postures for your bedtime routine.

Relieving pain

People with IBS have three common symptoms – constipation, diarrhoea and pain. A common misconception is that exercise increases pain, and when you have pain you should stop all physical activity. But in fact the exact opposite is true. When you don't move your muscles they quickly become weak and out of condition (the old 'use it or lose it' adage comes to mind). Deconditioning, in turn, can lead to even more pain. Being inactive leads to lost muscle tone and strength and less efficient heart action. It simply becomes harder and harder to exercise, setting up a vicious circle. Your sleep suffers, and you feel more fatigue, stress, and anxiety. Just reading about this decline is tiring!

Exercise releases chemicals called endorphins that block pain signals from reaching your brain. Endorphins are your body's natural pain-relieving chemicals that in many cases are more powerful than morphine. Getting morphine is pretty is a rather extreme way to cope with pain, yet you have a ready-made supply of endorphins just waiting to be released. We encourage you to do the exercise rather than finding a dealer!

Taking the First Steps

IBS is a complex condition. As we discuss in Chapter 10, the type of diet you need depends in part on the type of IBS you have. The same is true with exercise: People with diarrhoea-predominant IBS need to keep their exercise programmes close to home. People with constipation-predominant IBS-, on the other hand, can go on that long-distance run with impunity.

Checking your attitude

The first step in starting an exercise programme is getting the right attitude. We live in an instant gratification society, and exercise does not always give us immediate results. In some cases, exercise can actually make you feel a little bit worse when you start a programme.

You can easily reframe exercise as a mini-holiday from your work and daily chores. And you can remind yourself that a bit of muscle ache is, in this case, a good thing.

Getting – and staying – motivated

Maybe you've never been a regular exerciser. Or maybe you exercised regularly in the past but experienced some major stress, time constraints, or physical pain that stopped you exercising and you're having trouble getting back on track.

The more you exercise, the more the benefits build. But only your willpower and effort can get you off the starting block. We want your exercise programme to give you the incentive to begin your exercise adventure. Here's how to make your programme work for you:

- ✔ **Check with your doctor to make sure that it's safe for you to start an exercise programme.** Very few conditions mean *all* exercise is banned – usually you need to find an appropriate activity and build up slowly. But we recommend being on the safe side and getting your doctor's approval first.

- ✔ **Identify your major symptom(s) and focus on the exercises that can help the symptom(s).** In this chapter, we specify yoga exercises for IBS constipation, IBS diarrhoea, and pain.

- ✔ **Set a long-range goal.** For example, give yourself six months to reach a goal of exercising for 30 minutes each day.

- ✔ **Set a short-range goal.** A short-range goal can be to simply do five minutes of exercise today. Take one day at a time.

- ✔ **Take baby steps when you start your exercise programme.** Overdoing it at the beginning can set you up for defeat.

- ✔ **Vary your activities.** Do aerobic activities, strength training, and stretching. Walk one day, and do yoga the next.

- ✔ **Find activities you enjoy.** You can choose between hundreds of different sports. The more you like doing something, the more likely you are to keep up the exercising.

✔ **Get advice from the experts in the sport you want to try.** Whatever you choose to do, take some tips from those who know how to do it properly and can help you improve your technique in order to achieve your goals.

✔ **Exercise with friends or take your dog for a walk.** Company, even of the canine variety, can help you stay engaged and pass the time more quickly.

✔ **Don't be disheartened if you've a 'bad exercise day'.** Everyone has a day now and then when they can't do very much or things don't go well.

✔ **Develop a travelling exercise plan.** Take a DVD of your favourite exercises when you go on the road, or find a new sport to try locally.

✔ **Keep an exercise diary.** Tracking your progress can be very helpful. Unless you write it down, in three months you won't remember that you couldn't even exercise for five minutes when you began.

✔ **Pat yourself on the back**. If you feel good about the effort you're making, you're more likely to make it again. So polish your halo and keep reminding yourself just how much you're doing to improve your health.

Researchers found that a group of people who suffered from symptoms of IBS experienced a significant decrease in constipation, abdominal pain, and gas after they began a running programme. If nothing else motivates you, focus on getting rid of those symptoms!

Exercising Choices

We don't have enough space in this book to list all the possible sports, activities, and exercises that may be just the thing to inspire you into action. Only you know what appeals and, when you try the exercise, whether it's something you like and can stick at. Enjoying yourself is important – you won't make a success of your exercise efforts if you hate the activity. And you certainly won't come back the following week.

So think about which exercise options appeal to you. Talk to friends and relatives about what they enjoy doing, read about local activities on offer, and draw up a short list of activities you want to try.

As well as the sport itself, think about the following points:

✔ **The environment you exercise in:** Cold, windy sports fields aren't everyone's cup of tea.

✔ **The company you keep while getting fit:** Training with your friends may be a chance to catch up on the latest news.

✔ **The ease of access to the sport:** Is it local? Is it expensive? Do you need special equipment?

Loving Yoga

Yoga is one of the best forms of exercise for IBS. However, to say yoga is just an exercise does it an injustice. Yoga is a practice that incorporates postures and meditation to help you reach a more peaceful state. Now that sounds like something that can benefit all of us!

Postures that compress and stretch the abdomen work best for IBS. Think of it this way – when a baby experiences colic or abdominal cramps, she curls her legs up and goes into the fetal position, probably to try to press out the gas and release the tension. You can relieve adult tummy pain in the same way.

In the following sections, we present several yoga postures that may ease IBS symptoms and describe how to do them.

Happy baby

Figure 11–1 shows how to do the happy baby posture:

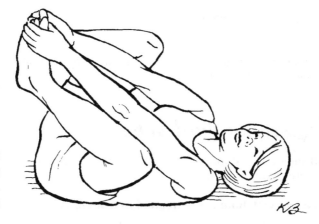

Figure 11–1:
Happy baby.

1. **Lie on your back on a mat.**
2. **Put your feet in the air.**
3. **Bend your knees and grab your toes with your fingers.**
4. **Pull your knees up and out to the sides of your abdomen.**
5. **From that position, rock back and forth or side to side.**

Ankles crossed, knees to chest

Figure 11–2 shows a posture in which you cross your ankles and pull your knees to the chest. Here are the steps:

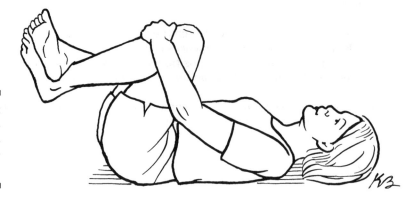

Figure 11–2:
Ankles crossed, knees to chest.

1. **Lie on your back on a mat.**

2. **Pull your knees into your chest.**

3. **Cross your ankles.**

4. **Wrap your arms around your knees and take deep breaths as you compress your abdomen.**

One-legged forward bend

Figure 11–3 shows a great forward stretch that can ease pressure in your abdomen. Here's how to do it:

1. **Sit on a mat with both legs extended in front of you.**

2. **Keeping your left leg on the floor, bend your left knee and pull your leg toward you so that your left foot touches your right thigh as close to the groin as possible.**

3. **Bend forward in that position over your right leg.**

4. **Take deep breaths as you bend further and both stretch and compress your abdomen.**

5. **Repeat the sequence on the other side.**

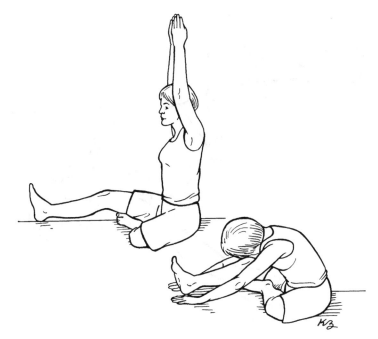

Figure 11–3:
One-legged
forward
bend.

Supine twist

Figure 11–4 shows a great stretch that can help ease tension in your abdomen and relieve gas.

1. **Lie on your back on a mat.**

2. **Keeping your legs together, roll your legs over to the right and, keeping the legs on the floor, bend the knees up.**

3. **Look to your left side and twist your upper body to the left.**

4. **Take deep breaths as you stretch your abdomen.**

5. **Repeat the sequence on the other side.**

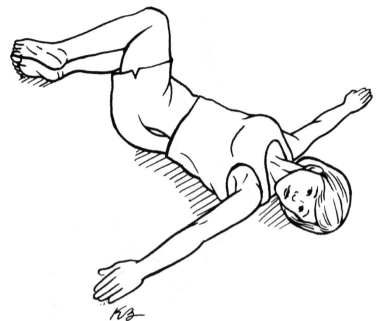

Figure 11–4:
Supine
twist.

Chapter 12

Managing Emotions and Stress

In This Chapter

▶ Staying in control of a rising tide of emotion

▶ Dealing with your feelings

▶ Talking about your troubles

▶ Finding the right person to help you

*I*n Chapter 4 we explain how little whirlwinds of stress are a perfectly normal part of daily life – the need to run for the bus, sudden demands at work, a screaming baby, a spilled cup of tea – your stress levels go up and down hundreds of times a day. Sometimes the stress is good, motivating and pushing you to get things done and giving you a sense of achievement. But sometimes stress is bad, resulting in exhaustion, frustration, and an unhappy gut.

Throughout this book, we discuss the fact that stress and IBS have an intimate connection. As we mention a few times in this book, although psychological disorders are common among people with IBS, stress does not actually cause IBS. Rather, IBS may be triggered by general mental distress of different sorts. Stress from major life events seems to be especially powerful as a trigger factor, but periods of generally excessive daily stress can exacerbate symptoms too. Episodes of IBS increase your stress level, setting up a vicious cycle. In this chapter we show you how to break that cycle.

We discuss some very useful stress-reducing and pain-reducing therapies in Chapter 13, which focuses on complementary therapies. In this chapter, we look at how your thoughts and emotions can rev up your mind up into a state of heightened anxiety, and what you can do to cut through this situation. We hope you keep an open mind and appreciate why stress-busting can be an important part of your daily routine.

Keeping on Top of Life

To take charge of your IBS, you need to stay in control of negative emotions. That means recognising negative thoughts when they invade your life, understanding how those thoughts generate symptoms of IBS, and developing a range of self-management tools to control negativity.

Research shows that almost half of people with IBS have significant psychological issues – stresses, anxieties, and low moods over and above the average we all face. But this research relates only to people who sought medical advice. Most people with symptoms of IBS don't seek medical attention – and these people actually have a similar psychological profile to healthy people. So it may be the psychological disruption that IBS causes for some people, such depression about being confined to the bathroom with endless spasms and diarrhoea, that quite understandably drives people to get medical help, rather than the severity of symptoms. Alternatively it may reflect that fact that if you can develop effective ways to keep on top of difficult times that life throws your way, you can also keep on top of your symptoms with less input from your doctor.

Many of those who seek medical help have had significantly negative early life experiences (perhaps the loss of a parent or bullying at school) and have a heightened state of anxiety about their health. So from an early age – often long before they were mature enough to understand and develop effective coping strategies – these people experience overwhelming stress that immobilises them. Conversely, those who only experience the usual drip, drip of small stresses that are part of normal life probably have more of a chance to build up some resistance to the effects of stress, find tactics that help, and develop self-belief that stress is something they can tolerate or overcome.

This means that people who work out how to deal with their stress or negative emotions themselves tend to feel more in control of their IBS, even if their symptoms are worse, and are less likely to feel the need for medical help. Keeping on top of your mental wellbeing means keeping in control of your gut.

Considering catastrophising and panic

A central idea about how the problem of stress links to bodily symptoms is that catastrophising (focusing on how bad things can be) and panic play a part. IBS often goes hand in hand with panic disorder – a condition where the person experiences episodes of intense anxiety, fear, or worry, associated with physical symptoms such as pain, palpitations, or dizziness. If you have panic disorder you may also experience a sense of imminent danger or impending doom, as well as a fear of losing control, going crazy, or dying.

One of the pioneers of self-help in psychology, Dr Claire Weekes, writes extensively on panic attacks and says that they consist of a *first fear* and a *second fear.*

The *first fear* is a group of sensations (usually without any trigger that the patient is aware of). Psychologists now call this state *arousal* or *dysautonomia*. For someone with IBS it may, for example, consist of a little rumbling in the intestines or a need to empty the bowels.

The *second fear* is a reaction to the first fear. Psychologists have some barnstorming arguments about why this second fear develops, but one of the strongest ideas (which Weekes believes) is that the second fear is a fear of the first fear and what it represents. The affected person misinterprets the signals from their gut as representing a threat to their health, a warning that dire things are about to happen (this is hardly surprising because people with IBS are used to their bowel doing fairly dire things that humiliate and embarrass them). People experiencing the second fear rapidly become anxious and anticipate a catastrophe. That *catastrophising* anxiety turns up the controls on the nervous system even higher, increases motility and secretions in the gut (hence people in desperately frightening situations feel an urgent need to open their bowels, as the body prepares to run), and – lo and behold! – symptoms of IBS appear.

People without IBS are more likely to ignore – or simply not even notice – minor sensations coming from their gut. They don't panic or catastrophise. If they do notice a rumble or a little twinge of cramp, they probably just think, 'Oh yes, there goes my baked potato and tuna mayo I had for lunch', in a calm, matter-of-fact way. But those with IBS think, 'Oh no! Here we go again, I'm going to have to dash to the loo in a minute. Everyone in the office will stare at me . . . I bet there'll be some really embarrassing farting . . . I just won't be able to stay at work . . . Much more of this and they're bound to fire me . . .'. They immediate anticipate the worst case scenario, and the stress quickly escalates.

This unhelpful pattern of thinking, with fear, panic, and catastrophising, is very treatable using cognitive–behavioural therapy (CBT), which we describe in the section 'Brooding over behavioural therapy', later in this chapter.

However, it's also very important to understand that those people with IBS who panic and catastrophise don't necessarily worry more in general. They seem to have a different neurochemistry – their enteric nervous system (the nerves that run between the gut and the brain) is wired differently and the sensations that lead to panic may feel very different to the rest of us, and be perceived differently by the brain.

Assuaging your anger

In Chapter 4 we explain that people with IBS may have increased activity in the nervous system of the gastrointestinal tract (the enteric nervous system) and that this can cause increased movement or motility in the intestines. Some research suggests that certain emotions – especially anger, aggression, and resentment – may act as switches that turn up activity in the gastrointestinal tract, generating engorgement of the mucus linings of the stomach and intestines, increased muscular contractions of the intestinal wall, and accelerated secretion of certain neuroendocrines (the hormones that carry signals between parts of the nervous system). This 'upregulation' happens in everyone but may be worse in those who have IBS. This isn't because people with IBS go around in a frenzy of bad temper (although you may feel that you've good reason to) but because when they do get angry (just like the rest of us) it seems to affect the gut more powerfully than it does in healthy people.

One group of scientists have even drawn out a map of what they call the *emotional motor system* linking the parts of the brain controlling feelings with the gut, and which they suggest is responsible for both the generation of emotional experience and gut dysfunction. Circuits involving fear inhibit upper GIT motility and stimulate the last part of the colonic function (so that you stop digesting food and empty your bowel). Anger is associated with enhanced contractions of the upper and lower bowel and increases in blood flow in the mucus-filled inner lining of the gut, as well as gastric acid secretion. In IBS this system goes haywire, like a badly wired house, as emotions in the brain trigger signals that cause excessive alterations in gastrointestinal motility and secretion from epithelial surfaces or, going the other way, signals from the gut travel up to change how the brain perceives bodily sensations.

Plenty of sources exist to help you manage anger, and you can find a lot of information online (try www.angermanagementstrategies.com, for example). But if you feel that you would like professional help you can talk to your GP and ask him to refer you for counselling, which we look at in the section 'Concentrating on counselling', later in this chapter.

Being assertive

When you battle with the sort of miserable symptoms that IBS can constantly throw at you, it can be difficult to keep up your energy and morale. Many people with IBS, especially when they've had it for years, feel ground down. Their emotions sink, they start to feel downtrodden, and their confidence ebbs away. As this happens it becomes harder and harder for them to make others aware of their needs.

After 10 years working for a small business providing technical skills around the clock to communication networks, Gerry's company announced that night shifts, previously a voluntary arrangement, would become compulsory. All the technicians would have to take a turn on the call-out desk. Gerry knew that this would make his life intolerable – his diarrhoea-predominant IBS was at its worst late in the evening, and he often avoided making social arrangements because he needed to be at home to cope with symptoms. A late night or disturbed sleep made his IBS much worse, and he had never found it easy to sleep during daylight. His heart sank at the thought of night shifts but he didn't want to make a fuss or explain about his IBS. Somehow, he thought, he must cope, or else he'd have to find another job.

To get on top of your emotions and aim for peace, harmony, and happiness, you have to be able to speak up for yourself, in order to get what you want and need – you have to be assertive. This doesn't mean being aggressive and loud, and beating everyone else into a pulp. But it does mean resisting those who try to dominate and manipulate you. It involves working on skills that enable you to communicate clearly, calmly, and frankly, so that the people in your relationships know where they stand and don't feel abused. This communication can help those who suffer in silence, which probably sums up a large proportion of people with IBS.

You can go on specialised courses known as assertiveness training to find out about these skills and other useful strategies such as working out how to get on despite feeling fearful, resisting manipulation, and coping with criticism. Assertiveness training can also help you to understand how humans interact and the roles that people play in relationships. If you're interested in finding out more ask in your surgery or local library to see if any courses run near you. Practitioners can help you to build assertiveness using a technique called transactional analysis (TA), which we consider in the section 'Trying transactional analysis', later in this chapter.

Dealing with despair

Sometimes, when IBS does its worse for weeks and months, seeing the way ahead is difficult. You may feel that your symptoms will go on forever, that with no real explanation for them you can't overcome them, and that your relationships, career, social life, or hobbies are all permanently blighted by the awful disruption. These feelings, where you have no hope, are those of despair.

So how can you get back a sense of hope when all around you – or inside you – seems hopeless? Hope means believing in possibilities ahead, and to believe that things can get better, you need to have realistic expectations. If you set yourself goals that unachievable, the likelihood is that you fail, become frustrated, and feel hopeless again. By setting achievable goals, which means recognising and accepting the limitations that your IBS places on you, your plans are more likely to come to fruition. As a result, you begin to gain control over your life again, and regain a sense of optimism.

For example, if you experience frequent loose bowel movements with ferocious farting, it may be hard work to simply get down to the supermarket and back. You may yearn to jet off to a relaxing holiday in the sun and yet utterly despair that this can never happen. You wonder how you would cope with the long journey to the airport, and then being packed in a plane for hours together with dozens of strangers and just a couple of tiny toilets, where everyone around you can hear and smell your gassy problem? Time to reset your expectations. You can find great British beaches, often with a good dose of sunshine, within a couple of hours of most places in the country. Alter your goal (initially, at least) to a weekend break on a British beach, or a couple of days holed up in a cosy country cottage with some good books and great DVDs (and a bathroom all to yourself!).

To create reasonable expectations you may need to do a bit of thinking around the issue that blocks you. You probably also have to compromise. But you can find achievable and fulfilling options if you look hard enough. It's worth keeping in mind that:

- ✔ Almost everyone with IBS finds that their symptoms fluctuate, with good weeks and bad weeks. If things are bad now, they'll get better at some point.

- ✔ IBS isn't a fatal condition. It won't get worse and worse until it kills you, Many of the years to come will be better than this one, so at some point you can get back to those ambitions and dreams.

- ✔ IBS doesn't destroy your independence – with a little planning you can still get out and about on your own, and do what you want to do without needing other people to do things for you.

Unravelling the Meaning of IBS

'Why me?' has to be one of the loudest cries you'd hear if you could listen to the thoughts of someone with IBS. People battling with any diagnosis – whether IBS, cancer, diabetes, or any other chronic condition – strive to comprehend that disease and what it means for them, and especially so when the problem is poorly understood by the experts. Knowledge and understanding are part of the journey of acceptance and healing. Most people have a variety of questions to which they want answers and, in conditions such as IBS where the explanation isn't always clear, it can be very frustrating.

Each person looking for a deeper meaning to their IBS eventually finds their own personal explanation that gives them a framework to look for ways to manage the condition. And remember that what is right and helpful for one person can be quite wrong for another. For example, some people take a hard scientific line – they may blame their genetic make-up, relate to explanations about aberrant wiring of the nervous system, or look for chemical additives in foods. Others take a spiritual view – they may see IBS as their personal challenge to accept and nurture the individuality that is a feature of all God's creatures. Or they may adopt a Zen approach and seek comfort through mindful awareness of the tiny pleasures in everything we see and do. Some look for meaning in their lifestyle – is IBS a signal from the body to put the brakes on a hedonistic way of life and get back to basics? And others blame society around them, whether raging about the stress of urban life or pollution of food sources.

Finding meaning in IBS is part of the personal journey we all make to find out who we are, why we are here, and how we can bring out the best in our life. It's a very personal, individual path. Healing is ultimately part of this inner path instead of just a mad rush to try new cures or search for ways to relieve stress.

Sounding Out Psychotherapy

Psychotherapy means 'mind treatment'. It's treatment that helps you to understand yourself and change ways of thinking or behaving. The British Psychological Society describe psychotherapy as 'the practice of alleviating psychological distress through talking rather than drugs'. This highlights an important point about psychotherapy – it's a talking treatment. With psychotherapy you spend lots of time discussing issues and exploring your thoughts with your therapist.

For many people the word 'psychotherapy' conjures up images of neurotic self-obsessed characters from American movies and TV series, who lie for hours on a leather coach obsessing and agonising about the minutiae of their lives, unable to take a step without consulting their therapist.

The reality is very different. Hundreds of thousands of people in the UK have some sort of psychotherapy. For most of these people, psychotherapy is a simple practical way of exploring the way they see life or getting to grips with problems that weigh them down, whether at home, at work, or in relationships.

Choosing the therapy for you

Psychotherapy comes in dozens of different varieties. For example, in *intensive psychoanalysis* the patient and therapist work together closely to explore past conflicts and unconscious motivations as the roots of current emotional and behavioural problems. And in *group therapy* a number of people with similar problems meet regularly with a therapist, who uses the emotional interactions of the group to help them understand and possibly modify their behaviour and find relief from distress – such as in Alcoholics Anonymous.

Couples' counselling, family therapy, cognitive–behavioural therapy, play therapy, self-help groups, pastoral counselling with spiritual advice from a faith leader . . . you can choose what feels right for you and your problems. Central to most psychotherapy is looking at and understanding your distress in the context of your own history and experience, personal coping strategies, and personality.

You may think that sitting in the hair salon talking over relationship problems with your stylist counts as a type of therapy – and in some ways you're right. But psychotherapists are highly trained individuals with the right skills to guide your thoughts and help you to consider their real meaning. Psychotherapy is team work: The therapist brings professional knowledge and expertise, and you bring knowledge and expertise about yourself.

Several things influence how much psychotherapy helps you.

- ✔ **Personal factors:** These include your motivation to confront difficulties and work to make changes. The more committed, motivated, and willing you are to work at a problem, the more useful your therapy may be.

- ✔ **Your relationship with your therapist:** This may be more important in deciding how helpful therapy is than the particular method the therapist uses. You need to open up and talk freely to your therapist, sometimes about very personal, embarrassing, or upsetting feelings. For psychotherapy to work, you need to feel that you can safely trust your therapist with this information and that your therapist understands and accepts you. If you don't like your therapist or you don't manage to establish a comfortable relationship, you may just as well talk to a brick wall. Try to explain to him that you feel that you're not making progress and would like to see someone else – people quite often change therapists, especially early in a course of treatment, so he should understand. Or talk to your GP about referring you to someone else.

- ✔ **The psychotherapist's methods:** Psychotherapy embraces many types, and even within one particular type the therapist may use a variety of different techniques and strategies. One of the therapist's roles is to find methods that seem to suit you or your problems.

- ✔ **Your optimism:** If you feel the therapy is going to be successful, then it's more likely to be so.

Brooding over behavioural therapy

Behavioural therapy involves looking at how your behaviour influences your condition, and how you can change that behaviour to improve symptoms. Several different methods are used such as relaxation therapy to identify and reduce stress; biofeedback regulation (this helps you to tune into the abnormal biological signals coming from your body, such as a raised pulse rate, which indicates tension – and then develop techniques to return them to normal); hypnotherapy aimed at controlling intestinal muscle contractions; cognitive therapy (this follows the idea that understanding about your disease and what causes it can help you to control it and feel better about it), and psychotherapy.

Relaxation therapy

Relaxation therapy may be useful when stress is contributing to your symptoms. You can choose from lots of different types of relaxation therapy, from formal techniques such as progressive muscle relaxation, yoga and meditation to massage, aromatherapy, or even simply making sure that you put your feet up and lie back on the sofa for at least an hour a day. Unfortunately you're unlikely to get any of these treatments on the NHS, but many of them are cheap and easily available.

Relaxation therapy can reduce general anxiety levels, which helps to reduce painful spasms and diarrhoea. For those with constipation-predominant IBS, lowering stress may improve bowel frequency. Some experts argue that a lot of the benefit of formal relaxation therapies comes simply from getting some attention from a therapist or teacher who is interested in your health, but if it works for you then why not! And if you can enjoy the therapy too, then even better.

Hypnotherapy

Hypnotherapy also gets a thumbs-up, especially as it helps people who don't get much relief from medical or other treatments. One particular advantage of hypnotherapy is that instead of just relieving a single symptom, it improves many of the features of IBS including quality of life and psychological wellbeing.

Hypnotherapy seems to be able to help you to reinterpret the sensations coming from your gastrointestinal tract so that you can accept them as normal instead of worrying about them – it works in a similar way to calm your brain's reaction to pain. Hypnotherapy also reduces contractions in the colon, and gives you a more positive outlook on your condition. Another bonus is that its effects are long lasting – for as long as five years after treatment.

Cognitive–behavioural therapy

The use of Cognitive–behavioural therapy (CBT) in IBS is based on the premise that IBS symptoms are initially triggered by stressful life events, daily hassles, or aspects of lifestyle. The affected person responds to these symptoms in unhelpful ways that don't address the underlying triggers and which may make the situation worse, for example, by imagining the worst or catastrophising. In CBT the therapist helps you to understand why your thoughts and actions are unhelpful and how you can break the vicious circle of harmful thinking and behaviour. Unlike other types of psychotherapy, it doesn't focus very much on your past, but looks at the 'here and now' of problems.

For example, the therapist works to help the individual break down problems into smaller parts. Starting with a particular symptom, such as excessive gas, you then consider thoughts, emotions, physical feelings, and actions related to that symptom, and look at how these can change.

The ultimate goal is for you to work out for yourself the most constructive way to see your problems, and take appropriate action. Treatment usually consists of up to 20 weekly sessions lasting from 30 minutes to an hour. Your GP should be able to arrange treatment for you although you may face a long wait on the NHS.

Research suggests that CBT may help you to cope with your symptoms without necessarily abolishing them. Benefits have been shown to include a general improvement in symptoms, especially bowel frequency, although there is little effect on abdominal pain, and improvements in work and social life. CBT often works better if it is used alongside many of the medical treatments, such as antispasmodic drugs, that we have already mentioned, not instead of them.

One of the great things about CBT is that you can do it using a self-help book or a computer programme, both of which act as the therapist would to ask you questions and guide your ideas. In England and Wales the NHS offers two particular computer programmes. Although the programmes aren't directly designed for IBS, you may them helpful or relevant to your situation. 'Fear Fighter' is for people with phobias and panic attacks (we talk about the role panic and catastrophising can play in IBS in the earlier section 'Considering catastrophising and panic'). 'Beating the Blues' is for people with mild to moderate depression – many people with IBS fall into this category. Talk to your GP about how you can register for these programmes.

If you want to know more about CBT, check out *Cognitive Behavioural Therapy For Dummies,* by Rhena Branch and Rob Willson.

Assessing psychoanalytical psychotherapy

Psychoanalytical psychotherapy, often called simply psychoanalysis, is a process that helps people to understand and manage their problems by increasing their awareness of the ways in which their inner world, or subconscious, influences their daily behaviour. It differs from many other therapies because it's usually a long-term treatment – often a number of years – that aims for deep-seated and lasting change within the patient's personality and emotional development.

The theory behind psychoanalytical psychotherapy is that we sometimes try to deal with problems by keeping them out of our mind as a way of getting rid of them. But the problems continue to affect feelings and behaviour. Early experiences help shape the way the mind works, but a large part of our mind operates outside of our consciousness. The therapist helps the patient understand these subconscious ways of dealing with experiences. As the patient becomes aware of the way their mind is working, it then becomes possible to bring about change.

It's not clear how effective psychoanalysis is in IBS – there simply hasn't been much research to prove how it can help although many individuals have found personal benefits. It may, for example, help people sort out particularly troubled aspects of their life and so generally reduce stress. Bear in mind too that psychoanalysis isn't usually available on the NHS. And as it generally involves therapy sessions several times a week for many months or, more often, years it is a huge financial commitment (as well as time commitment, too). However, some centres do offer reduced rates.

Be aware that many different schools of psychoanalysis exist, each based on slightly different ideas about how the mind works but most extrapolated from Sigmund Freud's initial work. These include Jungian analytical psychology, founded by Carl Jung, which has a more spiritual approach, and conflict therapy, which looks at emotional symptoms and character traits as an effort to resolve intrapsychic conflict. Research the topic and get a good idea of which school feels most comfortable to you or seems to reflect your own personal philosophy before you start looking for a therapist.

If you want to find out more, you can talk to your doctor or get in touch with the British Association of Psychotherapists (www.bap-psychotherapy. org), the British Psychoanalytical Society and the Institute of Psychoanalysis (www.psychoanalysis.org.uk) or The College of Psychoanalysts – UK (www.psychoanalysis-cpuk.org/).

Sussing Out psychodynamic interpersonal therapy

One type of psychoanalysis where there is some research to show an effect in IBS is Psychodynamic Interpersonal Therapy (PIT). PIT helps you develop insight into the development of your symptoms in the context of difficulties or changes in the important personal relationships in your life. So it looks for example, at whether symptoms are linked to marital strife or arguments at work.

Not only can PIT help you to understand how your emotional state relates to stress, but it can also demonstrate direct links between your emotions and bowel symptoms. According to some authorities, PIT can lead to significant life changes as well as an improved emotional state and IBS symptoms. Research has shown that this therapy is more effective than supportive listening and is cost-effective, causing a significant improvement in health-related quality of life and a reduction in healthcare costs. So it's good news for you and the NHS!

People with constant abdominal pain and constipation seem to do particularly well, and better than those with fluctuating symptoms. It also seems to be more effective among women than men, perhaps because women are more interested in, or willing to examine, the nitty gritty of their close relationships, If you want to try PIT you may need to do a bit of research to find a therapist who specialises in this approach but your GP, or the psychoanalysis resources we mentioned earlier, should be able to help.

Concentrating on counselling

It sometimes seems as though whenever anyone has a problem, the answer is a bit of counselling. Feeling low? Get some counselling! Worried about stress? Talk to a counsellor! Exhaust falling off your car? Well surely a counsellor can help! Counselling seems like the 21st century's solution to all known ills.

The counsellor gives you (the client) an opportunity to talk about your problems. By listening to what you have to say, the counsellor gains an understanding of your point of view and can help you to see things more clearly, possibly from a different perspective.

Counselling doesn't involve handing out advice or telling you how you must act. Instead, it enables you to make choices or changes. Counselling also provides an environment where you may feel more free to talk about difficult issues than with your family or friends, who you may not want to burden with your worries.

Your GP may refer you for counselling on the NHS if he thinks that it's appropriate. However, resources are limited. Some areas don't offer a counselling service, and even if they do you may have to wait months for treatment. So you may choose to pay privately for some sessions. Different schools or methods of counselling exist, and before you sign up to it we advise you to find out a little about the theory and approaches the counsellor uses to be sure that it's right for you.

Finding a therapist

Finding a therapist that meets your needs and with whom you feel you can develop a good working relationship may seem like a daunting process. Therapists tend to use terms that relate to the specific approaches or schools in which they're trained, such as 'psychodynamic', 'psychoanalytic', 'cognitive', 'humanistic', and 'person-centred' – all mind-boggling stuff, especially if your energy has been worn down by years of IBS.

One word to look out for is 'integrative'. Psychotherapists who use more than one approach describe themselves in this way and such a flexible approach may be best until you know what they're all about. We mentioned earlier that the factors linked to success with therapy have more to do with your commitment and your relationship with the therapist than the method they use. If you choose an integrative practitioner, you can focus on getting on with each other first and then choose a method that suits your view and problems.

Most doctors have some knowledge of the different types of therapy available. Try asking your GP what therapies may be most useful for you. Many therapists require your GP to formally refer you, just as a GP refers you to any other medical specialist. You can always try approaching some therapists directly, although they usually ask you to let them contact your doctor so that they're aware of your treatment and can provide any pertinent medical advice. (If the therapist doesn't ask you to tell your GP, or if they suggest specifically NOT telling GP, then you should hear alarm bells ringing and seek advice from the society with whom the therapist is registered.)

The following organisations provide lists of fully registered psychotherapists:

> ✔ **British Association for Counselling and Psychotherapy (BACP) (www. bacp.co.uk):** BACP is the largest professional organisation in the field of counselling and psychotherapy. It provides education and training for counsellors and/or psychotherapists, helps provide services within the NHS and offers information to the public about these treatments and how to find a therapist.

✔ **British Psychoanalytic Council** (www.psychoanalytic-council.org): this association represents the profession of psychoanalytic psychotherapy. It provides a register of therapist, sets training standards and produces a code of ethics.

✔ **British Psychological Society** (www.bps.org.uk): This society has a register of psychologists specialising in psychotherapy. It only includes chartered psychologists, so you can expect these therapists to have a certain level of qualification and competence.

✔ **UK Council for Psychotherapy (UKCP)** (www.psychotherapy.org.uk) The UKCP promotes research and education in psychotherapy and contributes to training and practice. It also holds a register of members.

Chapter 13

Evaluating Complementary Therapies

In This Chapter

▶ Exploring different treatments for your IBS

▶ Getting to the point of acupuncture

▶ Relaxing with massage

▶ Taking a holistic view of your body

Complementary and alternative medicine (CAM) therapies form such an accepted part of healthcare that drawing the line between them and conventional (allopathic) treatments is difficult. Whether you drink peppermint tea for indigestion, have aromatherapy massages for backache, or practise yoga for tension, CAM has become part of our daily lives.

Impressed by the effects and results of certain CAM therapies, increasing numbers of doctors and nurses study how to do these therapies and work with CAM therapists to recommend treatment. Nurses' basic training often includes massage therapy, and many GPs use techniques such as hypnotherapy and acupuncture in their surgeries.

Many NHS hospital units, especially cancer and palliative care units, and hospices incorporate CAM into their standard practice. The therapies that these facilities use tend to be those that involve touch, such as aromatherapy and reflexology, and techniques that target the mind–body link, relieve anxiety, and lift the mood, such as relaxation, visualisation, and hypnotherapy.

 Just like conventional medicine, CAM can have side effects too. Don't be fooled into thinking that a treatment is safe just because it has been used for centuries, seems gentle and pleasant, or is made from natural plant sources. Always check with your practitioner – or the person selling the remedy – for possible side effects before you go ahead with it.

With CAM, you also get the luxury of time — sometimes an hour or more – with your therapist, compared with the measly average seven to eight minutes with a GP. But of course the reason why CAM therapists can take a more considered interest in you is that you stump up the cash for the treatment – if you pay for a private consultation with a doctor you also get lots of time with them.

In this chapter we cover some of the most common complementary treatments used in IBS. For help with herbal medicine, take a look at Chapter 10.

Pregnant women and young children need to be particularly careful about using complementary treatments. They're more vulnerable than most to the side effects or complications of any therapy, whether conventional medicine or CAM. Treating a woman who is pregnant may cause harm to her unborn child. In addition very few research studies are done in these groups, for complex ethical reasons, so the effects of treatment may be less well known or difficult to predict.

Getting Started with Complementary Therapies

If you want to try some complementary therapies, you may be unsure where to begin. Doing some research and reading about a variety of treatments can help you work out what sounds useful to you. Ask your friends if they've tried, and recommend, any CAM treatments. But don't get carried away by anyone who has only good stories to tell – they may have their own agenda or be trying to sell you something, even if it's just their own rigid beliefs that CAM is good and conventional medicine bad.

Your GP is another good starting point for advice. Some doctors are sceptical about CAM, but remember that they work with your best interests at heart. So whether it's negative or positive, try to consider your doctor's view as valid. Many family doctors have some faith in acupuncture, osteopathy, chiropractic, homeopathy, massage therapy, and aromatherapy. And nearly 40 per cent of general practices in England provide access to some or all these CAM therapies (although you may have to pay for them). If you need a referral, your GP knows who has a good reputation in your local area, and may even be able to refer you directly (many GPs refer their patients with low back pain to an osteopath or chiropractor, for example). A few surgeries scattered around the UK have fully integrated conventional and complementary medicine, so if you're lucky enough to live near one of these you find that therapists are part of the team treating you. For more on integrated medicine, head to the section 'Integrating Complementary and Conventional Medicine', later in this chapter.

If you attend a gastroenterology clinic for your IBS, you may like to ask what information or links to particular CAM therapies they have that they think may be relevant to your situation.

When you try a complementary therapy, bear in mind the following:

- ✔ Always check that your therapist is fully trained and qualified, (ask her directly or check that she's registered with her professional organisation – most of these bodies act as regulatory authorities and require their therapist members to prove their credentials in order to achieve registration).

- ✔ If you have a serious illness, symptoms that persist, or any particular concerns about your condition, let your doctor know that you're using CAM therapies, especially if you take herbal or other types of medicine that can interfere with any conventional drugs you're taking.

- ✔ Don't give up conventional medicines for an alternative remedy without discussing this first with your doctor.

- ✔ Beware some treatments, especially herbal medicines, because very little quality control exists and you can't always be sure exactly what you're taking. For example, some Chinese traditional medicine mixtures imported to the UK recently were contaminated with heavy metals or mixed with prescription drugs. In the UK the Medicines and Healthcare products Regulatory Agency (MHRA) are bringing in safety legislation about the quality of herbal remedies but their rulings about products won't be compulsory until 2011.

- ✔ Buy products from a pharmacy or clinic, where the quality is more likely to be good and where you can get reliable advice, rather than a supermarket or market stall.

- ✔ Follow your therapist's advice and instructions carefully. If you've any doubts or questions, don't hesitate to go back and talk to your therapist.

- ✔ If symptoms persist or you have worries about the treatment offered, get a second opinion from another practitioner or talk to your GP.

Pondering the Placebo Effect

Numerous studies now demonstrate the 'placebo effect' where fake treatments, made from an inactive substance like sugar, distilled water, or saline solution, can sometimes improve a patient's condition. The improvement comes about simply because the person believes in the medicine and its power to heal.

Researchers don't have much idea about how mind and body link up, or how our thoughts can heal us. But scientists do think that our beliefs can cause the body to undergo actual biological changes. To make placebo effects even harder to judge, many chronic medical conditions wax and wane, with good times and bad. So is an improvement in a patient's condition due to the treatment, or was it going to happen anyway?

We believe that whether or not the results of some complementary therapies used to treat IBS are purely a result of their placebo effects doesn't really matter. If a treatment makes you feel better, and is safe to use, then these we must harness and accept these effects.

Helping with Homeopathy

As we discuss in Chapter 1 and elsewhere in the book, IBS is a *functional condition,* meaning IBS doesn't cause structural damage to your body and it has no single known cause or single effective treatment. Homeopathic medicine is safe and has a very good track record in the treatment of functional complaints. Many people who try homeopathy for IBS say their symptoms improve.

No scientific evidence proves that homeopathy has any effect in IBS, and sceptics attribute the success of homeopathy to the placebo effect (which we explain in the section 'Pondering the Placebo Effect', earlier in this chapter). However, the millions that benefit from homeopathy include infants and animals – unlikely candidates for the placebo effect. Then again, perhaps the close attention provided by a homeopathy therapist has a healing effect.

People use homeopathy widely in Europe and the US. Used correctly, it has very few side effects. You can even use homeopathy if you take conventional medications – but do check with your homeopathy therapist and doctor first.

Homeopathic remedies typically come in dosages of 6, 12, or 30 X or 6, 12, or 30 C potency. (The X stands for 10, and the C stands for 100, so the C potencies are much higher.) The higher the number, the greater the dilution, and the more potent the remedy. Usually, you take three pellets or four drops of a remedy several times a day. We recommend the liquid medications rather than the pellets because manufacturers make the pellets with lactose, which can cause problems if you have lactose intolerance.

Trying homeopathy for IBS

Unlike conventional medicine, which prescribes different drugs for physical and emotional problems, homeopathic remedies treat body, mind, and spirit. Moods and emotions, and even the preference for a certain season, colour, or climate, all go into the selection of the right remedy for you.

Homeopathic medicines are inexpensive and available in health stores and many pharmacies. You can simply try the homeopathic medicine that seems best suited to your symptoms, but we recommend visiting a trained homeopath. Your homeopath probably asks about your quirks and habits to find the remedy that suits your personality and your IBS symptoms. Your homeopath then prescribes a specific *constitutional homeopathic remedy* – a treatment that matches your personality and character traits and best suits your health problems.

For a very acute, painful symptom, you can take a remedy every 15 minutes. However, if after taking five or six doses of a remedy you experience no change in symptoms, the remedy is probably ineffective, and you should seek a new remedy. The following homeopathic medicines may help with mild to moderate IBS symptoms as a first-aid approach.

- **Argentum nitricum:** This medicine has the best results for anxious and nervous people who have the following gastrointestinal symptoms: bloating, rumbling flatulence, nausea, and greenish diarrhoea. Argentum nitricum also seems to help people who have diarrhoea immediately after drinking water or from eating too much sweet or salty food. These people may crave sugar and tend to have blood sugar problems.

- **Colocynthis:** Taking Colocynthis is useful when you experience cutting pains and cramping that pressure on the abdomen relieves somewhat. Eating fruit or drinking water triggers the cramps, which worsen just before an episode of diarrhoea.

- **Lilium tigrinum:** This medicine is useful if you have IBS symptoms of alternating constipation and diarrhoea. You may be constipated one day and then the next day be greeted by diarrhoea in the morning. You may also sense a lump in the rectum that can make you feel the unsuccessful urge to go. Lilium tigrinum can help to ease this sensation.

- **Lycopodium:** Homeopaths commonly use Lycopodium for people with chronic bowel problems who have a ravenous appetite and may get up at night to eat. Lycopodium can treat all the symptoms of IBS, including bloating, gas, stomach pain, and even heartburn. The people who benefit most from this medicine have symptoms that they can partially relieve by rubbing the abdomen and that are worse in the late afternoon and early evening.

- **Mag Phos:** Mag Phos (which is short for magnesium phosphate) is an antispasmodic medicine and the most commonly used magnesium homeopathic remedy. Mag Phos is effective in treating cramping and spasms in all muscle groups.

- **Natrum carbonicum:** People who may respond to Natrum cabonicum experience indigestion and heartburn when they eat an offending food. Dairy products seem to give them the most trouble, causing gas, explosive diarrhoea, and an empty, gnawing feeling in the stomach.

✔ **Nux vomica:** Often used to treat hangovers and overindulgence, Nux vomica treats abdominal pains and bowel symptoms accompanied by abdominal tension, chilliness, and irritability. The gripping tension in the abdomen may lead to soreness in the muscles of the abdominal wall (that you can somewhat relieve by putting pressure on the abdomen) and pain from trapped gas. Nux vomica is appropriate for both constipation-predominant IBS and diarrhoea-predominant IBS.

✔ **Podophyllum:** Homeopaths may give this medicine when a person experiences abdominal pain and cramping accompanied by a gurgling, sinking, empty feeling that is followed by watery, noxious-smelling diarrhoea. Alternating diarrhoea and constipation may also be present, or pasty yellow bowel movements containing mucus. The early morning is the worst time for this person, who experiences weakness, faintness, and headaches following episodes of diarrhoea and has accompanying stiffness of joints and muscles.

✔ **Sulphur:** This medicine is for people who wake up early in the morning with a sudden urge to evacuate the bowels. More episodes of diarrhoea can occur throughout the day, but this symptom alternates with constipation with accompanying offensive and odorous gas. A characteristic oozing around the rectum with itching, burning, and red irritation is a classic sign indicating that this medicine may help. Other features of a person who may benefit from this medicine include poor posture, back pain, and worsening of symptoms when standing for long periods of time.

Finding a homeopathic therapist

In some parts of the UK you may get homeopathic treatment on the NHS, although in many centres the NHS is stopping funding for this sort of therapy, because of the lack of solid evidence that it has any effect. If your GP can't offer it, you can try your nearest homeopathy hospital – there are five around the country, contact details can be found at www.homeopathyhome.com/directory/uk/hospitals.shtml. You can just phone up and make an appointment yourself, but be prepared to pay for the consultation and treatment.

The Society of Homeopaths (www.homeopathy-soh.org) has a list of registered homeopaths in the UK. The Web site of the British Homeopathic Association (www.trusthomeopathy.org) has lots of useful info, including details of clinical trials in homeopathy. Several good homeopathy books are available such as *The Complete Homeopathy Handbook* by Miranda Castro or *The Encyclopedia of Homeopathy* by Andrew Lockie.

Pinning Down IBS with Acupuncture

Acupuncture involves puncturing the skin with extremely thin needles that go into the underlying tissues at specific points. Experienced practitioners with very sensitive fingers can find these acupuncture points, and they can also use electrical measuring devices to detect them. The points lie along lines called *meridians,* which acupuncturists believe carry a stream of life force called *qi* (pronounced 'chi'). Inserting needles promotes the flow of qi. Your body has 14 principal meridians and 361 basic acupuncture points on the skin. Each meridian originates from, or flows to, a particular organ.

In the UK acupuncture is remarkably popular and supported by doctors too. According to a British Medical Association survey in 2000, almost half (47 per cent) of GPs arrange acupuncture for patients; 79 per cent think that it ought to be available on the NHS; and 86 per cent of NHS pain clinics already offer it.

Emotional freedom techniques (EFT) work on the same ideas of meridians and acupuncture points, but you can do these techniques yourself. See the section 'Evaluating Emotional Freedom Techniques', later in this chapter, for more information.

Achieving balance

In the West, we tend to think of acupuncture as a stand-alone therapy. In China, however, acupuncture is part of a larger system of healthcare called *oriental medicine,* which includes diet therapy, herbal medicine, medical massage (Tui Na), exercise (tai chi and qi gong), and moxabustion (which we describe in the next section, 'Healing with heat').

Acupuncture is very individualised. However, in IBS, what the practitioner looks for is an imbalance in various meridians, mainly the stomach, large intestine, spleen, kidney, and liver. These meridians can be overactive or underactive, suffering from dampness, heat, or stagnation. Inserting needles at the appropriate acupuncture points can help promote the flow of qi and regain balance in the meridians.

The practitioner reads the nuances of your body by holding your wrist and putting several fingers along the pulse. The practitioner identifies where imbalance lies in your body and uses acupuncture needles, moxabustion, and herbal medicine to correct that imbalance.

Most people feel understandably nervous about the idea of being stabbed with sharp needles, but almost all of those who have acupuncture express surprise at how little pain they feel, or at least how that pain is fairly easy to tolerate. The needles used are much finer than those used for injections, for example, and the sensation when they're inserted is often described as a tingling or dull ache. During a session that usually lasts up to an hour, the needles may be inserted and immediately removed, or left in place for 30 or more minutes. During treatment, patients commonly experience a heaviness in the limbs or a pleasant feeling of relaxation. The length of a course of treatment depends on the illness but it may involve one treatment a week for several weeks. Some people find their symptoms disappear completely while others need regularly course of treatment to keep symptoms at bay.

Healing with heat

Moxabustion involves burning a small cone of the herb *artemesia vulgarus* near an acupuncture point. In the past, acupuncturists placed cones of herbs on acupuncture points and ignited the herbs. When the herbs burned near the skin, the acupuncturist immediately swept them off. These days, acupuncturists light large sticks of pressed herbs, hold them near the skin, and then move the sticks away if the skin becomes too hot. Moxabustion is especially suited to treating the pain of IBS because the warmth seems to relax intestinal spasms by activating certain acupuncture points.

Heat from a hot-water bottle or heating pad can also be an effective way to turn off pain. Some people curl up with a hot-water bottle wrapped in a soft towel tucked into the abdomen. The pressure from the bottle and the heat combine to do the trick.

Finding an acupuncturist

Like a lot of CAM therapies, acupuncture has no single governing body in the UK. Many different organisations practice different versions of acupuncture, traditional Chinese medicine, and Chinese herbal medicine. Two of the main organisations are:

- ✔ **Acupuncture Society (www.acupuncturesociety.org.uk):** This society focuses on the original Chinese medical tradition of acupuncture, alongside Chinese traditional herbal medicine and other therapies.

- ✔ **British Acupuncture Council (BAcC) (www.acupuncture.org.uk):** This is the largest UK regulatory body for acupuncture. The Web site provides an online database of its 2,800 members and you can also contact BAcC to purchase a printed register. All BAcC practitioners complete a thorough training of at least three years in traditional acupuncture and bio medical sciences appropriate to the practice of acupuncture (you can spot these practitioners by the letters MBAcC after their name).

Ruminating on Reflexology

Reflexology practitioners believe that congestion or tension in the feet mirrors problems in the related body zones, and that reflexology helps the body to restore its own natural balance and heal itself.

When you have reflexology, the reflexologist first talks to you to assess your health problems and needs, and then she works with her hands to apply pressure to the feet in a unique way that addresses the problem areas of the body. The therapist detects subtle changes in small areas in the feet and by working on these can affect the corresponding parts of the body. The pressure applied during treatment should not hurt although it may be a little tickly. A session may last up to an hour and a course of several weekly treatments may be recommended. The way you feel after treatment – well and relaxed, or nauseous and lethargic – helps the reflexologist understand how you respond to the therapy and indicates how she can fine-tune the treatment.

Many doctors feel that insufficient scientific evidence exists to support reflexology as a treatment. But although no one has claimed that symptoms disappear altogether, plenty of people find they get relief from symptoms and keeping paying for more. In the end the choice is yours – if reflexology helps that's great, although you're very unlikely to get this therapy on the NHS. You can find out more from the Association of Reflexologists, Tel: 0870 5673320 www.reflexology.org.

Relaxing Your Way to Health

Stress plays a major part in IBS, and dealing with stress needs to be somewhere at the top of your list for coping strategies. Relaxing properly, and taking time out to do so, is an art that you must try hard to perfect.

Whatever relaxation is to you, you need to have some to look forward to every day. Many of the therapies we discuss in this chapter include an element of relaxation. But you may want to skim through Chapter 11 on exercise and IBS too, because exercise is a great way to relax and has important therapeutic powers.

Meditation conjures up images of people sitting in impossibly contorted positions for interminable lengths of time. You can certainly do that – don't let us stop you – but many other ways to meditate don't involve you twisting yourself into pretzel shapes.

One of the best-known ways of achieving a relaxed state was described in 1975 by Dr Herbert Benson, a professor at Harvard Medical School. This physiological state of relaxation is called the *relaxation response,* which is also the title of a book Dr Benson wrote in 1975 and updated in 2000. Dr Benson founded the Mind/Body Medical Institute, a behavioural medicine research and treatment centre in Boston. Dr Benson tells us that inducing the relaxation response is not difficult. You create the relaxation response in two essential steps:

✔ Repeating a word, sound, phrase, prayer, or muscular activity.

✔ Disregarding everyday thoughts that inevitably come to mind and returning to your repetition.

You can also initiate the relaxation response with the use of imagery, progressive muscle relaxation (where, while in a comfortable position you tense all your muscles and then gradually, from your toes up to your head, you relax your muscles), meditation, repetitive physical exercises, and breath focus.

Try following this relaxation routine, which combines some of the above techniques:

✔ Wearing loose clothes and with your shoes off, sit quietly in a warm, comfortable position. You'll find it hard to relax with a tight belt squeezing your intestines or a small toddler trying to shove a toy in your direction. So make sure that the children, dog, or other potentially noisy distractions are occupied elsewhere, and the TV or radio is turned off.

✔ Close your eyes.

✔ Tense all your muscles in your body, starting with your toes and progressing up to your neck and face until they're all clenched.

✔ Slowly relax your muscles again, unwinding from your feet to your calves, thighs, abdomen, shoulders, head, and neck.

✔ Repeat this sequence of tension and relaxation 2 or 3 times.

✔ With your muscles relaxed, breathe slowly and naturally, and as you do, say your focus word, sound, or phrase silently to yourself as you exhale. Don't speak out loud if you can help it.

✔ Assume a passive attitude. Don't worry about how well you're doing. When other thoughts come to mind, simply say to yourself, 'Oh well,' and gently return to your repetition.

✔ Continue for up to 20 minutes.

✔ When you think that you've done enough, don't stand up immediately. Continue sitting quietly for a minute or so, allowing other thoughts to return. Then open your eyes and sit for another minute before rising.

✔ Practice the technique once or twice daily. Good times to do so are before breakfast and before dinner.

A 2001 study on IBS at the State University of New York used the relaxation response. The researchers divided adults with IBS into two groups. They assigned one group to a six-week treatment programme and asked the group to practise the relaxation response twice a day. The researchers asked the other group to just monitor their symptoms. After the six-week period, participants using the relaxation response reported significant improvements in symptoms of diarrhoea, belching, bloating, and flatulence.

Homing In on Hypnotherapy

Hypnosis is one of the oldest remedies used to battle physical diseases and mental disorders, but conventional medical doctors don't practise it widely. However, one study showed that more than 70 per cent of family doctors thought that *hypnotherapy* (the use of hypnosis in the treatment of illness) may have a role to play in the management of patients with IBS. In fact, we found study after study showing that hypnosis – including self-hypnosis – is a scientifically proven tool that can modify gastrointestinal functions, such as mucus production, intestinal movement, and intestinal sensitivity, and how the brain perceives gastrointestinal symptoms.

Hypnotherapy is a treatment that involves getting a person into an altered state of awareness or trance, in which they become more responsive to suggestions or advice from others, in order to bring about some sort of change to their beliefs or behaviour.

Hypnosis acts on the physical level; it doesn't just erase your bowel from your mind. But it also functions on the psychological level, as the therapist can give suggestions that help you to cope with symptoms of anxiety and tension.

Directing the gut

In 1984 Dr PJ Whorwell developed gut-directed hypnotherapy (GDH) at the University Hospital of South Manchester specifically for IBS patients. GDH boasts a success rate of 80 per cent for improving symptoms of abdominal pain, bloating, diarrhoea, and/or constipation.

An effective GDH treatment programme can vary from 6 to 12 sessions that take place every week. Here's what to expect: At each session the therapist works to bring you into a state of extreme relaxation, and take you through a programme of suggestion. For example, she may ask you to imagine that a healing warmth is flowing through your digestive system, sorting out your symptoms as it goes. The programme varies each week, focusing on different symptoms or aspects of your life related to your IBS. The therapist records each session, and you listen to the recording every day until the next session.

In Chapter 20 we list a number of hypnotherapy resources in the UK to check out. Individual hypnotherapy practitioners may know about GDH and treating IBS; be sure to ask about it when you phone to make an appointment.

Hypnotising yourself

Studies show that hypnosis can reduce dependence on medication and decrease doctors' visits, which amounts to economic savings. But hypnosis administered by a professional obviously involves consultation costs. Self-hypnosis programmes, which put you into a state of hypnosis, or give you guidance on how to hypnotise yourself, provide affordable options that you may want to consider.

One study compared a group of patients who received hypnotherapy and a group who listened to a hypnotherapy audiotape. The results weren't surprising. There was an improvement in symptoms in the group that listened to the audiotape but more improvement in the ones who received a hypnotherapy session. The researchers concluded that the ease and economy of an audiotape makes it a useful treatment option, and people who don't improve sufficiently with an audiotape can then opt for hypnotherapy.

Finding a hypnotherapist

Anyone can train to be a hypnotherapist, so you may want to consider going to someone who is also a trained clinical psychologist or psychiatrist with a medical background – ideally, someone who knows about IBS. And remember, you need someone to do therapy, not parlour tricks. You want someone who practises *hypnotherapy* or clinical hypnosis and not just plain old hypnosis. Three different professional bodies represent and maintain registers of therapists, and contribute to education, training, and standards of practice:

- **The Hypnotherapy Association:** 01257 262124, or visit the Web site at www.thehypnotherapyassociation.co.uk
- **The National Council for Hypnotherapy:** 0800 952 0545; www.hypnotherapists.org.uk
- **The British Society of Clinical Hypnosis:** 01262 403103 http://www.bsch.org.uk

Appraising Aromatherapy

It doesn't take much imagination to see why aromatherapy may be a great stress reliever, knocking one of the main triggers of IBS for six and inducing a sense of peaceful calm. Aromatherapy uses volatile liquid plant materials, known as essential oils, and other scented compounds from plants in order to change your mood, reduce tension anxiety and other negative emotions, and so improve health. You can use aromatherapy oils in a variety of ways, such as:

- Diluted with massage oils, for an aromatherapy massage

- Added to baths (just add a few drops to warm water)

- As an inhalation (asthmatic people should avoid this)

Aromatherapy is especially effective in the treatment of stress-related conditions and may be helpful in a variety of persistent, difficult to treat conditions such as IBS.

You can choose between around 400 essential oils. Some of the most popular oils include chamomile, lavender, rosemary, and tea tree. Research shows that when you apply oils to the skin or inhale them, your body absorbs the oils into the bloodstream. This may explain how the chemicals in the oils directly affect the body but it also means a risk of toxicity exists and you must always follow instructions on the bottles of oil very carefully. For example, it is often necessary to dilute the oils down and mix them with creams or other liquids (alternatively you may want to get advice – or all of your treatment – from a trained aromatherapist).

Clinical trials demonstrate properties of individual oils – tea tree oil, for example, has antibacterial properties and peppermint oil may help to maintain a healthy digestive system.

Some of the oils we particularly recommend for IBS, because they may improve the functioning of the gut and calm problems such as painful spasms or bloating, include:

- Anise (*Pimpinella anisum*)

- Neroli (*Citrus aurantium bigaradia*)

- Peppermint (*Mentha piperita*)

- Ylang Ylang (*Cananga odorata*)

We think that aromatherapy is a fabulous therapy, but no scientific shows that it works in IBS. If you benefit from aromatherapy, you may be enjoying a placebo effect (which we explain in the section 'Pondering the Placebo Effect', earlier in this chapter), but if it works then why complain? Aromatherapy is rarely available on the NHS, however, unless you happen to come across a doctor or nurse with a particular interest in it and who has managed to persuade her surgery or health trust to fund the treatment.

Aromatherapists in the UK don't have to be registered to practise, so anyone can start up an aromatherapy business. But those registered with the Aromatherapy Council (AC) (www.aromatherapycouncil.co.uk) do have to abide by their code of conduct so you may want to check the AC Web site to find an AC registered aromatherapist.

Feeling Fine with Therapeutic Massage

People have used massage since ancient times. Many cultures use gentle massage of the abdomen to ease gastrointestinal problems such as colic and constipation. Many different schools and techniques of massage exist, and you can research these at your leisure. The therapeutic effects of all forms of massage are similar – freeing up tired and tight muscles and ligaments, relaxing tension, stimulating digestion, and sweeping calm across the body.

The theory behind massage in IBS is this: Stress makes IBS worse; massage makes stress go away; massage makes IBS better. However, studies of massage relevant to IBS remain few and far between, so you have to have faith in personal reports rather than science.

Manipulative therapy practitioners (which we explain in the section 'Opting for Osteopathy and Chiropractic') often use abdominal massage as part of their practice, and a number of reports suggest that massage given by trained osteopaths or chiropractors may be particularly useful in treating constipation.

It's probably worth investing in a massage from a trained therapist if you want one that is targeted at your gut symptoms, but you don't have to be a trained expert to give a good general massage helps with stress and relaxation – some people just have the knack and it is hard to go very wrong! The main thing is to find someone you trust and feel relaxed with, such as a good friend or partner, so that you don't feel embarrassed as they get to grips with your flesh. Then slip into comfy old clothes, slide onto a towel, and slop on the oil. Of course, you can read about and practise methods and techniques, but the main aim is to work your way across your body gently kneading, stroking, and stretching the muscles.

You can even give yourself a gentle abdominal massage, which may help to soothe pain and spasms, or ease constipation:

✔ Lie down on your back somewhere peaceful with a pillow under your head and another under your knees to bend your legs slightly (this flexes the body slightly and reduces pressure inside the abdomen.

✔ Pour a little oil or cream into your hands. Using each hand to cover its own half of the abdomen (ie left hand on left side, right on right side), start at the breast bone and gently but firmly stroke down and out along the edge of the ribcage towards the hips. Repeat this several times.

✔ Now you're going to massage your colon in the direction that your food flows through it. Place your right hand below and to the right of your tummy button, almost into the groin. Place your left hand just above it. Your hands now cover where the small intestine empties into the large intestine or colon. Move both hands, pressing down gently, in small circles. At the same time as making the circular movements, progress both hands up the right side of the abdomen, then across the top of the abdomen (beneath the ribs) and down the left side. This should take at least 5 minutes.

✔ If you find tender areas, move gently around them. Repeat the massage twice a day – or more often if it helps relieve pain. After each massage, place a warm pack on your tum for 10 minutes, close your eyes and daydream. (You can buy warm packs that can be heated in a microwave, in your pharmacy, or use a hot water bottle, but don't make it too hot.)

The most reliable way to find a good massage therapist is to ask for a recommendation from friends or your doctor's surgery. As there's no recognised professional organisation, you may prefer to ask an osteopath, chiropractor, or physiotherapist (if you know a good one locally) if they also do therapeutic massages – most do.

Opting for Osteopathy and Chiropractic

Osteopathy and chiropractic are types of 'manipulative therapy'. Interestingly, physiotherapists also practise manipulative therapy, but they're usually considered part of conventional rather than complementary medicine. Osteopaths and chiropractors apply manipulative therapies to the muscles and bones of the body, working with their hands on the bones, muscles, and connective tissue to diagnose and treat abnormalities of both the musculoskeletal system and other tissues and organs.

The evidence showing benefits from manipulative therapies in the treatment of conditions involving the internal organs, such as IBS, is very limited. Some research shows a significant reduction in symptoms and a general improvement in quality of life among a group of people with IBS treated by osteopaths, but sceptics may need more data to be convinced.

Osteopathy and chiropractic focuses more on problems of the musculoskeletal system, but a number of practitioners describe themselves as 'visceral osteopaths' and work with the soft organs of the body.

Osteopathy and chiropractic are the only two complementary therapies regulated by statute in the UK, so checking that your therapist is trained and qualified is easier than for other CAM therapies.

You can find out more about manipulative therapies from

- General Osteopathic Council (www.osteopathy.org.uk)
- General Chiropractic Council (www.gcc-uk.org)
- Manipulation Association of Chartered Physiotherapists (www.macp web.org)

Cracking Down on Colonic Irrigation

In recent years the idea of putting a rubber tube into your rectum and washing everything out (otherwise known as *colonic irrigation*) has caught on as a way to improve the health of the bowel, or at least make someone feel a bit better. Complementary therapists often recommend colonic irrigation for IBS.

Proponents of colonic irrigation depict the large intestine as a sewage system that becomes a stagnant cesspool if neglected. They suggest constipation causes hardened faeces to accumulate for months or years on the walls of the large intestine and stop it absorbing and eliminating properly. Their theory is that this causes food to remain undigested and the body to reabsorb wastes. But in fact the contents of the bowel have nowhere to hide – the bowel just doesn't work like that – and it immediately starts to fill up again as soon as the irrigation is over.

In Chapter 8 we talked about the use of enemas in constipation-predominant IBS. These enemas aren't the same as colonic irrigation. Most enemas consist of a small amount of fluid that contains a chemical that stimulates the bowel to empty. There are no tubes poking around in the bowel (other than a very small tube just to introduce the fluid), no large volumes of fluid poured in, and the bowel is stimulated to empty itself rather than being flushed out. Enemas can be very useful in constipation-predominant IBS, but only as a specific treatment to encourage movement in constipation. Occasionally, in severe constipation, a high enema is needed. This is more like colonic irrigation but is done by a doctor who is trained and experienced in the technique, and knows the risks.

Colonic irrigation has considerable potential to do harm. The intestines are delicate thin wall tubes and poking around in them too much risks puncturing the walls. The process of colonic irrigation can be very uncomfortable, causing severe cramps and pain, which may take weeks to settle. More importantly, if the practitioner doesn't adequately sterilise equipment between treatments, infection can pass from one patient to another.

Colonic irrigation also washes out the friendly bacteria that lie in the thin layer of mucus on the wall of the gut. These are the bacteria that we spend a lot of this book showing you how to cherish because they're so good for you and your gut. Wash these away and you wash away not only the main source of energy for the cells of the epithelial lining (see Chapter 2) but also one of the strongest barriers to infection in the body.

Astonishingly, therapists who offer colonic irrigation aren't legally required to have any training to do this powerful intervention. Colonic irrigation must be one of the most embarrassing therapies to undergo – none of the warm sweet smelling oils of aromatherapy or the Zen peace of yoga. Our view is that colonic irrigation isn't worth the humiliation. Far from being helpful, colonic irrigation delivers a huge insult to one of the body's most precious systems, and disrupts the harmony of the body's largest immune organ. Colonic irrigation is one complementary therapy we can't recommend.

Taking Control with Biofeedback

Biofeedback is a body-awareness technique in which you feel different physiological states in your muscles and nervous system. For example, you can develop awareness of your blood pressure changing, or levels of activity and tension within the muscles of the abdomen and gut. Biofeedback has the advantages of being non-invasive and completely painless, having very few side effects, and putting you in control.

During a biofeedback session you're hooked up to a monitor by a headband or a wristband, and you sit comfortably beside a computer. The computer either has a video screen that displays body activity such as muscle tension or brain waves, or you may hear a tone or bleep related to the body function. A trained therapist, who may be a doctor, nurse, or physical or occupational therapist, gives guidance on how to relax in order to change an abnormal response. It may be as simple as counting your breaths, breathing deeply, or repeating a word or phrase. This leads to changes in the body activity, which are shown on the video screen or in the audible tone, so that you can directly see or feel the results of your efforts.

You can discover how to gain control over the function of your gastrointestinal tract through this method. In most cases, biofeedback is a matter of retraining your bowel to work normally. Biofeedback proves useful in treating IBS. After biofeedback training, you can relax your gastrointestinal tract in stressful situations by remembering what you found out in your sessions.

The average number of treatments for IBS is six to eight 30–40 minute sessions held over a three-month period. When you've grasped the technique you can practise it at home, although you may need some simple equipment and access to a computer. A study from the Royal Free Hospital in London on gut-directed biofeedback using a computerised animation of the gut gave 40 IBS patients four half-hour biofeedback sessions. Eighty per cent of the patients achieved progressively deeper levels of relaxation and in 50 per cent the technique was helpful in controlling bowel symptoms on almost every occasion that they became troublesome.

You can find out more about biofeedback from the Association for Applied Psychophysiology and Biofeedback (AAPB) at www.aapb.org. Biofeedback may be available on the NHS but only in those clinics or hospitals that have a particular interest in it. You may find that the only way to get the treatment is to find a private practitioner. There is no professional body for therapists in the UK so to find a provider, ask at your local gastroenterology clinic at the hospital or talk to your GP.

Nailing IBS with Naturopathic Medicine

Naturopathic medicine looks at what can be done to promote wellbeing and treat disease without resorting to synthetic drugs or invasive surgery. It encompasses aspects of nutrition, lifestyle education, exercise, and psychological balancing. From the mind–body interplay in IBS to the effects of fibre and food supplements, naturopathic medicine has it covered.

One of the main aims of naturopathy is to support the body while it's own innate ability for healing sorts out the disease. Naturopathy gives a strong emphasis on holistic care, looking at the patient and their physical, mental, emotional, intellectual, and spiritual needs all together. A naturopath uses many of the approaches and therapies described in this book for IBS, except perhaps Chapter 8 on drugs.

Naturopathy was big in the 20th century until penicillin arrived, heralding a new age of synthetic drugs. But disillusionment with modern medicines and their side effects has now led to a resurgence of naturopathy. A number of colleges in America offer courses to train as a naturopathic doctor, but in the UK doctors train primarily in conventional medicine and then go on to study or take courses in naturopathic medicine after qualification. However, although interest in naturopathy is growing in the UK, the overall trend seems now to be towards integrated medicine, the ultimate combination of naturopathic and conventional ideas, as we explain in the section 'Integrating Complementary and Conventional Medicine'.

If you want to try naturopathy, the best plan may be to find a GP locally whose practice encompasses naturopathy. The practice may be able to offer this approach on the NHS. They may be able to select naturopathic approaches that are particularly relevant to IBS such as looking closely at your diet and finding IBS-friendly foods (which we cover in Chapter 10), or considering the balance of micro-organisms in your gut (which we discuss in Chapter 4) and the use of probiotics (foods full of helpful bacteria – see Chapter 10. If your own surgery can't point you in the direction of a GP who practises naturopathy, try The British Naturopathic Association (0870 745 6984; `www.naturo paths.org.uk`) who are the professional body for those practising naturopaths registered with the General Council and Register of Naturopaths in the UK.

Integrating Complementary and Conventional Medicine

We've called this chapter 'Complementary Therapies' because it looks at treatments that aren't part of conventional science-based medicine (also known as allopathic medicine) but which may be used alongside conventional medicine and complement it. However, a couple of decades ago the chapter may have been called 'Alternative Therapies' because in those days, when there was often a rather frosty antipathy between doctors and other therapists, people felt that they had to choose either one approach or the other. Nowadays, however, health professionals of all types tend to listen to what the others have to offer.

If you hang around for another couple of decades, you may find that Chapter 8 of this book, which is about drugs for IBS, completely merges with this chapter, under the title 'Integrated Therapies', because conventional and complementary medicine now work together even more closely.

Integrated medicine aims to use the safest and most effective combinations of different type of treatments from conventional and complementary medicine, as well as psychological therapies and self-help – that is, pretty much all the treatments we mention in this book. From conventional medicine, integrated medicine inherited the idea that treatment must be based on good science and solid statistical evidence to show how effective the drug or therapy is. From complementary medicine, integrated medicine embraces the holistic approach, which considers the patient as a whole, including their physical, mental, emotional, spiritual, social, and economic wellbeing (some doctors may argue that, especially in recent years, conventional medicine has become much more centered on the whole patient – this may be true but many complementary therapies showed it the way!) And integrated medicine draws on both types of medicine for their wide range of expertise, experience, and insight.

An integrated medicine specialist (or more likely team of specialists from different schools of thought) devises a programme of treatment that co-ordinates different therapies and medicines tailored to the needs, preferences, beliefs, and circumstances of an individual. These therapies may aim to cure disease or resolve underlying barriers to healing and optimal health. Patients play a central part in their healing process, and the programme provides them with information and skills to manage their own health.

Sam's girlfriend was treated for chronic back pain at a clinic specialising in integrated medicine, and she persuaded Sam to go along to the clinic for advice. At the clinic Sam saw a doctor (who was also trained in acupuncture) and a complementary therapist, who specialised in nutritional medicine and herbal treatments. Sam was surprised how long they talked to him for and the sorts of questions they asked – he was never in his GP's surgery for more than a matter of minutes. The doctor and therapist treated him as part of the team, checking all along on his views of the treatment they proposed. Finally, the two professionals wrote out a six-week treatment programme for Sam, which included an elimination diet (to look for dietary triggers), some work with a therapist to show him guided imagery (as a way to manage his abdominal discomfort), and yoga and simple meditation techniques to help him deal with his stress and control his diarrhoea-predominant IBS (and hopefully regain the calm personality he had before IBS turned him into an irritable grouch). Just six weeks later, Sam's IBS symptoms were becoming a distant memory.

So integrated medicine isn't just about treating symptoms or even curing disease – it's about helping a person to understand themselves and work out what they particularly need to improve their emotional, intellectual, social, and spiritual wellbeing as well as their physical health.

Already well established in the US, the idea of integrated medicine is catching on in the UK too, and some experts hail it as the future of healthcare. Two NHS general practices are even devoted to it, one in Marylebone, London and the other in Glastonbury, Somerset. If you don't live in these areas you may have to do a little research – asking friends or ringing around surgeries – to find a GP who practises integrated medicine.

You can find out more about integrated medicine from the British Society of Integrated Medicine (www.bsim.org.uk), the British College of Integrated Medicine (www.integratedmedicine.org.uk), and the Prince's Foundation for Integrated Health (www.fih.org.uk).

Certain factors make up an important part of integrated medicine:

> ✔ **Environmental medicine:** How often does your doctor ask you how old your house is and if it contains old (lead-based) paint? Does he enquire about the sorts of food you eat, the chemicals you come into contact with at work, or whether your sewers have played up recently? The answer is probably 'not very often', but these things may be very relevant to your visit to the surgery.

The world in which we live, sleep, and breathe has a powerful effect on our wellbeing. The list of environmental hazards in our industrialised environment is long, but here are a few examples:

- In our industrialised environment we face daily exposure to potentially toxic chemicals.

- A crowded, fast-paced cityscape can make us feel stressed and unhappy (and even lonely) and may limit the chance to get physical activity.

- Bad sanitation in cities can lead to infections that can cause or aggravate IBS, as well as many other diseases.

- Poor diet, or food that is nutritionally lacking, leaves us vulnerable.

- Atmospheric conditions (including erosion of the ozone layer) can expose us to the risk of malignant disease.

In integrated medicine, the patient's environment comes under close scrutiny, and practitioners may recommend efforts to change aspects of the environment.

✔ **Holistic health:** Holistic health is based on a simple premise – that a whole creature is made up of interdependent parts. The word holistic refers to the whole person and reflects the intricate connections between the interdependent parts – the body, mind, and spirit. When one of these parts doesn't work at its best, it impacts all the other parts of that person. Furthermore, this whole person, including all the parts, constantly interacts with everything in the environment that surrounds her.

For example, if you have constipation, a practitioner forming a holistic view of you may ask:

- What physical symptoms do you have? These may include bloated or painful abdomen, nausea, loss of appetite, or pain around the anus.

- What do you think about your constipation and how does it affect your mood? For example, does it concern you? Does it make you feel anxious or low?

- Have you looked for help or answers through prayer or a spiritual understanding of the meaning of their disease? (Some people see disease as a challenge provided by God as a test of their strength and commitment to him.)

Environmental factors to add in may include a very hot dry spell of weather that has left the person dehydrated. Holism wraps up all these aspects in order to get a better insight into what a person's disease means to them as an individual, and how it is best treated.

The British Holistic Medical Association (www.bhma.org) and the American Holistic Health Association (www.ahha.org) have lots of useful information.

✔ **Orthomolecular Medicine:** The Nobel-prize winning scientist Linus Pauling first described the concept of orthomolecular medicine in the 1960s. Orthomolecular medicine involves the use of optimal amounts of natural substances to prevent and treat disease. It centres around the idea that an individual's genetic make-up affects not only their physical characteristics, but also the chemical systems constantly churning away in the body.

Doctors associate diseases ranging from cancer to schizophrenia, or depression, with specific abnormalities in the chemicals of different body systems. By identifying these abnormalities through a series of tests on the blood and other tissues, doctors can give treatments based on natural molecules such as vitamins, minerals, essential fatty acids, enzymes, antibodies, and other plant-based supplements. Other therapies, including acupuncture, massage, or biofeedback, may also be used.

Despite the fact that orthomolecular medicines stakes a claim to a very strong scientific background, it remains a controversial topic among conventional health professionals, who aren't yet convinced that chemical supplements, whether natural or not, hold all the answers to IBS or other chronic conditions in people who don't have a recognised deficiency.

Part IV
Living and Working with IBS

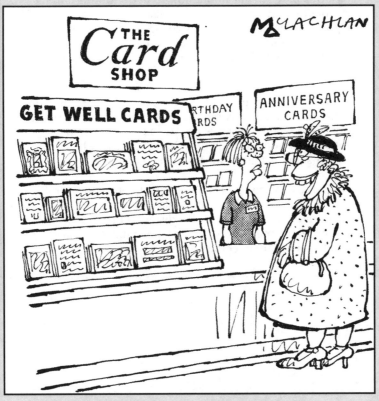

'Have you got a card suitable for
someone with Irritable Bowel Syndrome?'

In this part . . .

*I*n this part, we talk about how to live with this chronic condition every day. We recognise the frustration felt by people who are trapped in the house because of IBS symptoms, and we give you ways to cope. We also address how to deal with IBS when you have to go to work every day despite your symptoms.

Children with IBS are a special concern; perhaps if we can lighten their load early on, they may not continue to experience IBS when they grow up. We explain how to deal with the emotional strain of a chronic illness, which is the most important factor for helping children.

Finally, to continue to deal most effectively with your IBS symptoms, you need to know what's on the horizon in terms of treatment options. We discuss current research and potential breakthroughs that may improve your quality of life in years to come.

Chapter 14

Taking Responsibility: Reclaiming Your Life

In This Chapter

▶ Putting yourself in charge

▶ Considering the financial and emotional costs of IBS

▶ Coping with social situations

▶ Seeking the help and support you need

*M*any people with IBS suffer in silence. Although up to 11 per cent of the population have symptoms of IBS, most keep their condition well hidden. Unaware just how many of those around them would understand what they're going through, they find it easier to keep quiet and let their disease rule their lives, instead of finding ways to make their IBS fit around the life they want to lead. Perhaps you yearn for a job that takes you out and about in the fresh air but have opted for tedious but 'safe' office work where a toilet is always close at hand. Or maybe you would love to join your local Sunday Football team but can't make the commitment of a couple of hours mid-morning when your symptoms always seem to be at their worst. It's easy to let your IBS take charge of your life, but we would like to help you get your life – or the life you dream of – back again.

Living with IBS can be a real challenge. Working out how to manage the symptoms is a difficult task that we want to make much easier for you. We acknowledge that your spontaneity factor may be cut down several notches when you know that your symptoms can rear up at any time. (Boom! There goes the dinner party or trip to the zoo.) You have to be a quick-change artist because your plans are always changing.

IBS is one of the most unpredictable medical conditions. You may wake up in the morning and greet the dawn with a smile, and within an hour you're in agony with abdominal cramps and an urge to go to the bathroom. Or bloating can occur just because you go from a horizontal position in bed to a vertical position walking around your home.

In this chapter we give you more tools and the extra boost of confidence to encourage you out of the house.

Taking responsibility for your life is the first step to coping with your condition. Lifting up your head and looking around at all the available options empowers you to improve your quality of life and cancel out any notion that you're a victim of your illness. It also means that you're not a passive patient but an active participant in your healthcare.

Asserting Yourself

Taking charge of your IBS means that you need to stand up for yourself and what you want – in other words, you need to be assertive. To do this effectively you have to be able to express yourself clearly using direct, open, and honest communication that is self-enhancing and expressive.

If you normally let others persuade you into thinking their way, or you find it difficult to talk about your positive or negative feelings openly and honestly, then you may have problems with a lack of assertiveness. You may, for example, keep buried inside any dissatisfaction with the treatment your doctor offers for your IBS, or you may not have the courage to stand up and praise a nurse who really helps you. One result of lacking assertiveness is that you get pushed towards things that aren't right for you, and then you become angry or depressed.

Being assertive isn't about shouting loudly, ranting, raving, and demanding your rights while violating the rights of others. Assertiveness is about being strong and determined. Assertiveness (after you've got used to that feeling of power and control) can boost your self-confidence, improve your decision-making skills, and help others to see more clearly what is right for you.

To start being assertive you need to:

✔ Be clear about what you want

✔ Be in control of your emotions

✔ Be prepared for people to disagree with you

✔ Be ready to stand your ground

✔ Feel reasonably safe with the people around you

✔ Know your rights

Matt worked in a large garage where he had a reputation as being easy-going. But he often suspected that this really just meant that people could make him do what they wanted him to do – he was a pushover. It was good to be liked, but he rather regretted the fact that he always took the late lunchbreak that no one else wanted, or volunteered for extra hours. And being 'Mr Nice Guy' wasn't helping Matt to keep on top of his IBS. Stopping late for lunch, for example, meant hanging on desperately to get to the toilet to relieve his churning gut. One day, when his colleagues failed yet again to let him get away early, he decided it was time to put himself first. His workmates almost fell over in shock when he calmly but loudly announced that he needed a break. Amazed at the effect of his assertiveness, he even got them to agree to sort out a proper rota so that everyone took a turn at working though the lunch break.

Enjoying the Life You Deserve

The first step in sorting out your IBS is to get back in control and decide what you want from life. Take a deep breath and tell yourself (and anyone else who wants to listen – cats and dogs provide quite a good audience) that your IBS is no longer in charge – *you* are!

Take a long look at your career, your friends, your home – how much of your life is built around the demands of your insides? Remind yourself that that this life is no dress rehearsal and think about where you want to be. Are you happy in your job or do you yearn for something more thrilling, or just different? Are you stuck in a tedious routine because you're scared that change may upset your bowel? Do you get out and do the things you want to do, or is there a hobby or sport you've been burning to try? Do you see enough of your family and friends, or have the sort of relationship that you really want with them? Or has IBS got in the way of all your plans recently?

Tell yourself that if you're ever going to change things, then now is the time. You *can* change things, although you may have to accept going at a slow pace, a few steps at a time, and making some compromises for your condition. We offer some suggestions on how to cope with social situations when your IBS makes life difficult in the later section 'Tackling Social Situations'.

Make a list of those things you want to change in your life. For each point on the list make a note of what can help you achieve that change, how you fear your IBS may stop you, and what tactics you can employ to stay in charge of your IBS. You may have to do some research here to explore a new focus in your life and how to change things, but in this book we provide lots of ideas about tactics to stay in charge.

Dealing with Family and Friends

Dealing with your symptoms is just one part of coping with IBS – dealing with other people is an entirely separate problem. People react in very different ways to others' suffering and no doubt you've seen most sorts of reactions. Some see the whole topic of bottoms, gas, and belly ache as a vast reservoir of inane jokes. Others may be mortified, repulsed, or embarrassed and just don't want to know. Some well-meaning souls pour out endless advice, often without really listening to what you have to say and how your IBS affects you as an individual, and then feel affronted when you don't get too enthusiastic about their offerings.

So what can you do with family and friends? You can't give them a dose of IBS just to help them understand what your condition is like, so instead you have to invest a little time in showing the people in your life what IBS is all about.

Talking about the goings on of your bowel can be tough. Many people feel embarrassed and uncomfortable and prefer to keep their symptoms hidden. But explaining what is happening to you is essential in helping others to understand, and sharing your worries and troubles may even make you feel a little better. Here are some hints to help you get talking:

- ✔ Choose a suitable time (not over Sunday lunch, for example) and use measured words to begin to paint a small picture of your problem. Keep your comments relevant to the situation you're in and adapt what you say to match the person in front of you. Watch their reaction closely before you carry on and spill further beans. What's right for your mother to hear is likely to be very different to what your mates in the pub want to know, although you may be surprised when you discover who else shares your problem and is keen to swap notes (IBS is very common, after all).

- ✔ Accept that some people just can't face talking about health problems, and move on. Just knowing that you're unwell may be enough for such people, and they may find other ways to help, such as offering practical support or companionship without knowing the details of your IBS.

- ✔ Remember that humour works for some people but not others. A funny story about the misbehaviour of your bowels, or a good joke about farting or the squits, can be a dramatic and effective way to make a point – with the right person. But others may be offended by your efforts to make them laugh about something they see as very personal or embarrassing.

- ✔ Listen to others' views and accept all offers of advice. What they say may be rubbish but they're probably trying to help you and may have your interests at heart. Politely explain your view if you totally disagree with what they say, but otherwise chew over and swallow the information, making a mental note to spit it out later on after they've gone.

✔ Find some useful printed materials about IBS and leave a few (don't bombard people) scattered casually around. The loo may be a good place for some reading on IBS!

✔ Let people borrow this book, if you can bear to be parted from it. It's packed with useful information for friends and relatives of people with IBS. You may want to add a few page markers indicating the sections that would be particularly relevant for them to read.

✔ Try to keep your emotions in control, even if you feel upset or angry, when dealing with others. Calmly explaining that you're distressed is more effective than actually letting your distress pour out all over them.

Coping with Journeys

A busy life usually involves a fair amount of travelling around – few of us can find work, shopping, and all the other services and entertainment that we need on our doorstep (although the Internet has undoubtedly made life a lot easier and can save a lot of journeys).

So you need to find effective strategies to cope with the demands that a journey can make on your bowel. We suggest here some strategies you can try:

✔ When symptoms are bad, avoid unnecessary journeys – shop over the Net or chat with friends via messaging services (or get a Web cam).

✔ Prepare carefully for every journey. Work out your route and make a note of possible toilet stops, such as petrol stations, cafés, and fast food restaurants.

✔ Make a point of using the toilet before leaving the house.

✔ For a few days before a major journey, stick rigidly to the tried-and-tested IBS diet that works for you (we help you determine an IBS-friendly diet in Chapter 10).

✔ Before you leave on a long journey, stock up the car with a small travel bag containing extra underwear, pads (if you use them), wet wipes, toilet paper, and hand wash or alcohol gel hand cleaner. Keep an air freshener in the car, especially if you have passengers.

✔ Take loperamide or other medication that you use before you leave. Loperamide can be used on a regular basis for the long term if necessary, although it is worth reviewing your medication use every few months with your doctor.

✔ If you travel by public transport, use the toilet before you get on. If you plan to go on a long journey by coach, train, or plane, try to book a seat near the toilet.

✔ Try to keep your mind occupied on the journey – thoughts about your IBS, urgency, or accidents have a nasty habit of triggering bowel activity.

✔ If you suffer from faecal incontinence, wear a panty liner or incontinence pad, and carry adult wipes and a change of underwear (we explain these products in the section 'Experiencing faecal incontinence').

✔ If your gut functions better on small frequent meals, and you may not be eating while you're out, then make sure that you have a light snack before you go. But if any food stirs up symptoms, then you may be better off waiting until you return home before you eat.

Taking Steps Towards Better Health

In other chapters, we discuss the essential facets of taking responsibility for your illness, whether you choose to focus on exercise, nutrition, or yoga and meditation.

Throughout this chapter, we add to this list of ways to help your situation. But first, we want to acknowledge the impact that IBS may be having on you right now, so you realise that you aren't alone.

Surveying the effects of IBS

In 2002, the International Foundation for Functional Gastrointestinal Disorders (IFFGD) commissioned a nationwide survey of patients with IBS in the United States. The IFFGD talked to 350 patients and found that many live with the condition for years in isolation, trapped in their houses. And those people who try to find out what's wrong with them often see many doctors before getting a correctly diagnosis. The survey also found that participants had tried an accumulated 300 different types of prescription and over-the-counter medications in search of relief.

Although this was an American survey, many people with IBS in the UK and Europe can relate to the same issues. A postal survey carried out among more than 800 people in Britain a few years before, in 1996, showed similar findings.

Here are some results of the Surveys of the impact IBS can have show:

✔ Nearly half of the US survey participants reported having symptoms for five or more years before receiving a diagnosis of IBS. In the UK survey nearly a third of people with IBS experienced their symptoms for more than five years before doctors diagnosed IBS.

- Nearly 45 per cent of US participants reported severe symptoms, with another 40 per cent having moderate pain. Just over 70 per cent reported two or more episodes of IBS per week, and nearly half reported daily events.

- Participants described how their career suffered as a result of IBS. In the UK survey, over a third (39 per cent) of those in full employment had taken time off work because of IBS. But few felt able to tell their bosses about their problem – 43 per cent of those needing time off didn't give IBS as a reason for missing work. Instead, 82 per cent used the term 'a stomach upset' and 15 per cent said that they had a headache or migraine. And 71 per cent of those who needed time off work agreed that IBS had a negative effect on their job/career. Sadly, 21 per cent claimed work colleagues were unsympathetic to their symptoms.

Focusing on the financial costs of IBS

The frantic trips to the toilet that result from IBS can disrupt your home, work, and social life. The financial cost can be substantial, and the emotional cost includes a huge deficit in confidence that only adds to your burden.

A recent review of IBS in a medical journal listed the following costs of IBS:

- **Direct costs of medical care:** Direct costs include surgery and home visits, accident and emergency department visits, procedures, testing, medications, and hospitalisations. Economic data from 1997 estimated that the UK spent £45.6 million annually for IBS care, translating into approximately £90 annually in costs per patient. More recent estimates put the average direct cost per patient per year at £316. (But keep in mind that only 10 to 25 per cent of people with IBS symptoms seek medical care. If costs include the remedies that people buy or try themselves, they're going to be much higher.)

Some bean counters have worked out that, on average, medical expenses for people with IBS are more than 30 per cent higher than those for people without IBS. The more severe the disease, the more complex the care. Healthcare costs for very severely affected patients may be as much as six times those for patients without IBS.

- **Indirect costs to society from lost productivity:** This type of indirect cost results from absence from school, work, and other activities. The 75 to 90 per cent of people with IBS symptoms who *don't* go to doctors often stay home from work when symptoms flare up, or they can't produce at full capacity even if they make it to work.

- **Intangible costs:** These reflect the human cost and inability to contribute completely to your family and social circle because of IBS-related symptoms.

Paying for alternatives

When we consider the medical expenses associated with having IBS, we need to recognise that those expenses include payments for treatments that fall outside the scope of the NHS in most areas. Many people seek help from complementary or alternative medical professionals – those who emphasise using diet, exercise, meditation, herbal treatments, homeopathy, manipulation, reflexology, and other tools for improving your health.

People with IBS usually have to pay for complementary and alternative medicines (CAM therapies) themselves. Some stump up hundreds of pounds a year, or more. Other people want to try CAM therapies but simply can't afford them, perhaps because IBS directly hampers their ability to earn a living. Doctors also feel frustrated because many believe that their patients may benefit from CAM, but doctors just can't persuade their Primary Care Trust (the local governing authority who decide how the health budget for that area should be spent) to fund CAM treatments.

If the annual NHS bill for patients with IBS in 1997 (the last time anyone tried to add it all up) was nearly £50 million, it's probably significantly higher now, a decade later.

Obviously, absence from work and school adds to the costs of having IBS. And another price tag to consider is the amount of money people spend on changing their diets, taking supplements, and seeking complementary therapies for IBS, such as those we talk about in Chapter 13. The sidebar 'Paying for alternatives' offers some insight into what that price tag may be.

Emphasising the emotional costs of IBS

IBS can create some very strong reactions in sufferers, including anger, anxiety, depression, loss of self-esteem, shame, fear, self-blame, and guilt. Perhaps the biggest cost of IBS is your loss of confidence.

When you have daily pain and constipation or diarrhoea, you're probably always aware of your condition. But because of embarrassment, you may not share your concerns with others. You may feel as if a little devil with a pitchfork torments you all the time – not just sitting on your shoulder but actively poking your intestines – and you can't tell anyone!

Fearing public places

Perhaps you developed your IBS symptoms after an infection, but you periodically suffer from all the symptoms for no apparent reason. (In other words, you can't associate the symptoms with eating specific foods or experiencing some other specific trigger, so your symptoms are unpredictable.) If you have a severe attack of pain when you're out, that's one thing: You limp home and try to recover. But if you suffer the horrors of bowel leakage in public, you may think twice about going out again. The old adage 'Once bitten, twice shy' has IBS written all over it. We talk more about losing bowel control in public in the section 'Tackling Social Situations', later in this chapter.

Many people with IBS are afraid to go outside, but the reasons are very apparent. They get panicky in public places, terrified that they won't find a toilet or get to it before they have an accident. They're also afraid of passing gas in public, in case something else comes out along with it.

Fear begins in the mind as a concern, then becomes a worry, and can shift into a full-blown panic attack. For some people, the panic sets up a rumbling in the stomach. (As we explain in Chapter 3, an intimate connection exists between the mind and the gut, which is home to more neurotransmitters than your brain.) In people with constipation-predominant IBS, fear can cause spasms and pain. In diarrhoea-predominant IBS, fear can mean a frantic trip to the bathroom.

Fearing food

Another fear common to people who have IBS is eating. For people without IBS, this sounds bizarre. Eating is the most natural (and necessary) thing in the world. But people with IBS have an incredible burden: They're afraid to eat because just eating a meal can trigger a bout of symptoms.

This fear can rob you of one of life's greatest and most basic pleasures – the joy of devouring scrumptious food. Even if you manage to eat your meals, it becomes a mechanical exercise, a necessity to get sufficient nutrients in – any satisfaction is tempered by desperate anticipation of the cramping and churning that follows.

Fearing eating can cause havoc with your social life too. At home you can carefully stock the cupboard with things that don't seem to aggravate your IBS so much. And if symptoms do appear then you have the comfort and privacy of your own bathroom in which to deal with them. (Even so, people with IBS often have times when they choose to skip meals entirely or eat just tiny amounts because they cannot face the trouble that follows.) But when you're invited out for supper, or a working lunch is arranged in the staff canteen, the only choice you may have is between coping with symptoms in public, or going hungry. For the most severely affected, the very thought of eating can wind up stress and anxiety levels to such a pitch that their IBS is triggered. Food becomes an enemy that must be dodged and outwitted, rather than a basic pleasure or comforting friend.

Fearing the future

Fear of never finding a solution to your problem may prevent you from living life to the fullest. Here are some things that many people with IBS have come to believe about the condition:

- ✔ IBS is impossible to treat.
- ✔ Having IBS means that I am doomed to a life of misery.
- ✔ IBS is incurable.
- ✔ I can never eat a normal meal again.
- ✔ No one will love me because of this condition.
- ✔ My body is betraying me and rebelling.
- ✔ I can never have a normal bowel movement.
- ✔ My friends and family think that I'm a pain in the ass – literally.
- ✔ IBS controls my life.
- ✔ Nobody believes that I'm ill.

Complaints of this type are serious and genuine. Although there may be some truth to such concerns, we believe that in many ways you can take this condition by the scruff of its neck and shake out some very workable solutions. In the next section, we offer suggestions that can help you do just that.

Tackling Social Situations

'Where's the bathroom?' is not a great pick-up line. But if you're on a date and you have IBS, that question is probably on your mind constantly. (If your date thinks that he's the total focus of your attention, he's sadly mistaken!)

In this section, we discuss some topics that you may not feel comfortable talking about with anyone – unpleasant stuff such as faecal incontinence and nasty odours. We hope the information we provide here helps you realise that you aren't the only person in the world worried about such things and that you can take steps to minimise the impact that these problems have on your ability to get out and socialise.

Experiencing faecal incontinence

One of the most feared events in the world of IBS sufferers is faecal incontinence. This is not a symptom that you want to share with *anyone*. Face it: If you told people that you had these kinds of accidents, you'd fear that image would be on their minds every time they saw you or even thought of you. It's just too unbearable to imagine. After the age of three or four, society expects our stools to go in the toilet, so faecal incontinence carries a great stigma.

 We aren't going to try to convince you to tell everyone that you have this problem. However, you need to tell your doctor, who is sworn to secrecy and won't laugh at your troubles.

In one large study, researchers interviewed patients in the waiting room of family doctors and gastrointestinal specialists about faecal incontinence. Anonymously, about 18 per cent of the patients admitted that they experienced faecal incontinence. However, only 25 per cent of them had ever talked about the problem with their family doctor, and only 50 per cent of them had ever discussed it with a gastroenterologist. And they were all people sitting in the doctor's office at the time! Please, do yourself a favour and find the courage to talk to your doctor.

You may think that only people with diarrhoea are affected by faecal incontinence. The pressure of liquid stool building up in the rectum and wanting release is sometimes too much to hold back. When a bubble of gas sneaks towards the anal opening and tries to squeeze out, sometimes more than a bubble of gas escapes.

But severe constipation can also lead to bowel incontinence. A large amount of stool can fill up the rectum, and because the poo is so hard and solid it can't pass through the anal opening. This condition is called *impaction*. The impaction can weaken the anal muscles, allowing liquid stool that's being pushed down from higher up in the intestines to ooze around the impaction and leak out. Occasionally, impaction can cause the stool to harden like a stone, forming a *faecalith* that must be removed by forceps or surgery. If you have such a blockage, and your gut is still trying to do its job and send its contents in the right direction, diarrhoea is the only type of stool that can pass around it.

 Keeping a diary of episodes of incontinence can help you sort out what may be causing the problem in the first place. Take special note of

✔ When the incontinence occurs

✔ Possible triggers, such as stress, food, and fluid

✔ Associated symptoms of pain, gas, and bloating

Using panty liners

You may find that wearing a small panty liner (the kind that women use for the light days of their periods) is all you need to boost your confidence. For you men out there, panty liners have an adhesive strip that attaches them to your underwear. They have absorbent material on one side and plastic on the other to prevent moisture from reaching your underwear. Panty liners are small and convenient to carry, even in your trouser pocket. If your problem is the loss of a little bowel content when you pass gas, this type of liner should be enough to prevent staining and embarrassment.

Considering incontinence wear

But panty liners may not provide enough coverage for everyone with faecal incontinence. Incontinence pads are the most popular product worn to protect against leaks, and they've come a long way in the last decade or so, taking advantage of everything that technology can offer.

Incontinence pads may be disposable or washable and reusable, and they come in a variety of shapes and sizes for children, men, and women (check out the Continence Foundation Web site at www.continence-foundation.org.uk for details and diagrams). Pads can be relatively slim and unobtrusive and slip inside your ordinary underwear, or inside special stretch or waterproof pants or special pants with a built-in pouch. At the other end of the scale they take the form of wrap-around all-in-one disposable padded pants (for those who need or prefer a lot of security).

Some people resort to inserting a tampon in the anus, or blocking the anus with a roll of gauze, to prevent bowel leakage when going out in public. We *do not* recommend this drastic measure because it can dry up normal anal mucus secretions that keep the lining of the anus healthy.

The layer of the pads worn next to the skin is usually made of a material that draws fluid through to a soaker layer of absorbent materials underneath. Drawing the fluid away means that, as far as possible, the surface retains a 'dry' feeling. This helps to reduce leakage of fluid faeces and protects the skin from sores. Most pads also have a waterproof backing or under layer to minimise leaks. You can use those without a waterproof backing as an extra booster pad.

We suggest that you try a range of types and makes of pad to see which suits you best. You may also want to mix and match – for example, choosing a smaller pad most days but a more absorbent pad when your IBS slips out of control.

Some people have little choice but to use the disposable padded pants option to deal with the unexpected if they want to have a social life. You may lament that those bulges won't do wonders for your hot new outfit. But if you want to get back to living a more normal life, you have to be willing to adapt – you may branch out into a whole new style of clothes, for example.

When you think of adult disposable underwear, you may associate it with elderly people who suffer from urinary incontinence. But younger people with IBS, an inflammatory bowel disease (Crohn's disease or ulcerative colitis, which we explain in Chapter 1), or bowel cancer wear them as well. Tell yourself over and over that disposable padded pants aren't just for babies (no matter what your mother used to say) but provide an invaluable resource for every person who needs them.

Manufacturers design many incontinence pads for people who are bedridden. But if you keep looking, you can find one that suits your needs. Look for products called *adult pants* – they come in various weights and sizes for light incontinence to heavy incontinence.

Many adult pads and pants have absorbent material that neutralises odour, and have anti-leak cuffs. And, of course, if you chose the disposable types, they can be thrown away as soon as they're soiled. You probably aren't looking for a product with a large capacity, or one that's made for overnight use. You mainly need something to wear at work or on social outings to feel safe. (Chances are you may not even need the pants, but they definitely act as a security blanket for your rear end.)

The Internet makes it especially easy to research, window shop, and order these products in privacy. You can call a manufacturer directly and ask them to send a catalogue, which means you can browse products in peace at home and find the best product for you. In fact, most chemists or supermarkets don't carry the best brands. Some brand names of products used for faecal incontinence include Molicare, Bodyform, Depend, Contisure, Lille, Kanga, and Tena.

Here are some tips for getting the best use out of incontinence pads:

- ✔ Change your pads and pants at frequent intervals, or as soon as you're aware that they've become soiled.

- ✔ Practice good skincare habits. Wash with mild soap and water or the adult version of baby wipes (called, appropriately enough, *adult wipes,* they're bigger and stronger than baby wipes but otherwise much the same) that you can buy at pharmacies and some supermarkets, or online at pharmacy sites.

- ✔ Use a cream that covers the skin to act as a barrier anywhere that may be exposed to irritating faecal matter, such as around the anus. The best ones contain zinc oxide (an ingredient used in babies' nappy cream, and safe to apply to delicate parts), which is also healing for damaged skin.

If you prefer, instead of disposable padded pants, you can wear washable plastic pants over your cotton underwear. (You don't want to use plastic pants directly next to the skin.) To cut down on the rustle and squeaking when you walk, wear another pair of cotton pants over the plastic pants.

You may be able to get incontinence products on the NHS instead of having to pay for them yourself at the chemist or through the Internet. Talk to your GP about whether he can prescribe them for you. However, the NHS range can be limited, so you may still have to pay yourself to get the type that suit you most.

Using fibre and diet to combat faecal incontinence

Most programmes for faecal incontinence focus on two ways to treat this condition: solidify the stool and slow the gut. These solutions assume that your problem is incontinence due to diarrhoea. Taking fibre is the most common way to firm up your stool. We discuss the benefits of fibre in Chapters 8 and 10. The key to success with fibre is to introduce it very slowly so that your intestines get used to it; if you take too much, you may cause gas, bloating, and irritation.

As we note earlier, incontinence can also occur due to faecal impaction. If you suffer from faecal impaction, treatment with fibre, fluids, and mild laxatives, as well as identifying the triggers for constipation, can help you overcome the problem (Chapter 8 contains detailed information about using drugs such as laxatives in IBS).

Identifying your food triggers and eliminating them can often reduce your IBS symptoms, including severe ones like faecal incontinence. Chapter 10 walks you through an avoidance and challenge diet that can help you figure out what your food triggers are.

Fasting is not a long-term solution for faecal incontinence, but it may help you get through a specific event. It works because food consumption triggers contractions throughout the gastrointestinal tract. In IBS, these contractions often create the need to defecate. If you have poor bowel control, urgency and incontinence may result.

Eating a large meal, especially one full of fatty foods, can stimulate gastrointestinal secretions that increase your bowel motility. So especially when you're in public, keep those portions light.

Taking medications for faecal incontinence

Using a medication before going out is one way to cope with the physical and emotional reality of IBS accidents.

Loperamide

Loperamide (which we discuss in Chapter 8) is useful for treating faecal incontinence because, in addition to slowing down your gut, it actually tightens the anal sphincter. It generally works best at night, but you may find it helps during the day as well. You have to try it to know for sure. You don't want to use it if you're prone to constipation, but otherwise the drug is safe to use to prevent episodes of faecal incontinence.

Take loperamide 30 minutes before meals if you often have diarrhoea and/or incontinence immediately following meals. If you have early morning urgency, watery stool, and incontinence, a tablet or two at bedtime may help.

Colestyramine

Colestyramine (see Chapter 8) is a resin that binds bile acids. This reduces stimulation of the colon and slows the movement of bowel contents through it, allowing more time for the body to absorb water. If you had your gallbladder removed and this resulted in watery stool after a meal, you may find this medication useful. However, gassiness and bloating are possible side effects.

Amitriptyline

Amitriptyline in high doses is used as an antidepressant. Doctors prescribe lower doses to treat chronic fatigue syndrome, fibromyalgia, and sleep disorders, or to help decrease chronic pain. However, the drug does have a constipating effect, and some doctors use amitriptyline to treat faecal incontinence when fibre and loperamide don't work.

Covering up odours

Every human on the planet produces gas from their intestines, emitting farts sometimes dozens of times a day – it's a simple fact about how our bodies work. Many farts are small and go undetected but they can also be loud and, worst still, smell extremely unpleasant. Most people feel at least slightly embarrassed when their gut erupts like this in the company of others. But if you have IBS, smelly farts can be a constant and mortifying problem. In IBS processes such as bacterial overgrowth and fermentation in the intestines may churn out large volumes of gas that race through the gut at speed and burst out under pressure, leaving everyone else around you in no doubt about where the nasty niffs are coming from. It may be possible to shrug off the embarrassment of an occasional fart, but a barrage of noxious odours are more difficult to ignore.

Products containing the plant chemical chlorophyll can help to control odours arising in the gut. People have used chlorophyll since the 1920s to help with problems such as halitosis and body odours, and hunters even use the plant chemical to disguise their scents from animals! Manufactured from natural plant sources such as the algae chlorella and spirulina, chlorophyll treatments were first developed for people with a colostomy or ileostomy (where surgery diverts the intestines so that they empty their contents through a hole made in the surface of the abdomen, into a bag attached to the skin) and faecal incontinence. But chlorophyll is useful in IBS too and available in tablet, capsule, powder, and liquid form. The popular health drink, wheatgrass, is also rich in chlorophyll.

The other agent used to mop up rumbling whiffy flatulence is charcoal, which you can buy as tablets to swallow or biscuits to chew. The charcoal disperses quickly in the intestines to form very fine particles with a large surface area. This allows them round up gases and bind to toxic particles very efficiently. Charcoal tablets relieve flatulence and put the dampers on bloating and abdominal discomfort. But many people find charcoal tablets unpalatable, and they can interfere with absorption of other medicines, so always check with your doctor if you want to take them regularly.

For people whose main trouble is flatulence, some innovative products and gadgets exist that may help to control those odours. One such product is a flatulence filter seat cushion with replaceable carbon filters, which supposedly absorbs both the sound and the odour. You can also buy charcoal pads to wear in your underwear, which supposedly eliminate the odour of flatulence. We haven't investigated the effectiveness of these products, but we like the idea that companies are creating products that may comfort people who are embarrassed, not entertained, by flatulence.

Connecting with Others

Connecting with other people is one of the most important steps you can take when dealing with IBS. Keeping this condition a secret from your friends and family can lead to all kinds of tension and misunderstanding. Being alone with your illness in your house is one thing, but being alone with it in your mind is even worse.

Supporting someone with IBS

This section is one to share with anyone you want to have a better understanding of how to help you.

The following are some things to do if you're supporting someone else with IBS:

- Listen, listen, and listen more.
- Commiserate.
- Believe what the person is saying.
- Offer help with chores, projects, and errands.
- Keep the person's IBS a secret from others if that's what she wants.

And here are some things not to do:

- ✔ Try to give advice.
- ✔ Tell horror stories about your own and others' bowel conditions.
- ✔ Act bored or restlessly when you're being asked to listen.
- ✔ Give this person more work to do.
- ✔ Make bowel-related jokes – unless the person with IBS initiates them.

Communicating with your partner

We assume that your partner knows about your illness (it can be difficult to hide), but he may not understand fully what it costs you physically and emotionally. You may hear an edge in your partner's voice when you've gone to the bathroom six times and he's still waiting his turn. But it also means that you need to take time periodically to have the *IBS Talk*.

The IBS Talk reminds your partner what IBS is all about, how it affects your body, and the kind of support you need to keep your life together. The IBS Talk is just a reminder about the nature of your illness. Your partner may have forgotten some of these things – lucky him. But IBS is with *you* every day, and you can't forget. If you sense that your partner's impatience is overriding his sensitivity to your issues, just say, 'It's time for the IBS Talk'. Even that one sentence may shift the mood and serve as the necessary reminder.

The IBS Talk doesn't give you the right to run the relationship based on your illness. You must be careful not to use your IBS to get your own way, no matter how tempting. Playing games like that is not a good relationship-builder, and crying wolf about your IBS gets you in trouble – when you have a serious bout of IBS and really need support, you may not get it.

The key to the success of the IBS Talk is to express what's going on without your partner trying to fix the situation. Most people, when faced with a problem, want to fix it. You just have to remind your partner every so often that you need him to listen – you aren't looking for a quick fix.

Having sex

IBS is not a sexy illness. Intercourse can be painful even when you aren't having an attack (pain during sex needs always to be checked out by your doctor, in case there is a different cause). And if you *are* having an attack – forget it:

- ✔ In the middle of a painful abdominal spasm, sex is the last thing on your mind.

✔ If you have frequent diarrhoea, you're absolutely not going to put yourself in the reclining position only to have to interrupt the proceedings to hop into the bathroom.

✔ Intercourse when you have constipation can be extremely painful – you don't want someone lying on you, and you don't want any pressure on your swollen intestines.

The IBS Talk that we describe in the previous section is really helpful to have when your partner wants to have sex and you – your body, your mind, and your intestines – are absolutely not interested. Your partner has to know that when your pain sensitivity is sky high, all the romance and sexual tension in the world can't overcome pain. If he doesn't want his feelings hurt, he needs to know when to back off and wait for a more appropriate time.

If your partner is feeling rejected in the bedroom because you're in the bathroom, be sensitive to those feelings. We recognise that it can be a long road from sick to sexy, but when you're feeling well, think about initiating sex. Don't use your IBS symptoms as an excuse to avoid intimacy. (One person told us that IBS is to her what a headache was to her mother.)

Telling your friends

A big faux pas in a relationship is when your partner blurts out to mutual friends that you have IBS, without asking your permission. That's usually a major breech of trust. Be blunt with your partner about what's private and what's public information.

If your friends need to know that you have symptoms because you're going out or travelling by car together, you need to make a decision. If they're close friends who you see often, you don't want to have to tell white lies all the time to avoid the topic. Plus, you may find that if you clue them in, you can get the support from them that you really need. However, if you go out with people you rarely see and don't know very well, you always have the option of simply saying that you have food poisoning. It's your call.

Nearly one in five people suffers from IBS, so when you tell your friends about it, you may find that you aren't alone in your suffering. While we wrote this book, most people we talked to knew at least one other person who had IBS.

Making Web connections

A good way to socialise from home is to connect with people electronically. Online support groups and chat rooms exist for almost every condition and disease you can imagine. In an age where you can barely get a nod from your next-door neighbour, if you send out an appeal to an online support group, you can get a dozen replies (and hundreds of people may read your message). Those replies in turn help others who have similar concerns. It seems to be a win–win situation. Chapter 20 gives the resources to help you connect online.

In surveys of people with certain diseases (including cystic fibrosis, diabetes, and amyotrophic lateral sclerosis), results show that those who participate in online support groups fare better physically and emotionally than those who don't. And finding a support group is easy: Just use the key words 'IBS support group' in a search engine and you may be amazed at what pops up.

Most moderated online support groups prohibit promoting businesses, but some participants may encourage you to take specific products to help your IBS symptoms. Be sure to look at the signature line of the person offering advice. If the signature line includes a Web site, check that site to see if it promotes the product they recommend. Be cautious of advice coming from someone who may benefit financially from it.

Taking Baby Steps

If you've read the rest of this chapter but you still aren't convinced that you're safe to leave the house, we've a few more suggestions to get you back on the path to being a social person:

- ✔ **Have at-home dates with your partner:** If you feel trapped in the house, your partner may feel that way too. To avoid letting that situation turn into a source of resentment, schedule fun activities that the two of you can do at home. Set up movie nights, play games, or find a hobby that the two of you can pursue from the comfort of home.

- ✔ **Invite people to your house:** As long as you know that your own bathroom is just up the stairs or around the corner, you can feel confident enough to ask friends to your house. If throwing a party for 30 people seems like too much, start small: Pick two or three people you know and trust, and ask them to come for dinner. When you see that you can enjoy yourself this way, you can gradually work your way up to hosting bigger events.

- ✔ **Take short trips to public places:** Even as you work on improving your social life at home, don't stop making the effort to get out of the house. If the thought of trying to sit through a movie gives you shivers, plan much shorter outings to start with. Ask your partner to make a quick trip to the shops with you, or spend 15 minutes walking in the park. When you discover that you can survive, and even enjoy, these shorter outings, you can gradually increase the amount of time you spend in public. With each success, you find it easier to walk out the door the next time.

Chapter 15

Working with IBS

In This Chapter

▶ Recognising how IBS affects your work life

▶ Making changes to improve your time at work

▶ Discussing your IBS with the people at work

*A*bout 11 per cent of the population have IBS, which means that if ten people work in your office, one of them probably has IBS. Oops, that's you! Okay, different example: If 20 people work in your office, 2 or more of them may have IBS. So chances are that at least some of your fellow employees – maybe your boss – already know about IBS.

IBS affects people during their most productive working years. People who have IBS are almost *four times* more likely to miss work than people who don't have IBS. For these reasons, IBS is the second most common reason for not showing up at work, right behind back pain.

Unfortunately, IBS tends to put a crimp – and sometimes a cramp – in some professions. It makes police work and skyscraper construction more difficult, for example, just because you don't have immediate access to a bathroom. Some people leave the workforce altogether because of IBS and live on disability allowance or a pension.

Our goal in this chapter is to help you consider less drastic options than getting out of the workforce completely. We start the chapter by looking at some blunt facts about how IBS impacts negatively on your productivity and your ability to seize certain work opportunities, but we don't stop there. We offer suggestions on how to cope better at work, and we encourage you to consider negotiating to work at home, at least for some of the time, if your profession allows.

Facing Facts about IBS on the Job

We're realists, and we know (especially from talking with many, many people during the course of writing this book) that IBS has a definite impact on your work life. In the following sections, we address some of the most common problems that people with IBS face on the job, so you realise that you aren't alone.

Producing less work

Don't you sometimes feel that scientists study anything that moves? A journal called *Alimentary Pharmacology & Therapeutics* reported on one study in which researchers gave a standardised questionnaire to a group of 135 people with IBS to see how they fared at work. The participants indicated that they lost an average of about 12 hours per week due to their illness. That means that someone with IBS may be losing two out of five days of work each week. The study also estimates that an employee with IBS costs a company 50 per cent more than someone without IBS. This isn't good news to an employer, so we can see why some people don't want anyone (especially the boss) to know that they have IBS.

Keep in mind that not all the hours lost result from physical absence from the workplace. Instead, this study took into account lost productivity on the job (due to time spent in the bathroom, for example).

If you have IBS, the last thing you want to hear is that you're a financial burden on your employer. Most people with IBS already feel that their illness is an imposition to friends and family. But our goal here isn't to make you feel guilty; we want to consider not only how your IBS affects your work, but how your work affects your IBS. Many people we have talked to can trace the onset of their IBS to coincide with a new job, an increased workload, a change in staff or management, or a reduction in job satisfaction. We discuss the connection between work stress and IBS further in the section 'Suffering from stress', later in this chapter.

Passing up promotions

If your new job description involves travelling, entertaining, or golfing with business associates, you may feel compelled to avoid the promotion if you have IBS. We hear stories like this all the time. The decision is perfectly justifiable for many people who don't have their IBS under control.

But we believe that better ways exist to handle the adventures of a new job and the stresses of work itself. We offer some specific tips in this chapter, and we encourage you to look at other chapters in this book to realise that you have a wealth of tools at your disposal – including diet, exercise, and stress-reducing techniques – that can help you handle travel and social events better and without incident.

Suffering from stress

If misery loves company, you may be reassured to know that lots of people feel high levels of stress on the job. (For proof, see the sidebar 'Stressing at work'.) But you have the added burden of having a condition that not only *creates* more stress for you at work but can actually be *triggered by* that same stress. (We discuss stress as a trigger of IBS in Chapter 4.) Most articles about stress mention IBS as one of the physical ailments that stress at work affects most.

Many psychologists indicate that women seem to be more stressed out at work than men. And, as we note in Chapter 5, women are much more likely than men to have IBS. Although factors other than work certainly play a part here (think hormones, for example), stress and IBS aren't a good combination.

Some of the stories we hear from people coping with IBS at work are nothing short of terrifying – vindictive supervisors denying people bathroom privileges, IBS sufferers called hypochondriacs by their co-workers, and given more work when they complain to the boss. These examples, which we'd like to believe are exceptions rather than the rule, appear symptomatic of an abusive work environment that places profits first and employees last. And they do nothing but heap additional stress on the person in question.

Making Your Work Day Bearable

We're optimistic that you can use the information in this book to help you better manage your IBS in the long run so that your symptoms improve. But, again, we're realists. The road to better health can take time, and in this section we aim to help you cope with work even when your IBS flares up.

Starting your day in the right way

Coping with the demands of work actually begins at home, as you anticipate the day ahead and make preparations. Many people with IBS have three or four bowel movements before they even leave for work. And diarrhoea isn't the only problem that can mean you head off to work unprepared, in a bad mood, or late: Pain and spasms because of gas or pain from the pressure of constipation can also interfere with the start of your day. (If you have constipation, you may feel the constant urge to go. In that situation, you know that you need to be near a bathroom just in case the next effort produces results.)

A combination of factors can create a morning attack of IBS:

✔ Your stress hormones get revved up with the activity of standing upright and moving around.

✔ Whatever you eat for breakfast sends your gut into action.

✔ You may fear having uncontrollable gut spasms and even an episode of faecal incontinence in the car on the way to work. (If you experience diarrhoea in the morning, your body may actually be attempting to empty your colon so you don't have this sort of accident.)

So how do you avoid any or all these triggering events?

✔ If you know that the simple act of getting up in the morning triggers IBS symptoms, set your alarm 30 or 60 minutes early. Give yourself enough extra time in the morning to work through those symptoms and still not feel rushed or panicked (which only makes your symptoms worse).

✔ If what you eat seems to cause symptoms, and if you're afraid that those symptoms may make themselves known during your drive to work, we have two suggestions:

• For a long-term solution, try the avoidance and challenge diet we present in Chapter 10 to determine which foods you need to avoid in order to reduce your symptoms. You may find that you need to eliminate milk, toast, or fruit from your breakfast menu, but you can also find safe foods that you can eat every day without triggering symptoms.

• In the short run, pack your breakfast and take it with you to work. If you're worried about getting diarrhoea, better to deal with it in the office than in the car.

Enjoying an accident-free commute

If your journey to work is a source of stress because you're afraid that you won't be able to find a toilet when you urgently need one, consider some of these tips:

✔ As we mention in the previous section, pack your breakfast and wait until you get to the office (and near a bathroom) before eating.

✔ Give yourself plenty of time to catch the bus or train, or make the drive to work. The last thing you need is to feel a rush of stress brought on by a traffic jam or a missed bus.

✔ If you walk or cycle to work, look for a route that takes you past a public toilet or garage with facilities, so that you know in advance where you can stop.

✔ Use the stress-relieving techniques we explain in Chapters 12 and 13. Choose simple methods that you can practise in the car or sitting on the bus, such as diaphragmatic breathing, progressive muscle relaxation, and chanting.

✔ If necessary, take medications to help you get to work safely. Taking loperamide about 30 minutes before you walk out the door may solve any concerns about diarrhoea. This medication, which we describe in Chapter 8, slows down the bowel, and for some people it tightens the anal sphincter during the day as well as at night.

Dealing with an attack at work

Prevention is the best medicine for IBS. We strongly encourage you to consider the suggestions we offer in other chapters:

✔ Eat an IBS-friendly diet, based on information in Chapter 10.

✔ Consider taking dietary supplements, which we discuss in Chapter 10.

✔ Exercise, even if you don't feel like it! We get you started in Chapter 11.

✔ Practise stress-reducing techniques, like the ones in Chapter 12.

We do realise that you're bound to experience an IBS attack at work sometimes, no matter how hard you work to keep the symptoms at bay. Perhaps that tiny sliver of birthday cake you eat at a staff party or the added stress of an imminent deadline works its magic. For whatever reason, if pain and bloating get the best of you or you find yourself going to the bathroom every half hour, we have a few tips for coping with an acute situation:

✔ Take several deep breaths.

✔ If diarrhoea is the problem, take loperamide.

✔ If you're bloated, take a peppermint capsule to relax intestinal muscles and lower the pressure in the bowel (Chapter 13 explains how peppermint works).

✔ If you have pain, take a simple antispasmodic or analgesic (we discuss these medicines in Chapter 8).

✔ Use the self-hypnosis technique that we explain in Chapter 12, or try a visualisation technique and picture yourself with a healthy bowel relaxing on a tropical beach.

Talking to Your Boss and Colleagues

If you're a full-time employee, you're entitled to annual paid leave that you can use to negotiate the time you need off. But before your use up all your leave, make a plan! If you take quite a bit of time off work, you may consider discussing your illness with your boss. Together, you may be able to come up with ways that you can keep your IBS from interfering with your productivity and comfort at work.

We certainly understand that some bosses and co-workers may be easier to talk with than others. And if you absolutely know that your boss is going to react negatively to what you have to say, we respect your decision to keep your IBS private and cope with the situation in other ways. But we certainly hope that the majority of people reading this page have a slightly better work situation than that. If you can muster the courage to tell the truth, you may find that you get a lot of support – perhaps even from people who have personal experience of what you're going through.

Deciding when to tell

Timing is everything, and one of your biggest decisions relates to when to discuss your IBS with the people in your workplace. Some options for you to consider include:

✔ **When you first interview for the job:** If you feel that your condition may interfere with carrying out the duties of a job you're considering, it may be a good idea to let the cat out of the bag early on. First, you want to know what kind of company you're working for. Some companies don't hire people with medical problems, even though that hiring practice is illegal. You want to know up front whether a company is tolerant of people with medical conditions; otherwise, your job may be an uphill battle. Also, if your company has to pay health insurance, it may come out in your application that you have IBS, and you may be chastised for not disclosing your illness.

✔ **When you're running out of holiday allowance:** Don't wait until you've used up your annual leave to tell your boss that you have IBS. The stress of not being able to take a day off only increases your symptoms.

✔ **When you feel that your work quality is suffering:** You probably don't want to have this discussion when a deadline is looming and everyone is too stressed to think about how to help you. Instead, talk about your condition when things aren't too busy at work and you can take the time to discuss options that can improve your performance on the job.

The Disability Discrimination Act (DDA) 1996 prevents employers from discriminating against people with a wide range of medical conditions that have a long-term substantial adverse effect on normal day-to-day activities (we have no doubt that IBS falls into this category). So you should be safe telling your employers about your IBS, but you may want to wait until you start the job before you let them know. Don't keep it hidden because if, later on, you're fired because of poor performance, you'll find it hard to blame your illness if you have never let them know about it.

✔ **When co-workers start to ask you what is wrong:** Despite your best efforts to hide or disguise that you have an illness, your co-workers are likely to be the first to notice your extra breaks, absences, and trips to the bathroom. You may want to tell them about your challenges before they decide that you're just slacking off.

✔ **When your trips to the bathroom become fodder for jokes:** Having to use an office bathroom that may inadequately camouflage sounds and smells can be embarrassing enough. You certainly don't need the added stress of insensitive comments from co-workers who don't know that you have an illness. Telling your co-workers may protect both you and your colleagues from the embarrassment of nasty bathroom humour.

Deciding what to say

When you make the decision to talk with your boss or co-workers, you may want to get across some of these general ideas:

✔ You have a chronic condition that can flare up with no apparent warning. Having printed material on hand or a note from your doctor to describe IBS can be very helpful.

✔ You're taking steps to deal with your IBS, such as watching what you eat or taking supplements or medications to reduce the symptoms.

✔ Despite these steps, you may still need to visit the bathroom several times a day, and some days are likely to be more of a challenge than others.

✔ Most importantly, despite these challenges, you remain a hard worker and committed to your job.

If your company has a human resources (HR) department, you may be in luck. Because IBS is a condition that comes up in articles on work-related stress, you may be able to talk to someone who understands your situation. All it takes is one knowledgeable person in a department, and you have someone to talk to about some basic ground rules regarding you and your IBS. For example:

- ✔ Your condition may make it difficult for you to be on time for work every day.
- ✔ You need to be close to a bathroom.
- ✔ You may have to rush out of a meeting suddenly.
- ✔ You may have really bad days when you need to stay home altogether.
- ✔ You're not the right person to make home visits to clients.
- ✔ You promise to work all your hours in exchange for flexibility at work.
- ✔ You'd love to discuss the possibility of working from a home office, even just on a part-time basis. (We discuss this subject in more detail in the section 'Working from home', later in this chapter.)

If you're a hard worker and sincere, telling your boss or HR representative about your condition may have very positive results. For example, it may get you a desk nearer the toilets or lead to you working from home part of the time.

Plus, when you start sharing your IBS story with other people, you may find that they too have physical, emotional, or personal issues that they deal with. Opening up may be the first step towards developing better relationships at work, which can ultimately ease part of your stress. But only you can decide when and how to have this type of conversation.

Working from Home

As we note elsewhere in this chapter, one of the things you may want to request when you discuss your IBS with your employer is that you have the flexibility to work from home, even if only part of the time. Obviously, this situation won't work for everyone. If you work in retail sales or any other job that requires your physical presence, you aren't going to get far if you ask to work from home.

But many jobs *can* be done from a home office; all you need is a phone and a computer. Writing, editing, phone sales, medical transcription, public relations, multilevel marketing, selling certain products . . . many possibilities exist. If your current job seems like a good candidate for some at-home work hours, draft a proposal that seems logical and fair for both you and your employer. (You may offer to make yourself available for activities that require your presence in the office, such as staff meetings or client meetings, for example.)

If your current job can't mesh with an at-home situation, you may want to consider whether it's worth the effort to change careers in order to have that option. If starting your own business seems intriguing, go to the Business Link Web site at www.businesslink.gov.uk. The Business Link service is part of the government's campaign to promote enterprise, and is funded by the Department for Business, Enterprise and Regulatory Reform. Its supported by a number of other government departments and agencies, and can put you in touch with local sources of help too.

The downside to working at home is that you don't get out and socialise with other people. As we explain in Chapter 14, that can also be a problem when you have IBS. Don't let working at home become an excuse to be a complete recluse. Be sure to read our tips in Chapter 14 so that you can continue to have a social life, even at times when your IBS is acting up.

Chapter 16

Helping Your Child Cope with IBS

- -

In This Chapter

▶ Understanding how IBS affects youngsters

▶ Helping your child deal with pain

▶ Comforting your kids

▶ Working through difficult emotions and behaviour

- -

Children aren't mini-adults, especially when it comes to IBS. Kids may have the same symptoms of IBS that adults have, but they don't have the coping skills that develop with maturity. In this chapter we address many of the frustrations that children with IBS endure, and we look at ways in which you and your child can together get to grips with the symptoms and stresses they face. But first there are a few things about IBS in younger people that are worth keeping in the back of your mind:

✔ Tummy pains are common in children, which means knowing when the problem is IBS and when it's something else is tough – for kids and their parents.

✔ Stress from an emotional upset or trauma (something of a daily event for most children, even if trivial and quickly resolved) can trigger IBS.

✔ Embarrassment about bodily functions makes it difficult for children, especially older children and teenagers, to talk about IBS.

✔ At school, children are often not allowed to leave class for any reason. If they leave for an urgent bathroom visit, they may be told off or taunted.

✔ Children with IBS may not want anybody at school to know that they have this condition.

✔ Children have little control over what they eat and may not make the association between food and IBS.

✔ No IBS medications are entirely safe for children. When kids do take drugs, they may experience side effects (just as adults may).

Realising That a Tummy Ache Is Something More

We all had tummy upsets and pain in our childhood. But some kids deal with more than the usual stomach ailments that result from picking up bugs at school and eating too many sweets.

Recurrent abdominal pain is the most common pain complaint of childhood. It affects 10 to 15 per cent of school children, resulting in absences from school and impaired quality of life. One study shows that one-third to one-half of children with recurrent abdominal pain continue to report abdominal pain and related symptoms (such as IBS) when they're adults.

You may not believe that a child as young as four years old can have IBS, but he can. IBS is more common in the late teens and early 20s, but that doesn't mean it can't strike earlier in life.

Be aware of how quickly your child can dehydrate and become very ill when he loses a lot of fluids with frequent bowel movements. Dry skin, not going to the bathroom to urinate, sunken eyes, and lethargy are common signs of dehydration.

Finding out what's wrong

Before you deal with IBS in your child, you have to find out what's wrong. But some children don't tell their parents what they're experiencing. So what do you do then?

The key is to pay attention. If your child has frequent bouts of abdominal pain and constipation, spends a long time in the toilet when he needs to open his bowels, or runs to the bathroom all the time, he may have IBS. If he doesn't talk with you about his symptoms, he's probably embarrassed or thinks that something is very wrong and is too frightened to talk about it.

Observe your child's behaviour. Then gently ask what's up and give him all the chances he needs to talk with you. When he finally opens up, reassure him of your unconditional love and support, and let him know that you can help him deal with this problem.

Next, find out all you can about IBS – this book is a great start. Get a proper diagnosis from your family doctor by ruling out other conditions, which we discuss in the next section. Then, work on making lifestyle changes involving diet, exercise, and stress-releasing tools (see Part III of this book). Encourage your entire family to participate in these changes so your child doesn't feel even more isolated. Reducing stress within the family as a whole can also help to reduce your child's stress.

Ruling out other conditions

When abdominal pain, gas, bloating, diarrhoea, and/or constipation occur in a child, your doctor needs to rule out the following conditions and diseases that cause digestive upsets:

- ✔ **Gastroenteritis:** Infections of the gut due to bacteria, viruses or parasites (especially with a micro-organism called *giardia*) are very common in childhood and can be very serious because small children can easily become dangerously dehydrated. If your child has abdominal pain and diarrhoea, especially if it persists, it is very important that he sees a doctor who can check the diagnosis and recommend the right treatment. See Chapter 7 for more details.

- ✔ **Inflammatory bowel disease:** Blood in the stool, along with more than ten copious watery stools a day and a slight fever, is an indication of an inflammatory bowel disease – Crohn's disease or ulcerative colitis. We discuss these diseases in Chapter 7.

- ✔ **Dairy allergy:** (see Chapter 7) Reactions to proteins in milk and other dairy products can cause symptoms very similar to IBS. As dairy foods are usually an important source of nutrients in childhood it is very important to be sure of the diagnosis before changing a child's diet.

- ✔ **Gluten enteropathy (coeliac disease):** As we explain in Chapter 4, people with this disease cannot tolerate *gluten,* a protein found in wheat, rye, oats, and barley. Symptoms may mirror those of IBS and the treatment is lifelong avoidance of wheat, rye, oats, and barley. Identifying this condition early can curtail a lifetime of misery.

   A blood test can help doctors to diagnose this condition. But doctors often recommend performing an endoscopy with a small bowel biopsy as the most reliable way to identify the disease accurately. See Chapter 7 for more on endoscopies.

- ✔ **Lactose intolerance:** We explain this condition in Chapter 7. Almost all babies make an enzyme in their gut called lactase – they need this enzyme to digest the sugar in milk called lactose. But when babies are weaned onto solid foods their lactase levels drop dramatically. In some ethnic groups, such as Asian and African people, children make very little lactase after the age of about five. Then, when they eat milk or drink dairy foods (as most kids do) they're unable to digest the lactose, which passes into the large bowel and causes wind, bloating, pain, constipation, and/or diarrhoea. This may be confused with IBS. Children who are lactose intolerant must either avoid dairy products, take lactase milk enzyme tablets when eating or drinking things that contain milk, or use special lactose-free products.

If your child has copious watery stools, the situation can be life-threatening because water loss can lead to dehydration and damage to organs such as the kidneys and the heart. Get advice from your GP as soon as possible or take your child to the accident and emergency department at your local hospital. After your child stabilises, the doctor finds out whether your child has a bowel disease by using these tests:

- **Blood tests:** These tests indicate if there may be an infection or inflammation in the intestines. A key test here is the full blood count, which includes a measure of the levels of white blood cells in the blood. A raised white cell count is a sign of inflammation or infection. Another important test is known as the *C Reactive Protein* level or CRP. This protein is produced during inflammation and infection, and so a raised level is a sign that these processes are going on somewhere in the body. Blood chemistry tests check for levels of sodium, potassium, calcium, and other elements that may be lost in diarrhoea, and low levels of albumin, which may be a sign of malnutrition.

- **Stool tests:** Your child's stool or faeces may have a greasy rancid appearance if fat is not being absorbed properly. Examination may also reveal micro-organisms and parasites, including worms.

- **Endoscopy:** By passing an endoscope, or flexible narrow tube with a camera on the end, into the intestines doctors can check the lining surface, or mucosa, for disease, such as the ulcerations typical of ulcerative colitis. We discuss this test in Chapter 7.

- **Barium enema:** This test may help to diagnose Crohn's disease, an inflammatory bowel disease that can affect any part of the intestines from the mouth right through to the anus. Barium, which shows up on an X-ray, is introduced through the anus and rectum with an enema, and may reveal ulcers, scarring, narrowing, and other features in the lower intestine or large bowel. Because the barium does not reach the small intestine when introduced through the anus, a barium meal and follow-through study show the top end of the gut.

Healthcare professionals with experience in looking after children perform endoscopies and barium enemas with the utmost sensitivity while your child is under sedation or a general anaesthetic.

Struggling with the pain

Doctors studying IBS in children have found that, because children haven't developed adult coping skills, they tend to struggle on with the pain rather than trying to do something about it. This is called *passive coping*. However, they can also feel victimised and overpowered by the pain, which is called *catastrophising*. Kids sometimes use the following phrases to describe their condition:

✔ There's nothing I can do, so why even bother trying?

✔ Nobody understands.

✔ I just can't talk about this with anyone; it's too embarrassing.

✔ I just can't stand this any more.

✔ There's something horribly wrong with me.

Adults with IBS often think these very same things and have the same feelings of isolation, but they're usually aware of some ways to deal with it or how to seek help. But for a child these thoughts are as overwhelming as the condition itself.

When your child is overwhelmed by the pain of IBS, the most important thing you can do is show him that you understand that he's having a tough time and that you're there to help him in any way you can. Give him time to talk about his feelings and explain the pain or other symptoms he's getting. Find out what his real worries are. Try to reassure him that together you can find ways to cope, and that you can both take steps to make things better. If he won't talk to you, ask them if there's someone else that he'd like to talk to instead. Find information – such as in this book – that you can look at with your child and offer to go with him to the doctor to talk about the condition.

Overcoming the Stress of IBS

Adults tend to forget that children's lives can be as stressful as theirs – maybe even more stressful. Here are some examples of the stress on a child who has IBS:

✔ I have to get up early for school even though I can't get to sleep because of the pain.

✔ My mum forces me to eat breakfast, which only makes me feel worse.

✔ Some mornings I have to go to the bathroom five times before I can leave the house.

✔ I'm always late for school and then have to stay behind after school in detention.

✔ There's no way I'm telling anyone at school what's wrong with me because they'll make my life even more miserable.

✔ I sit in agony in class because the teacher won't let anyone leave the room without a note.

✔ I farted once in class. I just couldn't help it – the pain was so bad. Six months later, the people in my class still bug me about it.

✔ I'm seriously considering asking my mum whether I can be home-schooled. I can't take it any more.

✔ After my grandmother died, I just couldn't stop going to the bathroom.

✔ I think I'll ask my mum whether I can go to the doctor by myself. There's no way I want anyone else in the room when I have to tell the doctor what's wrong with me.

✔ Every time my uncle visits, I feel sick to my stomach. He yells and makes stupid jokes, but my father says I'm being rude because I don't want to be near my uncle.

Protecting your child from her own sense of embarrassment is impossible, and you can't really protect him from other kids' harsh comments. But you *can* do many things to instil confidence in your child, let him know that his feelings are important, and show him that you support him.

In the following bulleted list, we provide specific suggestions for making your child's life a little easier. Using the preceding list, we walk through each item and offer solutions to consider:

✔ **I have to get up early for school, but often I have trouble getting off to sleep at night because of the pain so I don't get enough sleep.** This is a common complaint, and we offer two possible solutions:

- *Diet:* Watch what snacks your child has in the evenings. Offer him apple sauce and mashed potatoes, which rate high on the list of soluble fibre foods that soothe the tummy. (We talk about the importance of soluble fibre in Chapter 10.) Ice cream, which is high in fat, sugar, and dairy, is a no-no. Popcorn is also off the menu because it's hard to digest and can irritate the gut, making it one of the worst insoluble fibres.

- *Stress/pain relief:* Try simple techniques at night to comfort and reduce pain and stress like a warm bath, a gentle massage, a story for younger children, or yoga for older ones. You can also try a warm (but not too hot) water bottle or compress that your child can place on his tummy.

✔ **My mum forces me to eat breakfast, which only makes me feel worse.** Of course you want your child to eat breakfast, but you must make sure that the food you offer doesn't trigger IBS symptoms.

You may find that a breakfast of a soluble fibre food, like cooked oats or barley, along with diluted orange juice or apple juice is a good choice. Experiment to find out what affects your child in good and bad ways. Our advice in Chapter 10 can help.

✔ **Some mornings I have to go to the bathroom five times before I can leave the house.** Frequent bowel movements in the morning are common in IBS. Possible culprits are the food eaten the night before, worry about getting to school on time, fear of pain or having to go to the bathroom, or worry about having an accident.

First, make sure that your child wakes up early enough to allow for extra bowel movements. Giving him an extra 15 or 30 minutes to get ready for school may reduce some stress if he worries about being late.

Two other possible solutions are:

- *Diet:* The dietary advice in the previous two bullet points applies here. Make sure that your child is eating soluble fibre foods both at bedtime and for breakfast, and try to discover what foods are particularly good and bad for his symptoms.

- *Stress relief:* Help your child to get everything ready for school the night before so that he doesn't need to worry in the morning. Talk about any problems he may be having at school or at home, and make sure he keeps on top of his homework. Then, in the morning, encourage him to wake up gently with some simple stretching exercises before he bounds out of bed.

✔ **I'm always late for school and then have to stay behind after school in detention.** This can happen if your child refuses to tell his teacher what's going on. Your child may develop a rough-and-tough attitude to cover up the problem and be identified as a kid with a chip on his shoulder. He may even get into fights and bully other kids so that he won't be bullied.

When your child's school performance is being affected by IBS, you need to talk to someone at the school such as his teacher, tutor, headteacher, or school nurse. However, before you do, you must have their assurance that the information is strictly confidential.

✔ **There's no way I'm telling anyone at school what's wrong with me because they'll make my life even more miserable.** It seems that children have the uncanny ability to ferret out the weaknesses in other children and torture them with that knowledge. Telling your child not to worry about this quirk of human nature is pointless. We can't miraculously change people's behaviour, but we can offer a suggestion.

When your child expresses this fear, it's time to have a long talk about bullies. You want your child to understand that bullies are bullies because they're hiding weaknesses of their own. Bullies lash out at other kids so that no one can spot their weakness. Most kids understand this explanation. Ask your child to describe the bullies in his school. You may be able to figure out pretty easily what's driving their behaviour.

✔ **I sit in agony in class because the teacher won't let anyone leave the room without a note.** If this situation arises, you definitely want the teacher to know that your child needs access to the toilet on his schedule, not the teacher's. Some teachers find creative ways to acknowledge a child's needs. Instead of informing the whole class that a child has to go to the toilet, a teacher may ask him to pick up something from the secretary's office or do some other errand.

✔ **I farted once in class. I just couldn't help it – the pain was so bad. Six months later, the people in my class still bug me about it.** If your child shares an embarrassing moment like this with you, consider sharing some of the worst moments in your life – as long as they aren't too risqué. This helps to make your child feel less isolated. Dig out a few juicy facts about farts – some research shows that humans fart on average 154 times a day!

By chatting with your child, you may be able to help him understand that passing wind is natural and we all do it now and then. This may not go down well with some children but 'normalising' symptoms can be a useful tactic to prevent a spiral of rising anxiety that only aggravates problems.

It's also important to discourage your child from holding in painful gas or bowel movements and to make sure that he understands that doing so can lead to long-term bowel problems. This is another situation where you can have a conversation with your child's teacher to ensure that you child is able to leave the classroom when experiencing a lot of gas or urgency.

✔ **I'm seriously considering asking my mum whether I can be home-schooled. I can't take it any more.** Although home-schooling may be an option for a child who is severely ill with IBS, it may bring its own problems. Doing lessons at home can be an isolating experience – you have to work hard to provide your child with social activities that help develop interaction and communication with other children, and even harder to provide the education and teaching that he needs. A frank discussion with your child about the pros and cons is the only way to handle this question.

✔ **After my grandmother died, I just couldn't stop going to the bathroom.** A tragic event such as a death in the family can trigger an underlying bowel sensitivity. The symptoms of IBS and the grief become intermeshed and can provide an ongoing source of emotional irritation for a child. Here are some possible solutions:

- *Talking with your child:* Encourage your child to talk about the death of a family member. The whole family can participate in remembering the person who has died by spending time each day or each week talking about the person, looking at photos, and sharing memories. Such shared events can go a long way towards helping your child deal with the stress of his loss. Psychologists find that the biggest problems seem to occur when families don't talk about the death.

- *Counselling:* Your child may benefit from getting psychological counselling about death, dying, and dealing with grief. If you don't know how to find a counsellor, ask your GP for advice.

- *Checking for blame:* Children can be surprisingly ready to blame themselves when things go wrong – even when events occur that actually have little to do with them. It may sound illogical to you, but your child may feel that it's his fault that his granny died, perhaps because of some trivial thing he did or thought. Self-blame leads to pervasive stress, so check this possibility out.

✔ **I think I'll ask my mum whether I can go to the doctor by myself. There's no way I want anyone else in the room when I have to tell the doctor what's wrong with me.** This is a common sentiment expressed by kids with IBS. Ask your child whether he does or doesn't want you in the room, and make sure that you respect the answer. If he says he'd rather be alone with the doctor, don't be insulted. Your child does have a right to privacy, and yes, he's growing up!

✔ **Every time my uncle visits, I feel sick to my stomach. He yells and makes stupid jokes, but my father says I'm being rude because I don't want to be near my uncle.** If your child makes a statement similar to this, treat it very seriously. He shouldn't be exposed to verbal abuse, even if it's not directed at him. And in the worst case scenario, your child may be trying to tell you that he's being physically abused.

Never force your child to kiss, hug, or otherwise interact with someone he seems to be afraid of. He often has very good reasons for that fear.

Maintaining Balance at Home

Having a child with IBS, or with any other chronic illness, puts a strain on the family and can stir up some difficult family dynamics. We often hear that the poorly child in a family seems to get all the attention and other children feel left out.

Some children may feel that the only way to get attention from parents who are too focused on an ill sibling is by being unwell themselves or by acting up. You don't want either of these situations, which add considerable stress. Instead, try using preventive psychology: Acknowledge your other children, praise them, take them on special outings, and give them responsibilities that let them know that you trust them.

You don't have to ask to know that a child feels neglected, perhaps even abandoned, when you spend extra time with a sibling. Your healthy child may find it hard to rationalise that you have to spend more time with your poorly child. Instead, your healthy kid just knows how he feels – and he doesn't feel good. Most children who have ill siblings are actually scared that their parents don't love them as much. This is the dreaded fear that you have to dispel.

Your child with IBS also has his own emotions about his condition to deal with. He may feel that he's a burden and worry that you don't love him because he's such a handful. That's one reason most children with IBS don't want to share their symptoms with anyone – even their parents.

As if attending to your children's needs isn't tough enough, you also have to make sure that you and your partner don't go off track. For example, if Mum does most of the caregiving, Dad can feel left out. Try to guard against this happening – and no, that doesn't mean just telling Dad to grow up! Ideally, try to divide the caregiving as equally as possible between the two of you.

Other ways to make sure that your family sticks together when you're working out how to cope with IBS in your child include making lifestyle improvements everyone's goal, leading to a healthier family in general. For example:

- ✔ Eat better by planning and cooking meals together.
- ✔ Exercise as a family, such as by biking, walking, or swimming.
- ✔ Talk, talk, and talk some more. We cannot overemphasise the importance of talking, and keeping communication channels open, no matter what.

Working Through Your Child's Emotions

Stress and emotions play a key role in triggering IBS symptoms, as we explain in Chapter 4. As an adult, what do you do when you're overwhelmed with stress, depression, or anxiety? You may ask your doctor for a prescription to help you get back to feeling normal. And when your child experiences those same types of emotional problems, your first thought may be to get a quick fix in the form of a similar prescription.

But such drugs are usually not suitable for children (and they're often not the best solution for adults either!). Children's physical systems and emotional lives are too delicate. In 2005, the National Institute for Clinical Excellence (NICE) recommended that doctors should only give antidepressants such as Prozac to children over the age of 12 who had already tried psychological therapies such as counselling and cognitive behavioural therapy. Because of the risks in children under the age of 12, doctors should only prescribe antidepressants very rarely, when a child is very seriously depressed and not responding to other treatments. .

To be good parents, we need to understand why our children think the way they do, and how we can help them to deal with emotions when they're so extreme that they interfere with normal life. If your child has a chronic illness such as IBS, you may have to work that little bit harder than other parents to tie everything together and help your child to develop coping strategies. You can read books, talk to experts, and share ideas with other parents, but in the end many of the answers are right in front of you – in your child.

If your child has emotional troubles that you suspect may trigger his IBS symptoms, what can you do?

Being there for your child

First and foremost, just be there for your child. Quite often your child won't really want to talk about what's bothering him. He knows that he's bothered but just wants it to go away. He may feel that talking about his worries is just going to open up all the pain and make him face what he'd rather hide from.

Let your child know that you're around if he needs you, but then give him space. Find things to do in a different corner of the house, but pop your head around his door now and then to offer him opportunities to do things with you – kicking a football, making a cake – whatever he wants. However, don't put him under pressure to do something if he doesn't want to.

Hopefully, during one activity you'll eventually strike a chord and then, while you're both involved with it, he may begin to feel secure enough to start talking about his problems. This may be easier for him if you appear a little pre-occupied with something else (like mixing up some icing for the cake you're both baking), allowing him to avoid your gaze as he speaks.

Listening to your child

Find a peaceful moment when you can give your child all your attention, and then ask him gently and quietly about what is bothering him. Then turn your ears up to max and listen out carefully for what he has to say.

Be patient if your child finds it hard to tell you something or seems worried that what he says may upset you. Keep your questions open – use 'how', 'why', and 'what' questions that encourage him to say more, rather than closed questions that induce a yes or no answer. Use questions like 'And then what happened?' to keep the story going if he goes quiet.

Take your time, and let your child take his time too. Don't be judgmental or try to tell him what he ought to do – he needs to work this out for himself with a few nudges and nuggets of information from you to guide him. Try not to show shock or anger at what he says – if you feel these emotions, keep a lid on them and deal with them later separately.

Helping your child take action

After your child starts to open up and talk about his emotions, the next step is to help his develop strategies and skills to deal with these. Ask him directly what he thinks may help.

You may want to start the process with a bit of a brainstorming together. But remember that your child needs to come up with the ideas for strategies himself. Finding his own answer – and knowing it was his idea – is a real confidence booster. Confidence is a big issue in chronically ill children, so do what you can to make sure that your child is self-assured and feels supported.

Encourage your child's good ideas and elaborate on them. Talking, listening, and feeling understood may be all it takes to start washing away the negative emotions. Try to be practical and optimistic – if you're getting nowhere, change the subject and move on to something more positive and relaxing for now.

Nailing negative emotions

Anger, anxiety, depression, frustration, fear – all these negative emotions drain energy and sap your child's self-esteem. So your child needs to recognise and understand these specific feelings that he may be having.

Help your child understand and abandon the negative ways in which he may be dealing with negative feelings, including:

- Catastrophising (always expecting the worst)
- Filtering (focusing on negative things only)
- Personalising (blaming yourself for bad things)
- Polarising (seeing things as always good or bad, not shades of either)

Alleviating anger

Children often feel angry about what's happening to them, or the IBS symptoms they're having to put up with (just like adults really!). But unlike adults they're rarely able to recognise their feelings as anger or know how to channel feeling cross. They may act out their anger, becoming difficult or hitting out at others. Older children may internalise this feeling, becoming withdrawn or sulky. To cope with anger, try these approaches:

✔ Talk to your child, using examples that he can relate to, about his grumpy feelings, and how these relate to his IBS. He may feel ashamed of his anger, so try to help him understand that this emotion is a perfectly normal reaction, although not the best way to cope. He needs to know that it's okay to feel this way and that you love him unconditionally, but what matters is how he deals with his anger.

✔ Find sociably acceptable ways for your child to express his anger, such as physical outlets to let off steam. Let him know that he can express his anger in some places (in the garden where he can kick a football or swing high on a swing while singing loudly, for example) and not in other places (in the living room, for example).

✔ Encourage older children to write poems, stories, or songs as an outlet for their feelings.

✔ Use humour as a way to defuse anger.

✔ Try some standard de-stressing activities, such as massage or a soothing bath, to keep anger levels down.

Altering anxiety

Adults often tease children who appear overly anxious and worried. Of course, that's the worst thing to do. You need to show that you understand and want to help your child with these feelings, which are quite common even among children who don't have a condition like IBS. Tell your child about things that have made you anxious too, and how you coped. Try the following:

✔ Help your child to recognise the symptoms of anxiety, such as feeling breathless or having a racing heartbeat, so that he knows when it's time to take action.

✔ Look at how your child interprets the world and whether this may make his anxious – for example, he may feel anxious because he suspects that you're embarrassed or cross about his IBS. Try to change these mistaken beliefs.

✔ Keep an eye on your diary and consider what's coming up that may cause your child to worry. Your child can be very sensitive to excitement and upcoming events and may, for example, express a particular type of anxiety called *acute anticipation* that can make his IBS flare up. Take steps to defuse your child's anxiety before it has a chance to build.

Sensing sadness

People often romanticise childhood as a happy-go-lucky time, but children are sad for many of the same reasons as adults, and depression can certainly occur. When your child feels chronically unwell and limited by pain or embarrassment because of IBS symptoms, he may have sad feelings. Anticipate sadness by watching your child for symptoms of sadness such as not sleeping properly, losing interest in favourite hobbies, having difficulties concentrating at school, or low self-esteem. And if these signs sound familiar, consider these steps to show him that you care and are there to support him:

- ✔ Watch your child for symptoms of sadness such as not sleeping properly, losing interest in favourite hobbies, having difficulties concentrating at school, or low self-esteem.

- ✔ Communicate with your child. Don't give him an intensive grilling about his every thought or expect him to open up to you immediately – very rarely do children simply announce 'I am feeling depressed'. Listen for clues about his mood or feelings (for example, when he talks about friendships at school) and try to gently pick up on opportunities to probe a little further. Even talking about trivial things shows children that you're listening,

- ✔ Ask for help from your doctor or health visitor sooner rather than later – as soon as you feel that nothing you're doing is helping or that things are getting worse. Depression in childhood needs expert advice.

Chapter 17

Keeping Up-to-Date with IBS

In This Chapter

▶ Understanding how different groups raise awareness of IBS

▶ Using the Internet to research IBS

▶ Getting the latest news on IBS

*I*n this chapter we show how far knowledge about IBS has come in the past decade and how to find out where it's going. Magazine and Internet stories bring new awareness of the condition. Research into IBS is accelerating, along with hopes that new medications will surface. Existing treatments, such as diet and exercise, prove successful at tackling IBS symptoms. And with all this progress, you have lots of opportunities to continue finding out about IBS on your own, long after you put this book down.

Raising Awareness of IBS

The more a condition is openly and calmly discussed, the less stigmatised and alone those with it tend to feel. In order to raise awareness like this, IBS needs its supporters. After people get over the embarrassment of having IBS, many feel able to speak openly about their condition, although few celebrities (who can attract headlines that highlight the condition, or inspire magazine editors to publish their story) admit to the problem (IBS affects as many as 1 in 10 people from all walks of life so plenty of famous faces out there have the same problems as you).

Foundations, self-help groups, and high-profile fundraisers also have a role to play in offering support to people with IBS but these groups often battle with hundreds of other worthy causes to seek funding for publicity or research. Raising public awareness of the condition plays an important part in generating this funding and giving IBS-related charities a voice. So the public needs to know that IBS is a problem. In the following sections, we explain how IBS is coming to more and more people's attention.

Marketing medications

Often, public awareness of a chronic condition such as IBS increases when a drug company tries to get people talking about it in order to make money – the company hopes that increased awareness of the condition sends more people scuttling to buy their treatments, or ask their doctor for a prescription. The positive side of this is that raising awareness makes it easier for people with the condition to ask for help. The negative side is that the company that stands to make a profit has a specific agenda and may provide biased information to the public about treatment options.

So if you see a sudden flurry of media interest in the condition that you've battled for years, there may well be an ulterior motive behind the stories. Be on your guard and ask some probing questions before you believe everything you hear, especially if a campaign promotes wonderful new treatments.

If you've had IBS symptoms for a long time, you're likely to feel a certain amount of desperation about finding a treatment that offers relief. When you see television and magazine ads, and even what appear to be genuine feature articles, that seem to speak to you and your symptoms and sing the praises of a new therapy, you may hold out great hope for that treatment. We've talked to people who've fought to have access to a certain drug, only to find, upon taking it, that their symptoms worsened. We've also heard from people for whom a medication had miraculous results. Always keep in mind that IBS is an individual illness with symptoms and effective treatments unique to each person.

Rebecca suffered from severe constipation-predominant IBS for several years and had tried every over-the-counter medication she could find. When a friend told her about a medicine that had helped his constipation-predominant IBS, Rebecca asked her doctor for a prescription. She took the medicine exactly as directed the next morning. Within a few hours, she had a bowel movement. She took another dose at night and awoke with gas and bloating followed by diarrhoea. Initially it was a relief to get her bowels moving but the diarrhoea persisted for a full month and caused her to become light-headed and dizzy. Her friend didn't have diarrhoea when he took the same drug, but Rebecca figured that everybody was different, and she kept taking the medicine. However, after six weeks Rebecca stopped taking the drug because the diarrhoea was so severe that she was afraid to leave the house.

Sharing your knowledge with a self-help group

A great tactic for keeping up to date with IBS is to talk to others with the condition and find out what they've managed to glean from their sources. They may have read an article that you didn't see, tried a remedy that you've never heard of, or talked to a gastroenterologist who described research that you didn't know about. At the same time you can pass on your own news. In this section, we turn our attention to self-help groups, most of which tune in avidly to the IBS grapevine.

An online IBS self-help group is the first stop for many newly diagnosed people, and even for those who haven't yet received a diagnosis. This type of group is usually a free service that provides support, information, and contact with others who have IBS. In our healthcare environment, where time with your GP is very limited and accessing a specialist gastroenterologist is difficult, self-help groups play a vital part in providing information and psychological support.

Perusing the pros and cons of joining a self-help group

Studies confirm that if you participate in self-help groups, which are really mutual-aid groups, you may benefit in the following ways:

- You know you're not alone.
- You have a feeling of community with people who have similar problems.
- You receive professional advice if you participate in groups with skilled moderators.
- You experience a sense of belonging and less isolation. (This is especially important for people with severe IBS who feel confined to their homes due to symptoms – more on this in Chapter 14.)
- You acquire practical information about your condition.
- You hone your coping skills.
- You develop an ability to think and act positively about wellness.
- You have support in times of crisis.
- You gain a sense of empowerment.
- You feel more hopeful about your situation.
- Your self-esteem grows.
- You experience a decrease in doctors' visits and hospitalisation.

A very positive aspect of online self-help groups is that, because participants can remain anonymous, people tend to share their deepest fears about their illness. (Online, you're identified by your login name and your condition only, and that's that.) When you participate, you often find out that a hundred other people think the same way as you. This alone can be tremendously empowering to someone with IBS who is afraid or embarrassed to even talk to a doctor about these problems. Also, when you hear people talking about their symptoms and making jokes about their problems, it tends to lighten your load considerably.

One drawback of self-help groups is that some participants tend to fall into a complaining mode. The best self-help groups share experiences, hopes, strengths, and victories and try to focus on the positive. One survey of online support groups found that positive comments were seven times more frequent than negative ones, so if you find that a support group you're participating in feels too negative, search for another.

Another possible negative about joining a self-help group is that you need to be just a little wary of the quality of the information provided by the group. A group may be run by an individual who's delighted to have found that a certain treatment (maybe a herbal treatment, or a particular drug) has worked wonders for them. They may rave endlessly about this treatment, or heartily recommend a particular therapist who uses it, and fail to draw attention to research that questions its value. Similarly, they may dismiss a particular therapy because it hasn't worked for them, even if there is evidence that it helps others Always try to obtain a good balance of information from different sources to help shape your view on IBS matters.

Meeting some of the groups

Formed in 1987, the Irritable Bowel Syndrome (IBS) Self Help and Support Group was the first online IBS self-help group and it now claims to be the largest Internet community for people with IBS. Members communicate on its bulletin board to share knowledge and experiences with IBS. Although the site is American, most of the issues and topics are just as relevant to people in the UK and Europe – the condition affects people in much the same way, so you can talk about the same problems and you may even enjoy building connections across the pond. You can visit this group at www.ibsgroup.org and link to books, studies, medical tests, diagnostic criteria, and medications (but keep in mind that some aspects, especially medications, in the UK may be different).

The Canadian Society of Intestinal Research (CSIR) at www.badgut.com offers lots of useful information to help answer your IBS questions. It also runs support groups that meet regularly – it's probably just a bit too far for those in the UK to pop over and visit, but the focus for their groups is something worth keeping in mind whenever and wherever you talk to others with IBS (and even maybe when you decide to set your own group up!). CSIR groups work hard to focus on creating a positive, friendly attitude by making the following statements, which they've generously shared with us, as a commitment to their ongoing support of each other:

- ✔ I am in a group of people with a common bond, sharing my concerns, feelings, experiences, strengths, and wisdom.
- ✔ Discussions are designed to foster positive attitudes and are directed towards solutions.
- ✔ I share my problems but don't dwell on them.
- ✔ I don't prescribe, diagnose, judge, or give medical advice.

✔ I have the right to not use the recommendations of others.

✔ I respect that personal information shared is confidential.

✔ Our facilitator advances discussions but is not there as an expert.

✔ Most sharing of ideas come from the group.

✔ We each have the opportunity for equal talking time or the right to remain silent – we can share as much or as little as we want.

✔ I actively listen when someone is talking and avoid interrupting and engaging in side conversations.

✔ I'm going to stick to my own experiences and avoid generalities.

✔ The support group meetings supplement, and do not replace, medical care.

✔ I don't provide or receive specific medical advice within the group.

✔ I'm not a part of this group for any commercial purpose, nor will I try to sell products or services to group participants at meetings.

✔ I share equally with the other members of the group the responsibility for making the group run smoothly.

✔ Having benefited from the help of others, I recognise the need to offer my help to others.

This is one of the most comprehensive guides we've seen for ensuring a successful self-help group. Reading these principles periodically helps members of any self-help group – online or otherwise – to focus on the intent of their group.

The IBS Network is a great resource in the UK for advice, support, and information (`www.thegutttrust.org`). It also offers a telephone helpline, and runs a limited number of local support groups. The network is keen to see more IBS groups throughout the country, and offer to help anyone interested in starting one up. This may be your chance to get a local group going! Why not start a group to match your interests – a support group for young mothers with IBS, cyclists with IBS, or just an open group for anyone in your area?

Surfing the Net

The Internet is home to more than 100,000 health-related Web sites, with everything from university and hospital academic sites to sites run by individuals. In the past, only doctors had easy access to medical journals and medical articles, but now everyone can access more than 12 million medical papers online. Health problems regularly feature in the weekly top twenty search topics noted by internet search engines such as Google or Lycos.

But recent research looking at dedicated consumer health Web sites in the UK, such as NHS Direct Online and BBCi Health found that less than half of users thought that the information they found on the net had completely aided their understanding of their problem. As a result, many patients collect information from a variety of sources on the net and then take this to their doctor to talk through in more depth. Most doctors like to see their patients becoming actively involved in managing their own condition. However, the sight of a ream of papers that have to be checked to ensure that they're reliable, and then explained, can make any doctor with a waiting room full of patients, feel understandably pressured.

Impinging on your doctor's turf?

Many doctors worry about the quality of information freely available on the Net. They've witnessed on numerous occasions how patients have been be misinformed by incorrect or biased information, or simply got the wrong end of the stick when they've tried, without enough background knowledge, to interpret complex papers published on the web. But with only 8.4 minutes on average to spend with each patient, GPs may find it impossible to explain everything that their patient needs to know.

So not surprisingly, many patients choose to look elsewhere for information. But without an expert such as your doctor to interpret health information correctly and spot poor quality information, the consequences of going it alone may be dire.

We certainly don't encourage you to go it alone either. You can benefit greatly from doing your own research into IBS and reading everything you can lay your hands on, but that doesn't mean you should cut your doctor out of your circle of caretakers. Most doctors aren't threatened by patients bringing information from other sources to an appointment to discuss. In fact, many doctors encourage patients to do independent research on their health issues and come to an appointment prepared to ask questions about what they've found. But if you've a lot to talk about, be prepared to leave information with your doctor and come back for a second appointment when she's had a chance to check it over without several other sick patients lurking outside the surgery door.

Just don't expect your doctor to agree with everything you read. Bear in mind that she doesn't agree with everything her medical peers read or quote either – active debate and discussion is a normal part of medical practice and doctors often disagree with each other but respect each other's views. So if your doctor doesn't agree with you, don't immediately abandon your new ideas but do some more research before making up your mind about what may or may not work for you.

Knowing your source

Be sure to find out the source of your IBS information. If you search for IBS information online, make sure that you find out who writes the information on a particular Web site and who funds the site. This information should be readily available; if it isn't, e-mail the site's webmaster and ask for full disclosure.

Be aware that some IBS Web sites are funded by pharmaceutical companies. These sites may restrict their treatment recommendations to the drugs developed by the sponsoring companies. If someone is selling something on a Web site, that doesn't mean the site doesn't contain valuable information about IBS. It simply helps to obtain full disclosure about who is funding the site and who has written the information so that you can make your own choice about whether to believe the information, follow the advice, or purchase a product.

Seeking alternatives

If you want information about complementary and alternative medicine (CAM), the Internet can be a great resource. For example, you can look up information about supplements (such as those we discuss in Chapter 10) and stress-reducing techniques (such as those we discuss in Chapter 12).

Medical schools don't generally instruct doctors about these topics, so chances are you'll find information online that may be new – and possibly very interesting – to your doctor. And if you find that your doctor isn't open to discussing information about CAM, you may want to consider seeking another opinion, perhaps by talking to another doctor in the practice, or even moving to a different doctor who is more interested in CAM. You definitely want to give yourself the benefit of working with professionals who have open minds and a willingness to consider all possible means of treating your symptoms.

Reaping the benefits

The benefits of the Internet are many and keep people coming back for more:

- ✔ **Anonymity:** Nobody else needs to know that you're looking up the word *incontinence.*
- ✔ **Convenience:** You don't have to dress up, leave home, be far from a bathroom, or interact with anyone but your computer.
- ✔ **Self-empowerment:** You can find out first-hand about any subject.
- ✔ **Variety of information:** You have the ability to quickly check multiple sources, and hear different views.

Seeing Possibilities in Serotonin Research

The biggest news on the IBS front right now seems to be research demonstrating abnormalities in the serotonin signalling system between the gut and the brain. Normally a constant coordinated interplay occurs among the muscles of your gut, central nervous system, autonomic nervous system (the body's 'flight or fight' system), and enteric nervous system (the nervous system of the gut). The mastermind behind this interplay is the neurotransmitter *serotonin*. Impaired function or coordination of any of these systems, or the communication among them and the muscles lining the intestines, can disturb the way the bowel moves and alter sensory perception, leading to the characteristic symptoms of IBS.

An increasing number of studies show that people with IBS have abnormalities in serotonin. For example, some research shows abnormally low levels of serotonin in the cells lining the intestines and another study shows very high levels in people with constipation-predominant IBS. Several other conditions associated with IBS are believed to relate to low serotonin levels too, such as depression, anxiety, and sleep disturbances.

This research supports the production and use of new serotonin-modulating IBS drugs (known as gastrointestinal serotonergic agents), and people with IBS feel excited and hopeful that more effective treatments that really can make a difference to their symptoms, may soon be available. However, there is always a need for caution when using a brand new class of drugs, where side effects aren't yet known. (It's worth bearing in mind that one or two of these types of drugs have already been introduced – and then withdrawn – because of side-effect problems.) In the following sections, we present what we know so far about this research and these drugs.

Finding abnormal serotonin levels in the IBS gut

In 2004, the pharmaceutical company Novartis sent out a press release entitled 'Molecular Defect Found for the First Time in IBS Patients'. The subtitle was 'New Research Demonstrates that IBS is Not 'All in Your Head'. (But then, you knew that all along, didn't you?)

A gastrointestinal expert and contributor to the research, Professor Michael Gershon of Columbia University, said in the press release: 'IBS has long been classified as a purely psychosomatic condition. . . However, IBS is now associated with a very real abnormality in the gut and one that is as biochemical as any other'.

This new research, published in the journal *Gastroenterology* in 2004, identified a molecular defect in IBS that does not appear in people without IBS. This research correlates with other findings that show people with IBS that was first triggered by an episode of gastroenteritis (post-infectious IBS), also have an increased concentration of cells in their guts that contain serotonin.

The research was the fruit of intense efforts in recent years by researchers to explore the way that serotonin works in the gut. Research also shows, for example, that in order to regulate the signalling process, excess serotonin must be removed by the serotonin transporter (SERT) molecules in the cells of the epithelium that lines the intestines. Changes in the amount or function of SERT can affect serotonin levels and therefore may be relevant to IBS. Research shows decreased SERT activity in people with IBS compared with healthy volunteers. Another study found that that genetic variations in SERT exist that may be relevant not only to symptoms of IBS but also how well people respond to gastrointestinal serotonergic therapies.

Now that scientists have a better understanding of possible underlying mechanisms in IBS, they're scratching their heads to develop innovative drugs that work in different ways to previous treatments and target serotonin and related chemicals more closely. Pharmaceutical drugs that increase the action of one particular serotonin receptor (5-HT4) have been clinically shown to improve constipation, for example. However, the precise mechanism involved is not yet known.

Realising that your gut has a nervous system

Studies are slowly piecing together the ways in which signals pass between the gut and the brain (along a pathway known as the gut–brain axis). A few years ago, based on some of this research, Professor Michael Gershon of the Columbia University College of Physicians and Surgeons in New York, developed the idea that the gut has an independent nervous system driven by serotonin (known as the enteric nervous system). In 1999 he predicted that if research showed an increased concentration of serotonin in the lining of the gut in IBS, suggesting abnormal activity of the gut's nervous system, then the treatment of the condition can radically change. This prediction is now being proven by research.

At the same time as the concept of the enteric nervous system was being heatedly discussed, the use of a new group of antidepressant drugs known as Selective Serotonin Reuptake Inhibitors or SSRI's (which include fluoxetine – better known by its trade name of Prozac) was bringing serotonin to public attention. In fact, the flurry of news about these drugs in the past decade may have lead you to think that most of the serotonin in the body is directed at brain activity. That's far from the truth. We now know that 95 per cent of this neurotransmitter resides in the gut, and only 5 per cent affects the brain.

At work in the gut, serotonin binds to specific receptors on nerve cells to make the intestines move. If too much or too little serotonin is bound to receptors, researchers believe that the intestines in someone with IBS move too quickly, resulting in diarrhoea, or too slowly, causing constipation (but beware – this is a massive over-simplification of a complex control system and scientists have yet to work out the exact effect of serotonin).

Supplementing your serotonin

You may imagine that if IBS is a problem with serotonin, then topping up your serotonin levels may just help to keep your symptoms under control. Unfortunately, we know from other diseases that molecular mechanisms are rarely that straightforward. Scientists have not yet worked out the exact problem with serotonin in IBS and the way it masterminds the gut–brain axis. Some research points to too much serotonin in IBS, other studies to too little.

IBS may be the result of problems unrelated directly to serotonin itself but instead to the receptors that detect serotonin (in which case you can give as much serotonin as you like but the bowel won't respond) or to complex feed-back loops (raise serotonin levels high in this case and you may shut down important systems in the body). Or it may be that only certain selective types of serotonin receptor are relevant to the bowel, and by raising serotonin generally in the body you may set every receptor jangling, leading to all sorts of complications or side effects.

So taking supplements that influence levels of serotonin in the gut is a bit of a gamble. The effect is hard to predict or explain for now. Even so, driven to despair by your IBS, you may decide it's worth a go.

Two supplements, available at your local chemist or health food store, may have a positive impact on the serotonin in your gut. In the following sections, we explain the connection each has with serotonin.

Spicing up serotonin with 5-HTP

A compound called 5-HTP is a precursor to serotonin and may be helpful in the treatment of IBS. Supplements of 5-HTP are produced from griffonia seeds, which are rich in the compound. This serotonin precursor is a cousin of another serotonin precursor, the amino acid *tryptophan*. (We discuss tryptophan in the next section.)

Talking turkey (and tryptophan)

We all know the post-Christmas dinner sleep-fest that occurs after devouring huge quantities of our faithful gobbler. You may have heard that the sleepiness occurs because turkey contains high amounts of an amino acid called *tryptophan*. Tryptophan is one of the necessary ingredients for making serotonin. It helps the body produce the B-vitamin niacin (B₃), which, in turn, helps the body produce serotonin.

By 1989, a variety of tryptophan called L-tryptophan was a very popular supplement used as a sleep aid and also for treating minor depression and anxiety. Then, a very unfortunate series of events occurred. In Japan a manufacturer supplied a contaminated batch of L-tryptophan, which appeared to trigger an outbreak of a potentially fatal condition called eosinophilia myalgia syndrome (EMS). Although tryptophan had previously been used safely for 30 years, the Food Standards Agency in the UK advised that manufacturers must not supply the supplement or add it to foods in case it was to blame (although it remained available on prescription as a medical treatment).

However, by 2005 the government's Committee on Toxicology of Chemicals in Food, Consumer Products, and the Environment (COT) reviewed the issue and concluded that L-tryptophan as a dietary (food) supplement isn't an appreciable risk to health provided that it meets suitable purity and dosage criteria. So once again, you can find tryptophan on the shelf in pharmacies and health food stores.

Your eagle eyes may have spotted that there we just mentioned another source of tryptophan – basic foodstuffs that contain tryptophan that the body can process into serotonin. Carbohydrates such as cakes, pasta, and bread are good sources (in one survey wholemeal banana muffins came out top), but healthier options include black eyed-peas, walnuts, almonds, sesame or pumpkin seeds, and cheddar, gruyère, or Swiss cheese. But don't dash out just yet and start scoffing tryptophan-rich foods. The body takes tryptophan in more readily when levels of other amino acids in food are low. And protein can reduce serotonin production, so your body may not be able to use the tryptophan present in many protein-rich foods such as turkey easily. You need to work quite carefully to include more serotonin via your diet.

Expecting more research

It's still early days in the world of drugs that modulate serotonin in the gut. Research only really got going in the late 1990s and scientists are still doing a lot of basic research to define the different types of serotonin receptors in the body, where they're found, and what they do. Translating that knowledge into the development of new medicines, testing how well they work and how safe they are, and then bringing them to the market is a notoriously slow business – it takes an average of 12 years for a drug to progress from the research lab through to the patient.

New drugs for IBS, some based on the gastrointestinal serotonin system, are on their way and you'll undoubtedly hear much more about them in the near future. But 'on the way' may mean they're still several years away, and many may prove to be non-starters before they even manage to make their first appearance on the shelves of the pharmacy. For now, we need to make the most of those drugs currently available, which we discuss in Chapter 8.

Part V
The Part of Tens

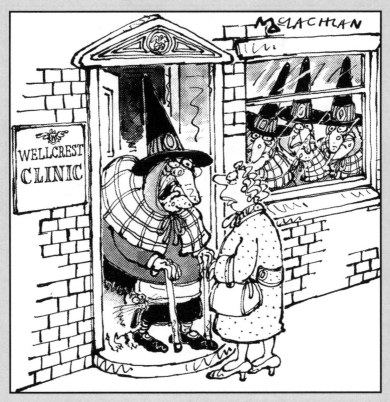

'You've got the wrong clinic — this one is
for Crone's Disease not Crohn's Disease.'

In this part . . .

Everybody loves this part of a *For Dummies* book. That's because the chapters are short and sweet, offering great nuggets of information you can easily digest (with no nasty side effects).

In this part, we present ten IBS triggers to be especially wary of. We also give you lists of do's and don'ts to help combat your IBS symptoms. We present ten key medical tests that you and your doctor should know about to get an accurate diagnosis of IBS. And finally, we offer a chapter chock full of resources you can consult to find out even more about IBS.

Chapter 18

Ten IBS Triggers to Avoid

In This Chapter
▶ Keeping your friendly bacteria happy
▶ Shunning harmful foods
▶ Coping with stress

*I*n Chapter 4, we discuss all sorts of possible triggers for IBS. One of the toughest parts of having IBS is that you can't rely on your doctor, a book, or your best friend to explain why you have symptoms. The answers aren't that clear-cut because everyone with IBS has a different set of triggers. That means you have to spend some time paying attention to your own body in order to sort through the triggers that affect you.

However, certain triggers are more common than others. In this chapter, we present ten of the biggest offenders, along with some pretty powerful ways you can avoid (or at least minimise) them. To find out more information about the topics we discuss here, flip back to Chapter 4.

Apprehending Your Alcohol Intake

Alcohol has important effects on the gastrointestinal tract (where it irritates the delicate layers of cells that line the gut), the liver, the brain, and the rest of the body, so we can make a pretty educated guess about what it does to someone with IBS. Most people can probably drink alcohol in moderation without affecting their IBS. But in larger amounts alcohol may well cause havoc – after all, even people with cast-iron guts find themselves with stirred-up intestines after a night on the tiles.

But how much is too much? Only you know. How sensitive you are to the effects of alcohol and at what level you start to feel unwell may be different for you than other people. You may be thinking, 'But I don't drink that much!

One glass of wine shouldn't be a problem'. Well, if you have IBS and know that you have a sensitive gastrointestinal tract, any amount of alcohol may be too much for you.

One study has found that among women in particular, alcohol can trigger IBS if they consume more than seven units a week of alcohol (that's an average of one drink a day). We also know that most people feel worse when they binge drink – so saving your units up to blow them all on a Saturday night is not a good plan, but one gin and tonic with dinner every night may be okay.

Consider too, that several medications prescribed for gastrointestinal conditions may react unfavourably with alcoholic drinks:

- **Non-steroidal anti-inflammatory drugs (NSAIDs)** such as aspirin that relieve pain cause microscopic bleeding in the stomach. Add alcohol, which directly irritates the cells lining the gastrointestinal tract, to these and you have a double recipe for gastric irritation, bleeding, and stomach ache.

- **Antidepressants** used in modest doses for slowing down bowel movements interact with alcohol, causing drowsiness, lack of concentration, and poor judgement.

- **Metronidazole** is used for gastrointestinal infections and is a very powerful drug that, on its own, can cause stomach upset and cramps, vomiting, headache, sweating, and flushing. Mixed with alcohol, the symptoms are intense, including relentless nausea, vomiting, and headache.

- **Opiates** used for pain control can cause diminished alertness and judgement, as well as reduction in brain function. Alcohol makes these side effects even worse.

Avoiding Antibiotics

Just about everyone takes antibiotics, whether for a serious infection or 'just in case'. Antibiotics have one purpose – to kill bacteria – and they don't discriminate between friend and foe. So whether you take them for a life-threatening illness or just in case your viral flu turns nasty, antibiotics kill off good and bad bacteria. The bad bacteria you can do without, but losing the good bacteria is a concern.

Good bacteria in the gut do a lot of beneficial things, which we discuss in detail in Chapter 2, When antibiotics kill off the good bacteria, the lining of the intestines becomes thin, vulnerable, and more easily penetrated. Some nasty new customers can move in instead and the bowel loses its natural harmony, which may trigger symptoms typical of IBS.

As well as damaging the mucosal epithelium, many antibiotics have the potential to lead to intense and life-threatening diarrhoea. They kill off the good bacteria that keep in check a criminal called *clostridium difficile* (*c. difficile*), which greatly irritates the lining of the intestine, triggering devastating bouts of diarrhoea. These can prove fatal in the weak and vulnerable.

We suggest seeking alternatives to antibiotics, because any amount of antibiotic use has the potential to cause intestinal irritation – or worse. We recognise that sometimes antibiotics are vital to treat bacterial infections, but many common illnesses, including colds, sore throats, ear infections, and stomach upsets, are caused by viruses, which don't respond to antibiotics anyway.

Always get medical advice from your GP when you're ill, unless your symptoms are very mild and recognisable. But be prepared to hear that your problem is viral and doesn't require antibiotics.

When you simply have to take antibiotics, make sure that you take probiotic supplements or eat organic, plain yogurt that contains *lactobacillus acidophilus* and/or *bifidobacteria* to build up your good bacteria and crowd out the bad guys. Take the probiotics two hours apart from the antibiotics. You can find more information on probiotics in Chapter 10.

Ending Erratic Meal Times

Sometimes it's not *what* you eat but *how* or *when* you eat that can save you a lot of aggravation and IBS upset. In particular, the work schedule that you put your bowel through can sometimes make the difference between pain and peace. A sensitive bowel may find it very difficult to cope with unpredictable or inconsistent demands on its machinery.

Every mechanism in the body moves to a natural intrinsic rhythm. These rhythms can adapt to the timetable that we set ourselves, but most are happiest when they're given a regular routine to follow. This means a constant pattern to the size and frequency (and sometimes contents) of the meals we eat. Eating puts the body into a state of major alert, ready to respond to the arrival of fluids and nutrients. If you suddenly wolf down a large cooked meal at 4 a.m. you're likely to find that your gut reacts by churning at great speed in a state of overexcitement (causing diarrhoea and cramps) or comes to a dead halt, simply refusing to budge any further (resulting in constipation and discomfort). In IBS, one mistimed meal can trigger a resurgence of symptoms that lasts for days.

We hope that by now you have a sense of how individual IBS and its management is, so you can see that no ideal meal routine exists for people with IBS. What seems to matter most is consistency: The IBS bowel doesn't like surprises.

Fathoming the Facts about Fibre

Fibre can be one of your great friends when you have IBS, but if you're not careful it can quickly become a formidable enemy. Two main sorts of fibre exist in food – soluble and insoluble. We explain about these different sorts of fibre and which foods contain them in Chapter 10.

As a general principle, you need to view dietary fibre as a scrumptious goodie – something to throw into your meals on a regular basis. But – and we have a few buts for you – you need to treat fibre with a degree of caution, rather like a firework-maker treats explosives. Eating just the right amount of the right fibre at the right time is an art. Not enough and you don't see much action; too much, too fast, and all hell breaks loose. Exactly what the right amount is varies from person to person – we can't tell you how much you need, or how much is too much, because the only way to find out is to test out the effects of fibre on your own body.

When you first start to increase the amount of fibre you consume, go gently. If you rack up your roughage too fast you may find your gut expands at a rapid rate, and excessive gas and bloating quickly make you miserable. Start slowly with small amounts and feel the effects on your gastrointestinal tract before you add more. Take your time: Firework-makers perfect their art over weeks and months – and you need to follow suit!

If you have diarrhoea-predominant IBS, you may be particularly susceptible to the effects of fibre and are more likely to find that it aggravates your symptoms, so go especially carefully. But if you have constipation-predominant IBS, you're likely to appreciate the benefits rapidly, as fibre adds bulk to – and retains moisture in – your stool, making life easier for the intestines. A large soft moist stool is much easier to push along than craggy rocks of the stuff.

The key question is: 'How much is too much fibre?' Between 3 and 10 teaspoons of fibre a day is often recommended in constipation-predominant IBS. But this is too much for some and not enough for others, and may work like dynamite in those with diarrhoea-predominant IBS. It also doesn't give a recipe for the proportions of soluble to insoluble fibre. Some people find insoluble fibre scrapes the delicate mucosa, causing pain and discomfort. Soluble fibre may be a kinder way to increase your fibre levels, although this isn't true for everyone. Only you can find out the magic mix for your bowels. In Appendix A we give a long list of the levels of soluble and insoluble fibre in different foods to help you work out what to eat.

Ferreting Out Fatty Meals

Fried foods soak up too much fat for an IBS stomach to handle and a number of foods such as certain cuts of meat are naturally high in fat, no matter how you prepare them. Biscuits, cookies, and cakes are usually laden with fat too. But the worst fatty food for a sensitive bowel may be ice cream because it has fat, dairy, and sugar all combined in one gooey mess.

Packaged and processed foods that claim to be sugar-free contain hidden fats. Fat-free products tend to be loaded with sugar and sugar-free products tend to be loaded with fat. Without either fat or sugar, food may seem much less palatable or satisfying, especially to a palate that's addicted to junk foods. So manufacturers tend to add one or the other of these to make you enjoy their products and come back for more.

Some people who have trouble digesting fat must go so far as to stop eating meat, egg yolks, and dairy. We encourage you to look at our suggested elimination and challenge diet in Chapter 10, which can help you determine which foods work for you and which don't.

We're not talking about the dangers of cholesterol when we speak of fat aggravating IBS. Instead, the problem is the way fat stimulates the muscles of the intestines to become more active and the various gastrointestinal sphincters to open, propelling intestinal contents at a rate of knots. In a particularly sensitive IBS bowel, the result is powerful cramps and explosive diarrhoea. This very strong reflex is best given only minimal stimulation.

Finding the Foods that Faze You

Food is a huge issue in IBS. The simple act of eating for some people is torture. That's why knowing your food triggers, and avoiding them at all costs, is important. We discuss food triggers in Chapter 4 and an IBS-friendly approach to finding your triggers in Chapter 10. We strongly recommend looking at those chapters for our suggestions.

Our eating habits haven't always been what they are now. Today's diet is a mish-mash of packet foods, pre-cooked meals and fast-food take-aways, packed with synthetic chemicals and ingredients alien to nature. Processed food laced with additives can't compare with fresh, organic home cooking. Your intestines know the difference!

Food upsets can be an *allergy* (where the immune system reacts to the food) an *intolerance* (where the body cannot digest the food properly) or a *sensitivity* (where the food triggers unpleasant symptoms).

Some foods – especially shellfish, nuts, and strawberries – can cause immediate, often severe allergic reactions, such as acute swelling of the neck and face, and breathing problems. But some experts believe that another type of allergic reaction to food exists that takes longer to develop and can produce IBS. As we explain in Chapter 4, the foods that probably cause this type of allergic reaction in the bowel are dairy and wheat.

If you suspect a specific food may be the culprit, you can try our avoidance and challenge diet, which we outline in Chapter 10, to identify your own food allergies. Alternatively, ask your doctor about having blood tests for food allergies.

Some people discover that their IBS is actually an intolerance, particularly to lactose or gluten. These intolerances are real diseases – they occur if you don't make the necessary enzymes to break down and digest the food in question in the small bowel. As a result, the food passes undigested into the colon where bacteria get their teeth into it, breaking it down by fermentation to produce gas, bloating, and symptoms like those of IBS.

You can identify most food intolerances fairly quickly by using an elimination/challenge diet, which we explain in Chapter 10. But medical tests can also help diagnose intolerances. The main test used is called a *hydrogen breath test,* which we describe in Chapter 7.

Food sensitivities are a bit more difficult to track down than allergies or intolerances, but probably account for most food-related symptoms in IBS. Again, we suggest following the avoidance and challenge diet in Chapter 10 to see what you can tolerate. And if you can't tolerate a particular food, try avoiding it altogether.

Handling Hormone Horrors

Women comprise up to 70 per cent of people with IBS, so we have to take a serious look at hormones as a trigger of IBS – and we do just this in Chapter 5. You can't just get rid of your hormones, but knowing that your most vulnerable time is around your menstrual period may help you to plan your life a bit better. It's not great to be reminded that PMS and IBS are going to hit you at the same time but at least it can help you plan your months.

Your IBS symptoms may well reduce when your hormones go into retirement at the menopause. (Plus, of course, PMS is only a bad memory then.) While other women moan about growing older, you can be looking on the bright side of no more IBS.

Losing the Late Nights

We've emphasised how your body needs routine, and suggested that you make a regular time slot for meals (whatever regular may mean to you) an essential part of your schedule. But the body also flourishes with a regular schedule of rest. Here are some that you can do to promote some fabulously restorative shut-eye:

- Avoid large meals late in the day.
- Create a haven of peace with a bedroom environment that offers the right sort of atmosphere, temperature, and noise levels for sleep.
- Eschew hot baths at bedtime.
- Get plenty of exercise earlier in the day.
- Hit the sack at the same sort of time every day.

During sleep, the blood flow to your gut usually drops and the activity of the gut muscles settles down. But if you stay up late, your gut has to stay up too. Without a chance to rest, the enteric nervous system may drive the gut to release digestive juices or churn unnecessarily. Meanwhile, as exhaustion sets in, your sensitive gut becomes even more sensitive and pain thresholds drop so that the spasms and soreness of IBS become even more intense.

Of course, we all need to stay up late now and then: But just be aware that a late night can keep the intestines in a heightened state of action that may have repercussions for days to come.

Stamping Out Stressful Situations

Stress may be the number-one enemy for someone with IBS – it's certainly usually up there among the top three most wanted criminals. Often, you can trace the onset of IBS as a chronic condition to an emotional upset or trauma, like a death in the family or a divorce. In other cases, stress may be the fuel that keeps the symptoms rolling.

We try to make the point throughout this book that stress is not the predominant *cause* of IBS, because we know that IBS is not a psychological condition. But you can see how intertwined IBS and stress really are. When you have a sensitive gut and add on stressful events, you can really escalate your symptoms.

The first step to avoiding stressful situations is to recognise how stress makes you feel and then ask yourself what situations usually bring these feelings or symptoms on. Make a list and ask yourself:

- ✔ How does stress affect me – do I feel angry, bothered, shaky, tired, upset, weepy, or suddenly at the mercy of my IBS?
- ✔ When do stress symptoms appear?
- ✔ What sort of situations do I dread, knowing that they aggravate my IBS?
- ✔ Do events at work or particular social events bring on symptoms?
- ✔ How do family or friends react when I'm unwell at certain occasions – do they understand and support me?

Then take a long hard look at your list of stressful situations and divide them into three categories: Those situations that you can avoid, those that you must face, and those that you can approach differently to reduce the stress involved. Try to think about how you can apply the techniques and strategies we provide in this book to reduce the stress that you face in these different situations.

Trying Not to Do Too Much

Whichever way you look at it, or experience it, trying to do too much can aggravate a sensitive bowel. Try to keep some space and time for calm quietness in your life. Maybe you can put your feet up for 20 minutes every lunch time and take stock. Be as positive as possible about what you've got done in the morning and convince yourself that you deserve a period of tranquility to calm your digestive system. Look at your life and prioritise what's important, while rejecting activities that waste your time and drain your energy.

If you want to slow down then you may want to research what has become known as 'The Slow Movement' on the Internet, to find out more about how you can get a better pace to your life. The Slow Movement doesn't abandon all the things that modern life has to offer but instead uses modern technology and knowledge to re-establish some of the best features of old-fashioned community life. Check out www.slowmovement.com to find out more.

Chapter 19

Ten Things to Do for Your IBS

In This Chapter

▶ Being responsible for your body and attitude

▶ Changing your eating and exercise habits

▶ Taking control of stress

*I*f you've read even just a couple chapters of this book, you probably realise that we feel diet and lifestyle are the most important aspects of treating IBS. Although IBS has been known for centuries, albeit under a different name (it was called mucous colitis during the 19th century and spastic colitis for much of the 20th century), the condition seems to have become much more prevalent in modern times. So what has happened in our society during the past few decades that is twisting up our intestines?

We say this change has something to do with a combination of bad diet, too much processed food, lack of exercise, and a massive accumulation of stress with no outlet.

We suggest lots of tools in this book to help address all these issues. In this chapter, we offer a handy summary.

Cutting Back on Medications

Natural dietary supplements often have labels that guarantee they don't contain sugar, wheat, corn, or dairy. However, drug companies don't seem to take into consideration the possibility of food sensitivities when they make their products.

That's one reason to cut back on medications. Another reason is the toxicity of many drugs, which can make them inherently irritating to the intestines or a cause of other bothersome side effects that can aggravate your problems. The *non-steroidal anti-inflammatory drugs* (NSAIDs), for example, that we often take for aches and pains, can cause so much gastrointestinal irritation that their major side effect is gastrointestinal bleeding. Most people are advised to take a type of drug called an H2-blocker which reduces stomach acid production (and so protects against irritation and bleeding) when they have to take NSAIDs regularly. Even the weaker NSAIDs that you can buy in your local pharmacy, such as aspirin and ibuprofen, can irritate your gut and cause small amounts of stomach and intestinal bleeding.

To find out whether a medication you take causes gastrointestinal irritation, chat to your pharmacist or GP. But if you take a prescription medication, don't stop taking it without going to see your doctor armed with information on side effects and talking it through.

Developing Regular Habits

Rest, food, and relaxation programmed into a reliable schedule help to protect you from exhaustion, hunger, and the stress of overwork. Of course, every day throws different challenges at us, so following a rigid routine is hard. Variety is definitely one of the spices of life: Some people are happy working shifts, grabbing food when they can, and spending all hours of the day at the office. But most people with IBS aren't.

If your meal times are erratic, hunger may sneak up on you, leaving you feeling irritable and likely to reach out quickly for a snack that may not be the best food for your intestines. Your body may also not cope well with unpredictable sleeping habits – late nights, unusually early mornings, or just a lack of adequate rest faze most people, so it's hardly surprising that these are famous aggravating factors in IBS.

Work on developing a fairly solid structure to your daily life:

- ✔ **Stick to a good sleep routine:** Listen to your body, not the TV schedule, when deciding what sort of bed-time suits you.

- ✔ **Schedule regular meals:** Regular hours and regular food can help your bowels to settle into regular habits. Get back to the good old-fashioned habit of proper meals. Make at least one meal each day a leisurely affair sitting at a table (rather than wolfing something down en route to work or balancing supper on your knees).

- ✔ **De-stress:** Finally schedule some serious down-time into your routine – find an activity you enjoy, whether reading, playing rock guitar or dancing the cha-cha and take a daily dose to counteract stress.

Eating a Healthy Diet

Call it a top ten list within a top ten list; following are ten good diet habits to follow for eliminating IBS (Chapter 10 is packed with details of all these tips):

- ✔ **Drink herbal teas.** Peppermint and chamomile are great choices.

- ✔ **Eat whole grains.** Quinoa, rice, corn, and barley are the best because they have the most soluble fibre.

- ✔ **Feast on fresh veg.** Avocados, beetroot, carrots, chestnuts, parsnips, potatoes, squash, sweet potatoes, turnips, and yams are ideal because of their soluble fibre content.

- ✔ **Focus on soluble fibre.** You find it in rice, pasta, sourdough bread, sweet potatoes, potatoes, parsnips, apple sauce, bananas, and papayas.

- ✔ **Keep an eye on what you eat:** Fill out a food diary to compare the contents of your meals with the appearance of symptoms, or go on an elimination and challenge diet, to pinpoint your food triggers.

- ✔ **Pick probiotic foods that contain 'live' healthy bacteria.** The beneficial bacteria in probiotic foods such as yogurt, for example, is very valuable for your gut.

- ✔ **Keep blood sugar levels constant.** Try to avoid wild fluctuations in the levels of sugar circulating around your body by avoiding sweet snacks and including plenty of slow burn carbohydrates in your meals.

- ✔ **Steer clear of spicy food.** For some people, spicy food is a distinct intestinal irritant.

- ✔ **Take care with fruit.** Some people with IBS find the natural sugars in fruit are a problem. Check which fruits suit you or stick to apples and pears, and only one or two a day.

- ✔ **Wolf down lots of water, especially if you are eating high-fibre foods.** Whether you have diarrhoea or constipation, you need lots of water.

Exercising Every Day

Exercise is one of the most powerful medicines known to science – it has dozens of benefits, its free and its available (in some form or other) to everyone. Exercise is particular beneficial in IBS because it helps in several ways. For example, regular activity of the muscles seems to stimulate the gut into more consistent action, reducing spasms and improving constipation. Exercise is also a great stress-buster, lowering tension and raising the threshold at which pain becomes a problem.

The problem with exercise is that you have to do it regularly and it's not like housework, which you can pay someone to do. We all know we should exercise, but it's usually the last thing on our 'to do' list.

Start small. Breathing – yes, simply breathing – can be good exercise. Taking three deep breaths is the way most relaxation programmes start, and taking lots of deep breaths is common in most forms of exercise. After you've taken some breaths, consider these simple options:

- ✔ Take a short walk around the block and enjoy yourself.
- ✔ Put on some upbeat music and dance around the house (and enjoy yourself even more).

When you get your blood moving and your muscles singing, you begin to feel the benefits within a short time. We suggest several forms of exercise in Chapter 11, but it doesn't matter what you do as long as you get moving. Thirty minutes daily does the trick.

Joining or Starting a Support Group

Try joining an existing support group if you find one that suits your needs. But if none is available, start your own. The IBS Network (www.thegutt rust.org) can offer you lots of help and advice to do this.

Start small. Maybe your first support group consists of your partner, your best friend, someone from work, and your sibling. But as you spread the word, more people with IBS and their support people join. If an invasion of your home is too much to contemplate, you can join or start an online IBS support group instead, which we discuss in Chapters 14 and 17.

Whether live or virtual, everyone needs to chat to someone who listens. But you have to start with a set of rules. If you just want to be listened to and don't want advice, make that clear from the beginning, or you may get inundated with advice that you may not want. Some of it may strike pay dirt, but often it's distracting if you just want to complain a bit and then move on.

Listening to Your Body and Taking Charge

We can't stress enough that IBS is a medical condition that's under *your* guidance and control. The more you listen to your own body the greater understanding you will develop about your condition, and how the way you live your life improves or aggravates your personal symptoms. IBS is highly individual and what your body is saying to you (maybe 'don't give me curries, they upset my intestines' or 'please give me more rest, I'm too tired to cope any more') may not be relevant to someone else with IBS.

The more information you have, the better you can take care of yourself. IBS is a condition that you experience and you manage; it does not necessarily require ongoing intervention by a doctor. (We discuss where your doctor fits into the picture in the section 'Working with a Doctor You Can Talk to', later in this chapter.)

Your doctor may not have the time to explain to you the elimination and challenge diet that we cover in Chapter 10, which is key to finding out what's triggering your sensitive gut. Your doctor may also not know about the value of yoga (head to Chapter 11 for the low-down on yoga and other exercise), or using herbal treatments, which we discuss in Chapter 10. Neither can your doctor be there with you every day when you choose what foods to eat. Only *you* can make those good food choices and lifestyle decisions.

Planning Your Next Move

When you have a condition like IBS, taking charge of it requires planning – lots and lots of planning. You have to plan where you are going and how you are going to get there without having an accident. You may need to plan what to eat when you go out, such as taking your own healthy snacks with you so that you don't end up eating something that your tummy can't handle. And you may learn the hard way not to eat bad foods before an important event but to save any favourite but troublesome foods for a peaceful night in, close to your bathroom.

We're not saying that all this planning ever becomes easy. In fact, this kind of organisation is one of the hardest things to do. When you leave home, you are not really thinking of your next meal or your next trip to the toilet: You aren't hungry, stressed or aware that your bowels will at some point need to open, so it's just not a priority. However, in a couple of hours you could find yourself starving hungry in the middle of a shopping centre and the only restaurants to choose from serve everything fried in gallons of grease.

Planning and preparation is the only way to keep things running smoothly and cope with the sort of problems that life constantly throws up which could make your IBS worse. Always visit the toilet before setting out, whether or not you think you need to go, check out in advance where the likely pit-stops are going to be, and always carry a healthy snack with you.

Releasing Your Anger

Throughout this book, we discuss the complex relationship between stress and IBS. The simple take-home point is that stress is bad for IBS, and you need to avoid it as far as possible. But how? Well, one way is to work on not letting yourself get worked up when bad things happen. Believe it or not, you can avoid getting angry. Here are some suggestions:

- ✔ Count to ten when you feel the steam rising – before it drops down into your gut.
- ✔ Take several deep breaths, and visualise feeling calm and peaceful inside.
- ✔ Practise singing the speech you have stored up for your boss, spouse, or child. Even if you don't get to deliver it to the intended recipient, we guarantee singing it makes you laugh and break through the cloud of anger.

If your anger is a consistent problem, try to find out why. Get a diary and write out the reasons. Here are some possibilities:

- ✔ I'm really angry that I'm stuck with a chronic disease.
- ✔ I'm even more angry that doctors can't help me.
- ✔ I'm frustrated that I have a disease with no cure.
- ✔ I'm livid that I have no control over my life, and my bowel is in control.
- ✔ It really bugs me that other people seem to live such a carefree life and I have to dance around my sensitivities.
- ✔ I'm really mad that I can't eat what I want, go out when I want, and party like most people my age.

If anger is a problem for you, write down what's bugging you and get it off your chest and off your gut. In the bright light of day, when these irritants are written down in black and white, you can slowly resolve some of them.

But if your anger is related to specific areas of your life, such as your job or a relationship, it may be worth talking to your doctor or other relevant people (such as your line manager at work or the relationship counselling service Relate www.relate.org.uk; Tel: 08451 30 40 16) about getting particular help to look into the causes more closely.

Weeding Out Worry

If you're a worrier, write down the reasons why. You can then prioritise them, to help you focus on what your main concerns are and how you can go about addressing them. The list may start with all your fears about your IBS:

✔ Will I ever be normal?

✔ Will there ever be a cure?

✔ Will I get worse?

✔ What if I have cancer and not IBS?

✔ What if I have Crohn's disease or ulcerative colitis and not IBS?

These are all perfectly acceptable worries to have, but worrying about them won't do your health any good. Instead, the stress of worrying makes your symptoms even worse.

Psychologists often say that you attract what's uppermost in your mind. So if you spend a lot of time worrying about something, you may be giving your body the impression that you are asking for that thing that you fear – and *voilà*, you have it! No, life is not always that simple. But the adage that you are living what you are thinking holds plenty of truth:

✔ Think positive thoughts and you can live a more positive life.

✔ Think negative thoughts and you can live under a dark cloud.

People with some of the worst health conditions sometimes manage to see their ordeal as a challenge, and they often say later that they wouldn't be who they are today if they hadn't gone through all that suffering and pain. These people are the inspiration you need when you face IBS. You have a chronic condition, and many people share the same symptoms and the same agonies that you do. Many of them get through the adventure and become better people.

The tools we present in Chapter 12 to reduce stress, such as meditation, the relaxation response, and deep breathing, all work equally well on worry. But just as with exercise, you have to practise them to get the benefits. Here are some de-stressing exercises to try:

✔ **Counting to ten:** This is a time-out tool that you can use whenever you feel your anxiety and tension levels rising. Counting is also a great tool to use if you think your tension is going to make you blow up at someone.

✔ **Laughing therapy:** This therapy is very easy to practise. When you rent films, get comedies. When you read, stick to the funny stuff. The endorphins produced when you laugh are actually therapeutic.

✔ **Meditating:** Something as simple as closing your eyes and counting your breaths can sometimes be enough to drop your anxiety levels. Your heart rate drops, your breathing rate slows down, and the tension in your body eases. Or try more formal mediation techniques.

Working with a Doctor You Can Talk To

Finding a caring doctor is just the start. For best results you need a doctor who you feel you can talk to, and who listens to what you have to say. Ideally your doctor is knowledgeable about IBS, but as long as you have a good relationship you may be able to explore new information together. To rule out inflammatory bowel disease (IBD) and other masquerading conditions, to diagnose IBS, and to identify the possible causes and triggers of your symptoms, you need a doctor who knows what tests to conduct for IBS (which we discuss in Chapter 7) and how to apply them to your case.

We think of your relationship with your doctor as a partnership. Your doctor has gone to medical school and done years of training, spending up to a decade learning about the human body. However, you have had a lifetime of experience with your own body. Your doctor needs to listen to your specific symptoms and concerns. Then, together, you can decide what's best for you.

IBS is not a defined disease with a clear-cut treatment protocol like a wound that needs to be stitched up and bandaged. IBS is a condition that affects every individual differently. Treating it properly with diet, exercise, stress management techniques, and a good attitude is a recipe for success, but it's a recipe that must be adapted in every case.

Chapter 20

Ten Ways to Get Help for Your IBS

In This Chapter
▶ Getting general information and support
▶ Finding resources to improve your lifestyle
▶ Investigating various therapies

A lot of help and information exists for people who have IBS. But sometimes finding that help and info can be a problem. Plenty of people also share your troubles and can support you through them, but again the difficulty may be spotting exactly who those angels are. The person sitting at the desk next to yours at work may know exactly what you are going through because they or their partner also have IBS. But if either of you are rather shy or embarrassed about the condition, you may never discuss IBS together and therefore not know that you have an ally just metres away.

In this chapter we provide pointers to the many free resources available to people who have IBS, from Web sites to local groups and worldwide connections. These resources can give you more information about your condition and allow you to share everything from recipes to companionship with people who know all about IBS.

We hope that you find these resources useful, but we want to be clear that our goal is to provide information – not endorsements. We encourage you to be discerning. A lot of information is available about IBS, especially on the Web. Carefully consider each piece of information or offer of help that you gather. And keep in mind that the information you get from these sources is not meant to be a substitute for a consultation with an appropriate medical professional.

Joining an IBS Organisation

Joining an organisation can bring you lots of benefits, from up-to-date info to opportunities to find out about, or even put questions to, experts in the field, hear about new ideas on triggers or treatments, and talk to other people similarly affected.

A number of organisations have an interest in IBS, either specifically or as part of a general coverage of gastrointestinal (GI) disorders. Only one or two are British, but don't let country borders hold you back in these days of the global information highway. You may discover, for example, that joining an American organisation brings a new perspective and some interesting contacts.

Here are some organisations to try:

- ✔ **American Gastroenterological Association (AGA)** (www.gastro.org) is dedicated to advancing the science and practice of gastroenterology. Although mostly for doctors, nurses and research scientists, it hosts a very useful "Patient Center" on its website, full of information.

- ✔ **British Society of Gastroenterology** (www.bsg.org.uk) is the professional organisation that represents and educates gastroenterology doctors. It has some limited information for people with IBS.

- ✔ **Canadian Society of Intestinal Research** (www.badgut.com) works to increase public awareness and understanding of GI disease as well as funding research.

- ✔ **CORE** (www.corecharity.org.uk) is the working name of the Digestive Disorders Foundation. The Web site has information on many GI conditions.

- ✔ **Gut Trust** (www.theguttrust.org) is the business name of the IBS Network, a UK national charity offering advice, information and support.

- ✔ **International Foundation for Functional Gastrointestinal Disorders** (www.iffgd.org) is a non-profit organisation dedicated to informing and supporting people affected by GI disorders, including IBS.

- ✔ **Irritable Bowel Syndrome Association** (www.ibsassociation.org) is a major US organisation for people with IBS, providing information and support groups.

- ✔ **Irritable Bowel Syndrome (IBS) Self Help and Support Group** (www.ibsgroup.org) claims to be the largest online patient advocate and support community for people with IBS. With blogs, forums, and pen-pals, it can put you in touch with other people who have IBS around the world.

Looking for Local Groups

Despite the wonders (and undeniable advantages) of e-mail, texting, chat rooms, online forums, and all those other ways to talk to people without making eye contact with them, most humans enjoy meeting real flesh and blood people and swapping notes and anecdotes on their IBS over a cup of tea or glass of beer.

Getting together in a local group is also a good way to explore facilities in your area for people with IBS. You may find out about shops that give you instant access to their staff toilet, restaurants with tasty food that isn't packed with ingredients you can't eat, or services at the local hospital. The group can also warn you about the local IBS black spots, where toilet services are limited or food is likely to upset your sensitive gut.

So how can you find a local IBS group, short of standing in the middle of the high street with a placard around your tum?

- ✔ Contact the IBS Network (`www.theguttrust.org`) and ask about your nearest group. At the moment they run only a few groups around the country, but the IBS Network wants to see a group in every major town and city in the UK. To meet this aim they will help new members of the IBS Network set up their own local group if necessary, and provide ongoing support.

- ✔ Ask your GP or practice nurse if they know of a local IBS or GI patient group.

- ✔ Visit your local library or Citizens Advice Bureau – they often stock info on local action/health groups.

- ✔ Chat to the PALS (Patient Advice and Liaison Service) staff in your local hospital about IBS or other GI disease groups. Just ring the hospital switchboard and ask for PALS. (Some hospitals give this service a completely different name, so be prepared to explain what you are looking for.)

- ✔ Inquire at the gastroenterology department at any large hospital (you don't have to tell them that you are not a patient of theirs). The consultants, nurses and possibly the secretary may have details.

Making Web Connections

When we did an Internet search for the term 'irritable bowel syndrome', we got more than one and a half million hits! We certainly didn't visit all those sites, and we don't suggest that you do. But you may like to get familiar with some of them, listen in to the buzz about IBS on the Net, and start to get a picture of how it affects people all over the world. In this section, we suggest some general IBS-related sites that you may find provide useful information, motivation, and support:

- ✔ **Bowel Control** (`www.bowelcontrol.org.uk`) provides information and support for people with faecal incontinence, from a gastroenterology consultant at St Marks, the UK specialist GI hospital.

✔ **IBS Tales** (www.ibstales.com) is an archive of personal tales from people with IBS, as well as other information on the condition. The site is run by a woman in the UK who has IBS.

✔ **National Institute of Diabetes and Digestive and Kidney Diseases (NIDDK)** (digestive.niddk.nih.gov) is part of the National Institutes of Health (NIH) in the USA, and has basic information about various digestive disorders and diseases, including IBS.

If you want to read up on the latest science on IBS, and you are prepared to get to grips with the jargon, try searching at some of the top journals or even at PubMed – a collection of *abstracts* (or summaries) of almost all the published reports on medical and scientific topics, provided by the National Library of Medicine and the National Institutes of Health in the USA.

Most journals offer only limited information for free and charge a lot of money to access a full report or research paper. Check with your local library or the British Library first – they may be able to get you the information cheaper. These journals can be useful

✔ **BMJ Clinical Evidence** (www.clinicalevidence.com) is the Web site of a branch of the *British Medical Journal.* It gives an excellent overview of the published evidence on which treatments do or don't work.

✔ **British Medical Journal** (www.bmj.com) is the leading medical publication in the UK. Published every week it contains a wide variety of articles on the clinical, scientific, social, political, and economic factors affecting health.

✔ **GastroHep** (www.gastrohep.com) is an online resource for all things gastroenterological.

✔ **Gut** (gut.bmj.com) is a specialist journal on GI disease from the *British Medical Journal* group.

✔ The **Lancet** (www.thelancet.com) claims to be the world's leading independent medical journal. Its coverage is international in focus and it extends to all aspects of human health.

✔ The *New England Journal of Medicine* (content.nejm.org) is a weekly general medical journal published in the USA that covers new medical research findings, review articles, and editorial opinion on a wide variety of medical topics.

✔ **Pub Med** (www.ncbi.nlm.nih.gov/sites/entrez?db=pubmed)

Signing up to a Mailing List Server

By joining a mailing list server, you can receive e-mails from people who are also dealing with IBS. Such lists give people opportunities to communicate about their illness and to offer moral support, tips, and remedies to each other.

The Yahoo! Web site is host to several e-mail lists that discuss IBS. Each list is owned or moderated by a different group or individual, and each has a different focus. Some are general discussions about IBS and others are limited to discussions about medicines for IBS. Following are some examples:

- **Careplace Irritable Bowel Syndrome Community** (`www.careplace.com/land/Irritable_Bowel_Syndrome/dhgd`) is an online community where people share information on different health topics.

- **IBS Patient Action Group** (`health.groups.yahoo.com/group/ibspag`) has more than 250 members and is dedicated to discussion about medication and social issues related to IBS.

- **Irritable Bowel Syndrome** (`health.groups.yahoo.com/group/irritable_bowel_syndrome`) is a general list with more than 500 members.

Informing Your Family

The people most able to understand you and your needs, and offer the sort of help you are looking for, are often right there under your nose – your family. But they may be blithely unaware of the daily struggle you have with IBS.

People frequently do a surprisingly good job of covering up their symptoms, keeping the burden of pain and a disruptive bowel to themselves, and putting on a display of coping because they worry about being a burden to their loved ones. But in order to understand your needs, your family need to hear it straight. They need to have a good picture of how your IBS affects you and the particular problems you have.

IBS is not the sort of topic that you can just blurt out over the roast on Sunday, so chose your moment carefully. You may start by leaving this book lying around – it won't take long before someone picks the book up and wonders who has left it there. You may even want to leave some coloured highlighter tape sticking out from the most relevant pages of the book.

But you may find it easier to explain face to face that IBS is giving you strife. Find a quiet time when you feel relaxed with your family. You may want to prepare beforehand by gathering together some information on IBS, and thinking about specific ways your family can help. You can make it easier for your loved ones by explaining simple things that will make life better for you, and how these things will make a difference – maybe changes in the family routine, or help with some of the domestic chores, for example. You may want to talk to different family members separately, or ask one member who understands best to explain to the others.

However you tackle it, your life will doubtlessly be better after your nearest and dearest are onboard with your mission to tackle your IBS.

Growing Your Own Support Network

A network, like a net, can catch you when you fall. We all need a support network, because we all have bad times that knock us down. But when you have a chronic condition like IBS, you may need a support network more than most.

Don't panic if you can't dredge up a dozen friends at the drop of a hat. What is important is not the size of your social circle but how reliable and trustworthy you think any one of your friends is. A network is ideal but one strong link is pretty good to hang on to.

Try to aim to have one person that you can lean on in each of the various different areas of your life – at home, among friends, at work, at school or college, in the pub or your local coffee shop, at the gym, or wherever else you hang out. Pick someone who understands. Knowing that wherever you are you have at least one ally can help to relieve the stress of IBS.

You may want to keep a special 'IBS address book' with names and numbers of those people who you can turn to if necessary. Add lists of professionals and places (such as shops and, of course, toilets) that may be helpful if your IBS flares up – therapists, doctors, and emergency services. Sketch out a map of your network – literally a map of the area you live – and plot lots of x's to mark the spots where you can find help. Look for gaps that need plugging – bleak spots where those with IBS dare not tread.

Unearthing Exercise Resources

As we discuss in Chapter 11, any exercise is good exercise, bringing a range of beneficial effects to help common IBS symptoms and also improving your general sense of wellbeing. So get your kit on and get out there! If you're not sure what sport is for you, take a look at the info and links at the Sport England website http://www.sportengland.org/.

In particular, certain types of exercise are helpful when you have IBS:

- **Pilates:** A great way to give your body a good all-round workout, Pilates improves your strength, flexibility, and balance. The Pilates Foundation (www.pilatesfoundation.com) has basic information on this form of exercise and details of where to find teachers and classes.

- ✔ **Pumping iron:** Most gyms have a range of good modern machinery to help you tone up specific areas of the body (such as building abdominal strength and tone to help control IBS symptoms such as bloating), as well as cardiovascular workout machines and a variety of exercise classes. Companies such as Cannons (www.cannons.co.uk) Virgin Active (www.virginactive.co.uk) LA Fitness (www.lafitness.co.uk) and David Lloyd (www.davidlloydleisure.co.uk) have gyms across the country, so go and road-test a few.

- ✔ **Swimming:** Power down the lanes for a good burn-up if you want to, but slow, gentle strokes are a great way to work those core abdominal muscles to help them control the bloating and distension of IBS. The British Swimming and Amateur Swimming Association (www.british swimming.org) have lots of information on the sport including details of local clubs.

- ✔ **Yoga:** Yoga can help IBS in many ways, from defusing stress to stretching out an abdomen tensed up by intestinal cramps. Yoga can also help alleviate conditions such as PMS and menstrual cramps, which are often worse when IBS is raging. Yoga Basics (www.yogabasics.com) is a great site to explore, while Yoga Journal (www.yogajournal.com) contains a lot of free and well-explained information for yoga beginners.

Stamping Out Stress Relief

The connection between IBS and stress is intricate and sometimes frustrating. If you experience stress, you can aggravate your IBS. But just having IBS increases your stress! That cycle is reason enough to check out these resources:

- ✔ **Stress Management.co.uk** (www.stressmanagement.co.uk) offers information and ideas on how to tackle stress and anxiety, and you can put questions to an expert.

- ✔ **Richard Ebbs Web Site** (www.feedback.nildram.co.uk/richard ebbs) has a useful section on meditation techniques from around the world.

- ✔ **Learning Meditation** (www.learningmeditation.com) offers simple guidance through techniques which will help you to relax and deal with daily stresses.

- ✔ **Massage Therapy UK** (www.massagetherapy.co.uk) is a Web site dedicated to massage, a great way to de-stress. The site is packed with information and descriptions of the main massage and holistic associated therapies, as well as a long list of massage therapists.

✔ **British Association of Therapeutical Hypnotists** (www.bathh.co.uk) provides basic information on Therapeutic Hypnotherapy and a list of therapists who are members of the association.

✔ **British Society of Clinical Hypnosis (BSCH)** (www.bsch.org.uk) is another professional body that aims to promote and assure high standards in the profession of hypnotherapy. The site provides a list of therapists and more info.

✔ **Hypnotherapy Association** (www.thehypnotherapyassociation. co.uk) is a British non-profit making independent professional body representing approved hypnotherapists in active practice. It offers information and details of therapists.

✔ **IBS Audio Program 100** (www.ibsaudioprogram.com) offers self-hypnosis tapes that may help you to reduce your IBS symptoms.

✔ **National Council for Hypnotherapy** (www.hypnotherapists.org.uk) is the professional body for therapists. The Web site has a list of practitioners.

Discovering Diet Data

As we stress throughout the book, what you eat makes a huge difference in how you feel when you have IBS. You may find that your doctor's surgery can refer you to a dietician for advice. Alternatively, the following Web sites cover the sort of dietary advice we offer, especially in Chapter 10:

✔ **Dieticians Unlimited** (www.dieticiansunlimited.co.uk) can supply a list of registered dieticians who work independently and provide nutrition and dietetic advice.

✔ **Foodreactions.org** (www.foodreactions.org) aims to simplify info on health problems related to the food we eat.

✔ **Help for IBS.com** (www.helpforibs.com) has some useful ideas about diet and IBS, and gives you the chance to exchange tips about diet with other people who have IBS through a message board. The site is run by an American woman with IBS. Beware – this commercial site flogs a variety of dietary therapies and supplements that are not proven to work, and you may find cheaper, simpler alternatives.

✔ **IBS Research Update** (www.ibs-research-update.org.uk) is the Web site of the IBS Research Appeal, a charitable research programme run by doctors and other health professionals who treat people with IBS on a daily basis at their clinic at the Central Middlesex Hospital in London. The site offers some very sound advice on diet.

- **UK Foods Standards Agency** (www.food.gov.uk/healthiereating) has heaps of information on all sorts of aspects of the food we eat, from labelling and packaging to GM foods. The agency's separate site at www.eatwell.gov.uk has advice on making healthy choices for your diet, including info about food allergies and intolerance.

- **Yeast Connection** (www.yeastconnection.com) can show you how to eliminate yeast from your diet. Most doctors don't believe in the theory that the yeast candida plays an important part in IBS, but if you do then this site offers a diet programme.

Taking Note from Other Diseases

Throughout the UK millions of people live with a chronic condition, whether arthritis, diabetes, high blood pressure, or IBS. People with these conditions share some common issues: They may have problems accessing the information they need, communicating with health professionals, getting on top of the stress that their condition brings, or understanding the implications for employment or benefits.

By looking at how people with other conditions manage, you may be able to develop valuable skills and find out how to cope better. Some conditions bring very similar issues to IBS, and we provide Web links for these conditions below.

But your first stop may be the Expert Patients Programme (EPP). This training programme was set up in 2002 by the NHS to help people who live with a long-term chronic condition develop new skills to manage their condition better on a day-to-day basis. See Chapter 9 for more detail on the EPP, and visit their Web site at www.expertpatients.co.uk.

Information on other diseases and conditions with symptoms or issues especially similar to IBS can be found at the Web sites explored in the following sections.

- **Coeliac Disease:** Coeliac UK (www.coeliac.co.uk) has general information about coeliac disease, as well as recipes, books, and gluten-free product listings.

- **Colitis and Crohn's Disease:** The National Association for Colitis and Crohn's Disease (NACC; Web site at www.nacc.org.uk) has support groups, information, experts' comments – in fact, everything you need on inflammatory bowel disease.

- **Lactose intolerance:** Food Reactions (www.foodreactions.co.uk) is a Web site run by a UK medical laboratory technologist, and includes information on lactose intolerance. Lactofree (www.lactofree.co.uk) contains everything you need to know about lactose intolerance, albeit from a commercial Web site run by manufacturers of lactose-free milk.

Part VI
Appendixes

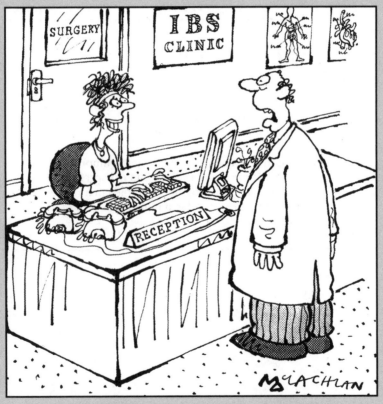

'My full name, and no jokes please,
is Ian Brian Smith.'

In this part . . .

*N*othing to do with the bit that sticks out of your large intestine, we promise. Instead, these appendixes are a couple of useful ready-reference aids which help you with the details of a complex subject.

The first appendix is a chart comparing the amounts of soluble fibre (which you want to eat lots of) and insoluble fibre (which you may want to limit or avoid) in a range of common foods. The second is a handy glossary of IBS-related terms.

Appendix A

Soluble and Insoluble Fibre Chart

● ●

*A*s we note in several chapters, particularly Chapter 10, increasing your intake of fibre (especially soluble fibre) can help alleviate symptoms of both diarrhoea and constipation. The following chart, based on a table produced by the US Department of Agriculture, helps you compare sources of soluble and insoluble fibre.

Food	Soluble Fibre (Grams Per 100 Grams)	Insoluble Fibre (Grams Per 100 Grams)
Bread, white, soft	1.26	2.13
Bread, white, firm	1.56	4.63
Bread, wholemeal, soft	1.26	4.76
Bread, wholemeal, firm	1.51	5.21
Tortilla, corn	1.11	4.39
Tortilla, flour (wheat)	1.51	0.85
Brown rice, long grain, cooked	0.44	2.89
Oatmeal, cooked	0.42	1.23
Pasta, cooked	0.54	1.33
White rice, long grain, cooked	0	0.34
Apple, raw, ripe, with skin	0.67	1.54
Avocado, raw, ripe	2.03	3.51
Banana, raw, ripe	0.58	1.21
Grapefruit, raw, white, ripe	0.58	0.32
Grapes, raw, ripe	0.24	0.36
Mango, raw, ripe	0.69	1.08
Oranges, raw, ripe	1.37	0.99

(continued)

Food	Soluble Fibre (Grams Per 100 Grams)	Insoluble Fibre (Grams Per 100 Grams)
Pears, raw, ripe, with skin	0.92	2.25
Pineapple, raw, ripe	0.04	1.42
Prunes, pitted	4.50	3.63
Raisins, seedless	0.90	2.17
Watermelon, raw, ripe	0.13	0.27
Chick peas, canned, drained	0.41	5.79
Lentils, dry, cooked, drained	0.44	5.42
Pinto beans, canned, drained	0.99	5.66
Red kidney beans, canned, drained	1.36	5.77
Split peas, dry, cooked, drained	0.09	10.56
Beans, green, fresh	1.38	2.93
Broccoli, fresh, cooked	1.85	2.81
Carrots, fresh, cooked	1.58	2.29
Corn on the cob, fresh	0.25	2.63
Peas, frozen	0.94	2.61
Potato, white, baked, with skin	0.61	1.70
Broccoli	0.44	3.06
Carrots, raw	0.49	2.39
Cucumber, raw, with skin	0.20	0.94
Tomatoes, red, ripe, raw	0.15	1.19
Spinach	0.77	2.43

Appendix B

Glossary

• •

*A*bdomen: The part of your body that extends from below your lungs in the chest to the top of your hips and pubic bone. The contents of the abdominal cavity are the stomach, liver, gallbladder, spleen, pancreas, small intestine, appendix, and large intestine.

Abdominal pain and abdominal spasm: A common component of IBS. Intestines stretched by gas or constipation can produce excruciating pain. However, not all abdominal pain is due to IBS.

Allergy: A reaction by the immune system against foreign substances, which may be any food or chemical that we ingest, inhale, or come into contact with.

Anaemia: The most common abnormal condition of the blood. It means that you don't have enough red blood cells or haemoglobin in your blood.

Anal fissure: A small tear or cut in the surface lining of the anal canal that can cause pain and/or bleeding, especially when you pass faeces (or stool) during a bowel movement.

Anal fistula: A tiny channel or tract that can develop in the presence of inflammation and infection. Fistulae are a common symptom of Crohn's disease, but not a feature of IBS.

Anus: Where faeces comes out – the final exit point of intestinal contents that's commonly referred to as the back passage. Faecal matter builds up in the rectum before the anal sphincter muscle relaxes, allowing elimination through the anus.

Appendix: An 8–10 centimetre long narrow tissue sac attached to the caecum. Some scientists suggest that the original function of the appendix was to break down seeds and other hard plant materials (it does this in animals such as rabbits), but as humans have evolved the appendix has become redundant, and just a cause of trouble if it becomes inflamed.

Ascending colon: The first section of the large intestine, located on the right side of the abdomen.

Aspartame: A low-calorie sweetener, also known by its trade name Nutra-Sweet and listed on food labels as E951. Aspartame is used in a variety of foods and drinks and is about 200 times sweeter than sugar.

Barium: A chalky liquid that coats the inside of the gastrointestinal tract when swallowed or used in an enema. Because it shows up on X-rays as a white shadow, barium can be used to check the gastrointestinal tract for abnormalities.

Bloating: A sensation of fullness or expansion of the abdomen, usually due to the build up of gas in the intestines. Bloating causes increased pressure and pain within the sensitive bowel. For fear of passing stool along with gas, some people with IBS are reluctant to allow the gas to escape through the anus, which may cause a worsening of symptoms.

Borborygmi: Gurgling and rumbling sounds caused by gas moving through the intestines. The name (pronounced *BOR-boh-RIG-mee*) almost sounds like what it describes, and is a much more aesthetic name than stomach rumbling or growling.

Bowel: A general term for the small intestine and the large intestine – two hollow tubes in the abdominal cavity through which food passes.

Bowel incontinence: The inability to control defecation, also called faecal incontinence. When control of the anal sphincters is lost, faeces escapes from the rectum and anus.

Bowel movement: The passage of waste matter from the process of digestion through the large intestine and out through the rectum and anus.

CA-125 test: A blood test designed to detect an elevated level of a protein antigen called *CA-125*, which may indicate ovarian cancer, among other disorders. It may be an important test in the investigation of IBS in women because it can rule out ovarian cancer, which also causes symptoms of abdominal pain and bloating.

Caecum: The area of the intestines where the small intestine and large intestine meet.

Candida albicans: A yeast that can infect the mucus membranes of the mouth or vagina in people who have weakened immune systems or who take antibiotics. Very rarely, Candida can cause a serious blood infection. Overgrowth of this yeast in the intestines was once thought by some to be a cause of IBS (and a number of other chronic conditions), but doctors have generally discarded this theory due to a lack of any reliable scientific evidence, along with better understanding of other changes in IBS.

Carbohydrates: The sugars and starches in food. *Simple carbohydrates* are sugars found in fruit and table sugar. *Complex carbohydrates* comprise a large number of sugar molecules joined together and you find them in grains, beans, peas, legumes, and vegetables like potatoes, yams, and squash.

CEA test: A medical test that looks at levels of a chemical known as carcinoembryonic antigen. This is a chemical produced by a cancer that is found in the blood for a number of cancers, including cancers of the colon and rectum. The CEA test may be important in the investigation of IBS to rule out a tumour as a cause of symptoms.

Coeliac disease: A condition also called *gluten intolerance* that is often misdiagnosed as IBS because it produces symptoms of diarrhoea, bloating, and fatigue. Gluten intolerance damages the small intestine, leading to malabsorption of nutrients from food, and is caused by sensitivity to a protein found in wheat called gluten.

Chronic fatigue syndrome (CFS): Associated with severe, debilitating fatigue for which the cause is unknown. Doctors diagnose CFS if fatigue is present for at least six months and the patient has at least four of these symptoms that resemble a low-grade flu or viral infection: fever, impaired memory or concentration, sore throat, lymph node swelling, muscle pains, joint pains, headaches, poor sleep, and post-exertion exhaustion. Thirty to 60 per cent of people with CFS also have symptoms typical of IBS.

Colitis: A general term that means inflammation of the colon. (Note that *ulcerative colitis* is the name of a specific inflammatory bowel disease with physical signs of inflammation and ulceration.)

Colon: Another name for the main part of the large intestine or large bowel. This hollow tube runs from the small intestine to the rectum and has three major jobs to do: absorb any remaining water and salts into the body, ferment and break down indigestible food particles, and form and store faeces ready for elimination.

Colonoscopy: A test performed by a doctor to view the rectum and colon. After the intestines have been cleared out with an enema, the *colonoscope* – a long, flexible, narrow tube with a light and tiny camera lens on the end – can be passed into the back passage. The doctor can then see the inside of the bowel and take samples of the bowel lining if necessary.

Constipation: Not passing stool as frequently or as easily as normal. Doctors now use the Rome III Diagnostic Criteria that defines IBS constipation purely on stool consistency (passing hard stools rather than loose stools). The previous criteria also rated stool frequency as well as symptoms associated with defecation, but these criteria have been abandoned because doctors found them too complex to use to identify every case of IBS-constipation. Other symptoms of constipation include straining during a bowel movement, as well as having painful bowel movements, gas, bloating, fatigue, and lethargy.

Crohn's disease: An inflammatory bowel disease that affects any part of the gastrointestinal tract from mouth to anus. The disease most commonly affects the lower end of the small intestine (known as the *ileum*), with ulcerations, scarring, strictures, and symptoms of fever, diarrhoea, abdominal pain, and bleeding. In the very early stages, Crohn's may be mistaken for IBS.

Descending colon: Part of the large intestine that lies on the left side of the abdomen between the transverse colon above and the rectum and anus below.

Diarrhoea: Loose stool: mushy, runny or watery. The Rome III Diagnostic Criteria define IBS-diarrhoea very simply as loose stools (the previous criteria also included stool frequency and other symptoms related to bowel movements, but doctors became concerned that these criteria were so complex that they missed some cases). Other symptoms often associated with IBS-diarrhoea include urgency (having to rush to have a bowel movement); a feeling of having incomplete bowel movements; passing mucus (white material) during a bowel movement; pain or discomfort in the back passage (known as *proctalgia*), and/or abdominal fullness, bloating, or swelling.

Digestion: The breakdown of food in the body into small units that can be used for growth, energy, and repair.

Digestive system: The tissues and organs in the body that help break down and absorb food and liquids. The digestive system is also called the *gastrointestinal tract* and includes the mouth, oesophagus, stomach, small intestine, large intestine, rectum, and anus. Ancillary organs that also help with digestion are the tongue, teeth, salivary glands in the mouth, pancreas, liver, and gallbladder.

Digital rectal examination: An important medical procedure, also known as a per rectum (PR) examination, that allows a doctor to examine the anus and rectum for signs of hemorrhoids, polyps, or tumours. With the patient lying on their side, the doctor puts on a rubber glove, covers it in lubricant jelly, and gently inserts a gloved finger through the anus and into the rectum to feel for abnormalities. In men, the examination allows the doctor to examine the prostate gland too.

Diverticulosis: A medical condition, diagnosed with a barium enema X-ray, that occurs when small pouches (*diverticula*) occur at weak spots in the wall of the large intestine. When the pouches become infected or inflamed, the condition is called *diverticulitis*.

Dysentery: An infection of the intestines that causes watery diarrhoea (which sometimes contains blood or mucus), nausea and vomiting, abdominal pain, and fever. Two main types of dysentery exist: One is caused by a bacteria (usually a type called Shigella), and the other by an amoeba. After an episode of dysentery, some individuals may develop IBS.

Dyspepsia: An older, vague term for indigestion that describes all sorts of problems that cause abdominal pain or discomfort. Dyspepsia is not always caused by too much stomach acid; it often occurs when stomach acid is able to reflux back up from the stomach into the gullet or oesophagus, where it irritates the delicate lining. Dyspepsia also describes the pain from gas trapped in the stomach. The majority of people with IBS (about 75 per cent) suffer from indigestion for no known reason.

Endoscopy: A diagnostic procedure involving an *endoscope* – a fibre-optic tube through which a doctor can inspect the inside of the gastrointestinal tract. The different types of endoscopy procedures are named for the parts that they visualise: sigmoidoscopy (which views the sigmoid colon and rectum), colonoscopy (which views the colon or large intestine), and oesophago-gastro-duodenoscopy or OGD (which views the oesophagus, stomach, and upper part of the small intestines).

Eructation: A fancy name for the process of expelling gas through the mouth that has built up in the stomach – in other words, burping or belching.

Faecal occult blood test: Looks for microscopic amounts of blood hidden in the faeces, which may be a sign of a cancer of the bowel. The doctors wipes a small amount of stool on specially treated paper, which changes colour in the presence of blood.

Fibromyalgia (FMS): A disorder of the musculoskeletal system associated with pain, fatigue, and insomnia, for which the cause is unknown. *Fibro* relates to fibrous tissue of muscles, ligaments, and tendons. *Myalgia* means pain. So *fibromyalgia* means pain in the muscles, ligaments, and tendons.

Gallbladder: A ball-shaped organ that hangs beneath the liver. The gallbladder stores a greeny-yellow liquid called bile that is made in the liver, and releases it to aid in the digestion of fats.

Gas: Created in the intestines from swallowing air, food digestion, or as a waste product of bacterial fermentation. You release gas as burps or flatulence (farting).

Gastroenteritis: Any infection or irritation of the stomach and intestines. Gastroenteritis is mostly caused by an infection that may be due to a bacteria, virus, or parasite.

Gastroenterologist: A doctor whose specialty is disorders and diseases of the gastrointestinal tract (much classier than *gut doctor*).

Gastrointestinal tract (GIT): The muscular tube that runs right through the body from the mouth to the anus. Food and drink passes through the tube and the body digests, absorbs, and eliminates the contents.

Gastro-oesophageal reflux disease (GORD): A digestive disorder in which the lower oesophageal sphincter, which normally controls the passage of food and liquid between the oesophagus and stomach, is unusually relaxed. This allows highly acidic stomach contents to flow back up into the oesophagus where they damage the mucosa. A higher incidence of GORD exists in people who have IBS.

GIT: See *Gastrointestinal tract.*

Gluten intolerance: See *Coeliac disease*

Heartburn: A common gastric disorder that makes you feel burning or pain behind the sternum or breastbone. Heartburn may be associated with Gastro-oesophageal reflux disease (GORD). A higher incidence of heartburn exists in people who have IBS.

Haemorrhoids: Swollen, painful, itchy varicose veins in the blood vessels around the anus and lower rectum. Haemorrhoids, also called piles, may cause bleeding from the anus. People with IBS-constipation have a high incidence of haemorrhoids.

Hiatus hernia: A condition in which the opening in the diaphragm (a horizontal muscular sheet that divides the chest cavity from the abdominal cavity) is weakened to the point that the stomach slides upward above the diaphragm, into the chest. The condition causes pain and discomfort that is made worse by bending over or lying flat.

IBD: See *Inflammatory bowel disease.*

IBS: See *Irritable bowel syndrome.*

Inflammatory bowel disease (IBD): Two conditions in which the intestines are chronically inflamed, leading to episodes of fever, abdominal pain, weight loss, diarrhoea (which may be bloody), and complications such as fissures, abscesses, and strictures. *Ulcerative colitis* and *Crohn's disease* are both IBDs.

Insoluble fibre: Dietary fibre that comes from plants, especially roughage foods with skins, husks, and peels. Sometimes described as 'nature's broom', gut bacteria does not easily break down this fibre and therefore it mostly passes thorough the gastrointestinal tract undigested. But insoluble fibre can hold up to 15 times its weight in water and it therefore helps to soften and bulk up the stool. This fibre can aggravate symptoms for some people with IBS.

Intestinal flora: Microscopic organisms, predominantly bacteria, as well as fungi or yeasts, that live in the intestines.

Intestinal mucosa: The inner lining of the intestines, that absorbs food in the small intestine and water in the large intestine.

Intestines: The narrow tube in the gastrointestinal tract that runs from the stomach to the caecum (called the small intestine or small bowel) and the wider tube from the caecum to the anus (the large intestine or large bowel).

Irritable bowel syndrome (IBS): A functional condition that affects the gastrointestinal tract with symptoms that include diarrhoea and/or constipation, abdominal pain, bloating, and gas.

Kidneys: Organs located at the back of the abdominal cavity on both sides of the spine that filter waste from the blood and excrete it in the urine. The kidneys also help to control the amount of fluid in the body.

Lactobacillus acidophilus: One of the types of 'friendly' bacteria found in the large bowel that helps to digest food and keep the intestines healthy by supplying energy to the cells of the lining mucosa. You can eat some foods that contain the bacteria or take a supplement.

Laparotomy: An operation in which a doctor makes cuts into the abdomen in order to examine or operate on the intestines or other organs in the abdominal cavity.

Large intestine: Part of the gastrointestinal tract that runs from the end of the small intestine to the anus.

Laxatives: Medicines used to induce bowel movements and relieve constipation. If you use them too often, your gut can become dependent on them to work properly.

Liver: The most important organ in the body for detoxifying drugs, chemicals, and foreign materials. It also has hundreds of functions that include making bile, hormones, and cholesterol.

Lower oesophageal sphincter: A muscle that forms a ring around the bottom of the oesophagus, which closes off the oesophagus and keeps the acidic stomach contents contained.

Lower GI series: The series of pictures a doctor takes during a barium enema X-ray that show the large intestine and the end part of the small intestine.

Malabsorption syndrome: A condition in which the small intestine is unable to absorb nutrients from foods. Symptoms include gas, bloating, stools that contain fat and undigested food, failure to thrive, weight loss, and anaemia.

Mucous colitis: One of the original names for IBS.

Mucus: A viscous, clear liquid that coats and protects the underlying membranes and tissues. Cells that line the gastrointestinal tract make mucus.

Neurotransmitters: Chemicals in the brain and body that carry messages between the cells of the nervous system to conduct or inhibit nerve activity. Serotonin is a neurotransmitter that conveys messages to make the bowel speed up or slow down.

Occult bleeding: The loss of tiny amounts of blood into the stool. Doctors can't seen the blood (occult means hidden), but it shows up on a special occult blood test. Blood in the stool may be an indication of bleeding from the surface of an inflamed or irritated gut as a result of aspirin use, ulceration, or cancer.

Oesophagus: A narrow tube, about 25 centimetres long, that is more commonly called the gullet. The oesophagus forms the first part of the gastrointestinal tract and joins the mouth and throat to the stomach.

Pain threshold: The level of stimulation that an individual perceives as pain. Some people have a high threshold or high pain tolerance. Researchers say that people with IBS have a low threshold for pain in their intestines and feel it much sooner and more severely than people with a high threshold.

Pancreas: An organ that lies behind the stomach. The pancreas produces insulin that regulates blood sugar and pancreatic enzymes that digest protein and fat.

Peristalsis: Rhythmic muscular contractions of the entire digestive tract (from oesophagus to rectum) that push food through the gut and then eliminate the waste products through the rectum and anus.

Peritoneum: A protective lining around the inside of the abdominal cavity that wraps around all the organs.

Polyp: An abnormal growth shaped like a ball on a stalk. Polyps are common in the lining of the large intestine, where they are painless but may cause bleeding into the gut. Doctors advise that polyps be removed because they can turn cancerous.

Proctoscopy: A test used to examine the anal canal. The doctor inserts a lubricated metal or plastic instrument called a proctoscope into the anus to look for inflammation, fissures, fistulae, haemorrhoids, and tumours in the anal canal.

Radiation colitis: Inflammation caused by treating cancer of the colon with radiation. The inflammation can have symptoms similar to IBS and may be treated with dietary restriction and lifestyle changes.

Rectum: The collecting pouch for faeces at the lower end of the large intestine, connected to the anus. When enough pressure from collected faeces builds up, the body triggers the rectum to empty and the person feels the urge to open their bowels.

Rome III Diagnostic Criteria for IBS: The criteria used widely by doctors to diagnose IBS. IBS diagnosis must be based on at least three months (with onset at least six months previously) of recurrent abdominal discomfort or pain that has two or more of the following features:

- Improvement with defecation
- Onset associated with a change in frequency of stool
- Onset associated with a change in form (appearance) of stool

Serotonin: A neurotransmitter found throughout the body, including the brain and blood platelets, but 95 per cent of it exists in the bowel.

Small intestine: There are three parts to the small intestine: the duodenum starts where the stomach empties, then becomes the jejunum, and then the ileum, which connects to the large intestine. The small intestine is crucial in the absorption of nutrients from food into the bloodstream.

Soluble fibre: A type of dietary fibre that dissolves and swells when mixed with water. Soluble fibre helps to regulate bowel movements, lowers cholesterol, and controls blood sugar levels. You find this fibre in many fruit and vegetables, including oranges, apples, carrots, and dried beans and peas, as well as oats, oat bran, barley, flax seed, and psyllium husk.

Spastic colitis/colon: Previous names for IBS.

Sphincter: A circular muscle that constricts a tube or closes a natural opening. In a relaxed state, a sphincter opens and allows materials to pass through the opening. When closed, the muscle blocks material from passing.

Stomach: An organ in the shape of a pouch with a large upper end and a tapered lower end. The stomach attaches to the oesophagus at its top end, and to the *duodenum* (the first part of the small intestine) at its bottom end. The stomach continues the action of the teeth in breaking down food and starting digestion.

Stricture: Abnormal narrowing of a body opening, tube, or canal, usually due to a tumour or scar tissue.

Sugar: Refined sugar comes from beets, sugar cane, or corn. Eating sugar can be detrimental to someone with IBS, causing gas and bloating.

Tumour: An abnormal mass of tissue that may be cancerous or benign.

Ulcer: An eroded area of tissue in a mucous membrane that can bleed or cause pain.

Ulcerative colitis: An inflammatory bowel disease of the large intestine that causes fever, abdominal pain, ulceration, diarrhoea, mucus, bleeding, and complications such as abscesses, fistulae, and strictures.

Yeast: See *Candida albicans*.

Index

• A •

abdomen, 119, 343
abdominal pain/spasm
  children's symptoms, 286–289
  constipation symptoms, 59
  defined, 343
  less frequent IBS symptoms, 16
  medications, 163–167, 235, 236
  men versus women, 97
  overview of, 56–57
  primary IBS symptoms, 14
  Rome III Diagnostic Criteria, 12–13
  urgent care signs, 110
  women's misdiagnosis, 99–100
  yoga postures, 213–216
abnormal gut motility, 46
activated charcoal, 167
acupuncture, 237–238
Acupuncture Society, 238
acute anticipation, 297
addiction, to medication, 149
adrenaline, 80
adult pants, 267
adult wipe, 267
aerobic exercise, 206
air, toxins in, 48–49
air-contrast study, 137
alcohol
  drug interactions, 314
  food record, 184
  IBS triggers, 91, 313–314
  leaky gut, 48
  liver function, 30
  sleep problems, 180
allergy, food
  cause of IBS, 45, 318
  children's symptoms, 287
  coeliac disease, 77
  defined, 73, 343
  dietary control, 74
  differential diagnosis, 142, 143
  questions for doctor, 118

  testing for, 80–81, 140
  vomiting, 52
alosetron, 152
alpha galactosidase, 167
alternator, 13
alverine, 163, 164
American Gastroenterological Association, 330
American Holistic Health Association, 251
amitriptyline, 166, 269
amoebic dysentery, 141
amylase enzyme, 25, 201
anaemia, 110, 133, 343
anal fissure, 119–120, 343
angelica root, 200
anger, 220, 296–297, 326
anise, 200, 243
ANS (autonomic nervous system), 83
antenatal care, 95
antibiotic medication
  drawbacks of, 315
  effects on bacteria, 34, 71
  IBS triggers, 69, 314–315
  leaky gut, 48
  overview of, 86
  reason for symptoms, 115
anticholinergic medication, 163–164
antidepressant
  alcohol interactions, 314
  cause of IBS, 87
  children, 294
  diarrhoea, 59
  overview of, 165–167
antimuscarinic medication, 149, 163–164
antispasmodic drug, 56, 163–164
anus
  anal fissure, 119–120, 343
  barium enema procedure, 136–137
  defined, 343
  endoscopy procedure, 134
  lubricant enemas, 162
  proctalgia fugax, 63
  rectal exam, 119–120, 131
  suppository use, 162

anxiety
  children's feelings, 296, 297
  control of feelings, 218–222, 326–327
  exercise benefits, 208, 210
  faecal incontinence, 62
  hypersensitive gut, 43–44, 83
  psychological therapies, 225–226
appendix, 343
arachis oil, 162
areca seed, 200
Argentum nitricum (medication), 235
aromatherapy, 243–244
Aromatherapy Council, 244
arousal, 219
artificial sweetener, 186, 196
ascending colon, 22, 343
aspartame, 186, 344
assertiveness, 220–221, 256–257
associated condition, 66
Association for Applied Psychophysiology
    and Biofeedback, 248
Association of Reflexologists, 239
atropine, 148, 149, 163
autonomic nervous system (ANS), 83

• *B* •

bacteria
  cause of IBS, 67–69, 70–71, 86
  colonic irrigation, 247
  diarrhoea treatment, 153–154
  dietary fibre, 79
  gas reduction tips, 54
  good versus bad types, 32–34
  large intestine function, 31
  leaky gut, 48
  post-infectious IBS, 67–69
bacterial implantation, 154
baking food, 198
barium
  defined, 344
  enema, 88, 136–137
Beano (medication), 56, 167
beans, 79, 186, 195
beetroot test, 39
behavioural therapy, 225–226
Benson, Herbert (doctor), 240
betaine hydrochloride, 201
bicarbonate, 30
bifidobacteria, 202

bile
  binding agents, 150–151
  cause of IBS, 73
  digestion process, 28, 29
  protective functions, 40
biofeedback, 225, 247–248
biological stressor, 84
biopsy, bowel, 138–139
bisacodyl, 160, 162
bitter herb, 200
black stool, 36
blame, 296
bleeding
  emergency conditions, 18, 109–110
  faecal occult blood test, 131–132
  stool colours, 36
bloating
  cause of IBS, 47
  defined, 344
  elimination diet, 193
  IBS triggers, 91
  incidence, 55
  less frequent symptoms, 16
  overview of, 54–55
  primary symptoms, 14
  tips for reducing, 55–56
  urgent care signs, 109
blood sugar, 79–80, 138, 323
blood test, 132–133, 288
BMJ Clinical Evidence (Web site), 332
boiling food, 198
borborygmi, 344
bowel, 138–139, 344
Bowel Control (Web site), 331
bowel incontinence
  defined, 344
  medication, 268–269
  overview of, 61–62
  social situations, 264–269
  travel plans, 260
bowel movement
  common symptoms, 15
  defined, 344
  healthy habits, 178
  mild cases of IBS, 16–17
  nausea reduction, 52
brain–gut axis. *See* gut–brain axis
bran, 78, 151, 157
Branch, Rhena (*Cognitive Behavioural
    Therapy For Dummies*), 226
breakfast, 278, 290

breathing, 53
Bristol Stool Form Scale, 3
British Acupuncture Council, 238
British Association for Counselling and
    Psychotherapy, 229
British Association of Psychotherapists, 227
British Association of Therapeutical
    Hypnotists, 336
British College of Integrated Medicine, 250
British Dietetic Association, 122
British Holistic Medical Association, 251
British Homeopathic Association, 236
British Medical Journal, 332
British Nutrition Foundation, 189
British Psychoanalytic Council, 230
British Psychoanalytical Society, 227
British Psychological Society, 230
British Society of Clinical Hypnosis, 242, 336
British Society of Gastroenterology, 330
British Society of Integrated Medicine, 250
bromelaine, 201
bulk-forming laxative agent, 151–152, 156–157
burping, 35, 53
Buscopan (medication), 163
Business Link (Web site), 283

• C •

C reactive protein (CRP) test, 132, 288
cadaverine, 33
caecum, 344
CAM. *See* complementary and alternative
    medicine
Campylobacter jejuni, 68
Canadian Society of Intestinal Research,
    302–303, 330
cancer, 95, 133, 142
Candida albicans
    cause of IBS, 72
    defined, 344
    questions for doctor, 117–118
    women's misdiagnosis, 100
caraway seed, 200
carbohydrate, 187, 345
carcinoembryonic antigen (CEA) test, 133,
    344
career
    disclosure of IBS, 280–282
    effects of IBS, 276–277
    home office, 282–283
    lifestyle issues, 261
    men versus women, 97
    morning routine, 277–279, 325
    overview of, 275
    scheduled meals, 315
    workday attacks, 279–280
Careplace Irritable Bowel Syndrome
    Community, 333
cascara, 160
Castro, Miranda (*The Complete Homeopathy
    Handbook*), 236
catastrophising, 83, 218–219, 288
cause, of IBS. *See also* irritable bowel
    syndrome
    candida, 72
    chemicals, 85–90
    common triggers, 66–67
    defined, 65–66
    digestion problems, 45–46
    food-related causes, 72–81, 87, 318
    genetics, 84–85
    holistic theories, 90
    immune system, 69–70
    infection, 67–69
    leaky gut, 48–49
    motility issues, 46
    overview of, 1, 11–12
    questions for doctor, 117
    stress, 82–84
    trapped gas, 46–47
CBT (Cognitive Behavioural Therapy),
    62–63, 226
CDSA (comprehensive digestive stool
    analysis), 141
CEA (carcinoembryonic antigen) test,
    133, 344
Celevac (bulking agent), 151
cell replacement, 29
cerebrospinal fluid, 51
CFS (chronic fatigue syndrome), 95, 345
chalky stool, 36
chamomile, 200
charcoal, 167, 270
chemicals
    cause of IBS, 85–90
    environmental, 48–49, 250–251
    foods, 23–24, 45, 49, 87
    laxatives, 160
    stressors, 84

chewing food, 24–26, 53, 69
childhood experience
  causes of IBS, 60, 85
  control of feelings, 218
  culture of upbringing, 101
  gender gap in diagnosis, 96
children
  abdominal pain, 286–289
  balanced home life, 293–294
  complementary treatment, 232
  diagnostic process, 288
  emotional support for, 294–298
  incidence of IBS, 93
  overview of, 285
  stressors, 289–293
Chinese medicine, 233, 237
chiropractic, 245–246
chlorophyll, 269
chocolate, 203
cholecystokinin, 38, 60
chronic fatigue syndrome (CFS), 95, 345
chyme, 28
cilansetron, 152
clinical trial, 147–148
clomipramine, 166
coconut oil, 189
codeine, 59, 154
coeliac disease
  children's symptoms, 287
  defined, 345
  differential diagnosis, 143
  gluten-free diet, 140
  Internet resources, 337
  investigations, 138–140
  overview of, 77
  questions for doctor, 117
coffee, 28, 180, 186, 196
Cognitive Behavioural Therapy (CBT), 62–63, 226
Cognitive Behavioural Therapy For Dummies (Branch and Willson), 226
colestyramine, 150–151, 269
colic, 167
colitis, 337, 345
College of Psychoanalysts – UK, 227
Colocynthis (medication), 235
Colofac (medication), 163
colon
  abdominal pain, 57, 58
  cancer, 142

  defined, 345
  gut motility, 46
  illustrated, 22
  immune system malfunction, 70
  large intestine function, 31
colonic food, 33
colonic irrigation, 246–247
colonoscopy, 134–136, 345
comfort food, 203
communication, 270, 271, 280–282
commute, to work, 278–279
complementary and alternative medicine (CAM). *See also specific CAM treatment*
  children and pregnant women, 232
  doctor's attitude toward IBS, 112
  integrated medicine, 249–252
  Internet sources, 305
  medical expense, 262
  overview of, 231–232
  placebo effect, 233–234
  referrals and information, 232
  selection, 233
  therapists, 122
The Complete Homeopathy Handbook (Castro), 236
complex carbohydrate, 187, 197, 345
comprehensive digestive stool analysis (CDSA), 141
computed tomography (CT) imaging, 137–138
conflict therapy, 227
constipation
  accompanying pain, 57
  bloating incidence, 55
  causes of, 59–60
  defined, 345
  dietary remedies, 60, 157, 158
  exercise, 162
  faecal incontinence, 265
  gastroenteritis symptoms, 69
  incidence of, 6
  medication, 36, 151–152, 154–162
  overview of, 59
  primary symptoms, 14
  sex issues, 272
  stool consistency, 37
  treatment options, 36, 162
  women's hormones, 98
constipation-predominant IBS (IBS-C)
  causes of, 59–60
  common symptoms, 59

defined, 13
high-fibre diet, 78
overview of, 59
treatment options, 60
constitutional homeopathic remedy, 235
Continence Foundation, 266
cooking food, 197–198, 199
co-phenotrope, 148–149
coping skills, 103
CORE (Digestive Disorders Foundation), 330
corticosteroid, 49
corticotropin-releasing factor (CRF), 70
counselling, 228–229
co-worker, 281
cramp. *See* abdominal pain/spasm
Crohn's disease
    children's diagnosis, 288
    defined, 346
    differential diagnosis, 142
    versus IBS, 18
    Internet resources, 337
    investigations, 137
    questions for doctor, 118
CRP (C reactive protein) test, 132, 288
CT (computed tomography) imaging, 137–138
culture, of sufferer, 101–102
cure, for IBS, 94, 146, 147, 173
cyst, 133
cytokine, 70

● *D* ●

dairy product
    allergies to, 142, 287
    children's symptoms, 287
    gluten-free diet, 140
    history of eating habits, 5
    lactose, 74–76
    overview of, 186
    substitutes, 79, 195
dantron (danthron), 160
DDA (Disability Discrimination Act), 281
death, 292–293
deconditioning, 210
dental problem, 25
dental product, 89
depression
    children's feelings, 297–298
    control of feelings, 221–222
    medications, 165

descending colon, 22, 346
desipramine, 166
detoxing, 192–193
diagnosis. *See also specific exams/tests*
    in children, 288
    diagnosable disease versus functional
        disorder, 44
    differential, 141–143
    evidence-based medicine, 11–13
    process of, 129–130
    questions for doctor, 117
    uncertainty of, 10–11, 45
    women's pain, 94–96, 99–100
diarrhoea
    accompanying pain, 57
    antibiotic drawbacks, 315
    children's symptoms, 287–288
    defined, 346
    differential diagnosis, 141–142
    faecal incontinence, 265
    gastroenteritis symptoms, 69
    medication, 59, 148–154, 235, 236
    nausea reduction, 52
    overview of, 37, 58–59
    primary symptoms, 14–15
    sex issues, 272
    travel plans, 71
    urgent care signs, 110
diarrhoea-predominant IBS (IBS-D)
    antidepressant research, 166
    defined, 13
    dietary fibre, 78, 316
    overview of, 57–58
    symptoms, 58–59
diary
    detoxing tips, 93
    exercise programme, 212
    food record, 52, 125–126, 184–185
    incontinence, 265
    life events, 174–177
dicyclomine, 163, 164
dicycloverine, 163
diet. *See also* eating habits; food
    cooking tips, 197–198
    disastrous foods, 186
    elimination plan, 190–194
    food combinations, 187–188
    food shopping, 196–197
    guidelines, 323

diet *(continued)*
    Internet resources, 336–337
    problems with healthy foods, 189–190
    records, 184–185
    stress interactions, 203
dietitian, 121–122, 336
Dietitians Unlimited (Web site), 336
differential, 133
digestion
    cause of IBS, 46–49
    defined, 346
    herbal aides, 200–201
    process, 24–32
    transit time, 39, 187
Digestive Disorders Foundation (CORE), 330
digestive enzyme
    digestion process, 24, 25, 26, 28
    gas reduction, 167
    gastroenteritis, 68
    lactose absorption, 75
    overview of, 201
    protective functions, 40
    supplements, 201–202
digestive juice, 24
digestive system
    controlling systems, 37–38
    defined, 346
    illustrated, 27
    transit time, 39
digital rectal examination, 346
diphenoxylate hydrochloride, 148, 149
Disability Discrimination Act (DDA), 281
disaccharide, 74–75
disposable underwear, 266–267
distended abdomen, 54–56
diverticula
    barium enema procedure, 136
    constipation complications, 60
    defined, 346
    endoscopy procedure, 134
diverticulitis, 136, 346
doctor. *See also specific types*
    attitude toward IBS, 111–112
    children's stress, 293
    diagnosis in women, 95–96
    exercise programme, 211
    first appointment, 123–127
    GP versus specialist investigations, 130
    incidence of IBS, 94
    medical limitations, 10
    misdiagnosis, 100
    overview of, 107
    physical exam, 118–120
    purpose for visit, 108
    referral to specialist, 120–122, 232
    relationship with, 112–118, 328
    selection, 111
    symptoms warranting visit, 108–111
    urgent care signs, 18, 109–111
docusate sodium, 160, 161
double-contrast study, 137
doxepin, 166
drug abuse, 30, 149
duodenum, 50, 351
D-xylose sugar, 138–139
dysautonomia, 219
dysentery, 141–142, 346
dyspepsia, 54, 347
dysphagia, 16

• *E* •

e. coli bacteria, 68
eating habits. *See also* diet; food
    avoidance of *candida,* 72
    bloating-reduction tips, 55–56
    bulking agents, 151–152, 157
    cause of IBS, 45–46, 72–81
    children's stress, 290, 291
    common symptoms, 14–15
    constipation treatment, 60
    detoxing tips, 192
    diarrhoea treatment, 153–154
    digestion process, 24–31
    digestion time, 39
    effects of IBS, 263
    effects on bacteria, 71
    food record, 125–126, 184–185, 190
    food substitutes, 195–196
    gas reduction, 54
    gluten intolerance, 140
    good versus bad bacteria, 33–34
    history of, 45
    IBS triggers, 315–318
    importance of, 23–24
    lactobacillus consumption, 100
    less frequent symptoms, 16
    life-events diary, 175

mild cases of IBS, 17
morning routine, 278
nausea reduction, 52
overview of, 183
reasons for symptoms, 16
serotonin research, 309
sleep tips, 181
symptom management, 173, 177–178
travel plans, 71, 259
elimination diet, 190–194
ELISA test, 81
EMA (endomysial antibody), 139
embarrassment, 54, 61, 113–114, 291
emotional freedom technique, 237
emotional motor system, 220
emotions, of sufferer
children's feelings, 293–298
control of feelings, 218–222, 326–327
diary entries, 175, 185
doctor visit, 113
effects of IBS, 262–264
emotional healing, 222–223
exercise benefits, 208, 210
mind-body relationship, 19, 82–83
psychological therapy options, 223–230
stress–diet interaction, 203
typical feelings, 10
Encyclopedia of Homeopathy (Lockie), 236
endocrine system, 38, 70
endometriosis, 142
endomysial antibody (EMA), 139
endorphin, 206, 208, 210
endoscopy
children's diagnosis, 288
defined, 347
overview of, 134–136
enema
barium enema procedure, 136–137
children's diagnosis, 288
colonic irrigation, 246–247
constipation remedy, 159
endoscopy procedure, 135
overview of, 162
enteric nervous supply, 38, 219, 220
environmental medicine, 250–251
eosinophilia myalgia syndrome, 309
eructation, 347
erythrocyte sedimentation rate (ESR)
test, 132
essential fat, 188
essential oil, 243

evidence-based medicine, 11–13
exercise
benefits of, 179, 207–210, 323
bloating-reduction tips, 56
constipation remedy, 162
defined, 206–207
diary entries, 175
digestion process, 29
digestion time, 39
general guidelines, 324
large intestine function, 32
options, 212
overview of, 205–206
programme creation, 210–212
resources, 334–335
sleep tips, 180
yoga, 213–216
Expert Patients Programme (symptom management programme), 171–172, 337
explosive fart, 47
eye exam, 119

• **F** •

faecal incontinence
medication, 268–269
overview of, 61–62
social situations, 264–269
travel plans, 260
faecal occult blood test, 131–132
faeces
colour and consistency, 36–37
digestion time, 39
explosive fart, 47
good versus bad bacteria, 33
investigations, 141
large intestine function, 31–32
overview of, 35
stool softeners, 160–161
tests, 131–132, 288
faecolith, 15, 265
family
balanced life, 293–294
children's stress, 293
communication issues, 271
genetic predisposition to IBS, 84–85
lifestyle issues, 258–259, 273
medical history, 126
social situations, 264–273
support of, 270–271, 294–298, 333

family planning, 95
fart. *See* gas
fasting, 268
fat, dietary
  abdominal pain causes, 57
  bloating-reduction tips, 56
  cause of IBS, 73, 76–77
  constipation treatment, 60
  digestion rate, 28
  IBS triggers, 317
  menu plan, 196, 197
  overview of, 187
  reduction of, 188–189
  stool consistency, 37
FBC (full blood count), 133
FBD (functional bowel disorder), 10, 44
fear
  control of feelings, 218–219
  effects of IBS, 262–264
  emotional motor system, 220
fennel, 201
fermentation, 35, 138, 187
fever, 67, 110
fibre, dietary
  bloating-reduction tips, 55
  bulking agents, 151–152, 157
  cause of IBS, 78–79
  constipation treatment, 60, 155
  digestion time, 39
  faecal incontinence, 268
  food sources, 341–342
  good versus bad bacteria, 33
  IBS triggers, 90–91, 316
  nausea reduction, 52
  overview of, 186
  problems with, 189
fibroid, 133
fibromyalgia (FMS), 95, 347
fig, 158
financial issues, 261–262
5-HT4 partial agonist, 56, 159
5-HT receptor, 152
5-HTP supplement, 308
fizzy drink, 56
flatulence. *See* gas
flatulence filter, 270
flexibility, 207
fluoride, 89
FMS (fibromyalgia), 95, 347

food. *See also* diet; eating habits
  additives, 87
  diary, 52, 125–126, 184–185
  fried foods, 196, 198, 317
  intolerance, 73, 318
  labels, 23–24
  poisoning, 126
  sensitivity, 73, 318
  substitutes, 196
food allergy. *See* allergy, food
Foodreactions.org (Web site), 336
fried food, 196, 198, 317
friendship, 272
fructose, 74
fruit
  constipation remedy, 158
  diet guidelines, 323
  digestion rate, 28
  leaky gut, 49
  menu plan, 196
  questions for doctor, 117
  substitutes, 195
  sugars, 74, 188
full blood count (FBC), 133
functional bowel disorder (FBD), 10, 44
functional condition, 66
fungus, 49
future, fear of, 264

• G •

gallbladder, 28, 40, 347
gas
  abdominal pain causes, 57
  bloating causes, 55
  bulking agents, 157
  cause of IBS, 46–47
  children's stress, 292
  common symptoms, 15
  defined, 347
  elimination diet, 193, 194
  faecal incontinence, 265–266
  food sensitivity, 73
  IBS triggers, 91
  lactose digestion, 75
  medication, 167
  overview of, 35, 53–54
  social situations, 269–270
  sources of, 35

trapped, 46–47
types, 53–54
yoga postures, 213–216
gastric acid, 26, 27, 40
gastrin, 38
gastroenteritis
  children's symptoms, 287
  defined, 347
  IBS causes, 67–69
gastroenterologist, 121, 130, 347
GastroHep (Web site), 332
gastrointestinal serotonergic agent, 306
gastrointestinal tract (GIT)
  basic facts, 22
  defined, 346, 347
  digestion process, 24–32
  hypersensitive gut causes, 43–44
  illustrated, 22
  overview of, 21
  protective forces, 40
  transit time, 39
gastro-oesophageal reflux disease (GORD),
    50, 348
General Chiropractic Council, 246
General Osteopathic Council, 246
genetics
  cause of IBS, 84–85
  orthomolecular medicine, 252
  serotonin research, 307
giardia lamblia, 142, 287
ginger
  nausea reduction, 52
  overview of, 201
GIT. *See* gastrointestinal tract
globus hystericus, 16
glucose, 79–80, 158
gluten, 139, 186, 287
gluten intolerance
  defined, 345
  differential diagnosis, 143
  investigations, 138–140
  overview of, 77, 78
  questions for doctor, 117
gluten-free diet, 140
glycerol, 162
goal setting, 211, 222
GORD (gastro-oesophageal reflux disease),
    50, 348
grain
  bloating-reduction tips, 55
  digestion rate, 28

elimination diet, 194
leaky gut, 49
menu plan, 197
grief, 292–293
griffonia seed, 308
group therapy, 224
gut motility, 46
Gut Trust (IBS organisation), 303, 330
Gut (Web site), 332
gut–brain axis
  cause of hypersensitive gut, 41–44
  defined, 19
  incomplete evacuation, 62–63
  overview of, 41
gut-directed hypnotherapy, 241–242

• *H* •

haemorrhoid
  bleeding, 109
  constipation complications, 60–61
  defined, 348
  rectal exam, 119–120
  stool colours, 36
hair, 119
happy baby posture, 213
health insurance, 280
Health Protection Units, 126
heartburn
  defined, 348
  less frequent IBS symptoms, 16
  medication, 235
  overview of, 50
Help for IBS.com (Web site), 336
herbal treatment, 199–201, 238
hiatus hernia, 348
holiday allowance, 281
holistic health, 251
home office, 282–283
homeopathy, 234–236
hormone
  constipation treatment, 60
  digestion process, 28
  digestive controls, 38
  IBS triggers, 91, 318–319
  leaky gut, 49
  men versus women, 97–99
human resources department, 282
humour, 258, 281, 327
hunger, 235, 322

hydrogen breath test, 138–139, 318
hydrolysed protein, 24
hyoscine, 163
hypersensitive gut
  cause, 41–49, 66–72
  overview of, 41
  stress effects, 83
hypnotherapy, 225, 241–242, 336
Hypnotherapy Association, 242, 336

• *I* •

IBD. *See* inflammatory bowel disease
IBS. *See* irritable bowel syndrome
IBS Audio Program 100 (Web site), 336
IBS Network, 303, 330, 331
IBS Patient Action Group, 333
IBS Research Update (Web site), 336
IBS Tales (Web site), 332
IBS-C. *See* constipation-predominant IBS
IBS-D. *See* diarrhoea-predominant IBS
IgA (immunoglobulin A), 40
ileocecal sphincter, 26, 31
illness, accompanying, 71, 209, 276
imagining symptoms, 19
immune system
  cause of IBS, 69–70
  exercise benefits, 208, 209
  gluten effects, 77
  good versus bad bacteria, 33
immunoglobulin A (IgA), 40
impaction, 265
incomplete evacuation, 59, 62–63
incontinence. *See* bowel incontinence
indigestible foods, 31
indigestion, 54
infection
  abdominal pain causes, 57
  children's diagnosis, 288
  destruction of good bacteria, 153
  FBC test, 133
  reason for symptoms, 115
  urgent care signs, 110
inflammation, 67–69
inflammatory bowel disease (IBD)
  children's symptoms, 287
  defined, 348
  versus IBS, 18
  symptoms, 15

insoluble fibre
  bulking agents, 152
  defined, 348
  effects, 78
  food sources, 341–342
insomnia, 180, 210
Institute of Psychoanalysis, 227
insulin, 30, 80
integrated medicine, 249–252
integrative therapy, 229
intensive psychoanalysis, 224
International Congress of Gastroenterology, 12
International Foundation for Functional Gastrointestinal Disorders, 11, 330
Internet resources, 303–305, 332–337
interview, job, 280
intestinal flora. *See* bacteria
intestinal mucosa, 68, 349
intestine
  cause of IBS, 46–47
  defined, 349
  gastrointestinal infection, 68–69
  trapped gas, 46–47
intrinsic nervous supply, 38
investigation. *See also specific investigations*
  children's diagnosis, 288
  defined, 129
  food allergy test, 80–81
  overview of, 130
involuntary muscle, 32
Irritable Bowel Syndrome Association, 330
irritable bowel syndrome (IBS). *See also* cause, of IBS
  defined, 44, 349
  incidence of, 1, 9, 93
  subtypes, 13
Irritable Bowel Syndrome mailing list, 333
Irritable Bowel Syndrome Self Help and Support Group, 302, 330
irritant laxative, 160
ischaemic colitis, 152
isolation, of sufferer, 270–271, 283
ispaghula, 78, 151–152

• *J* •

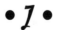

jaundice, 119
jejunum, 75

joint health, 207
joke, workplace, 281
Jungian analytical psychology, 227

• K •

kidney, 349

• L •

lactase, 75
Lactobacillus acidophilus
  defined, 349
  supplements, 34, 100, 202–203
lactose intolerance
  children's symptoms, 287
  differential diagnosis, 143
  IBS triggers, 72
  Internet resources, 337
  investigations, 138–139
  overview of, 74–76
  questions for doctor, 117
lactulose, 158
Lancet (journal), 332
laparotomy, 349
large intestine
  defined, 349
  digestion process, 30–32
  good versus bad bacteria, 32–34
  gut motility, 46
  IBS symptoms, 16
laxative
  barium enema procedure, 136
  constipation treatment, 60, 154–162
  defined, 36, 349
  endoscopy procedure, 135
  IBS triggers, 91
  overview of, 156
  sorbitol effects, 76
leaky gut, 48–49, 57, 69
Learning Meditation (Web site), 335
lifestyle, of IBS sufferer
  assertiveness, 256–257
  family issues, 258–259
  life changes, 257
  overview of, 255–256
  pace of life, 320
  recent research, 260–261
  sex issues, 271–272
  travel plans, 259–260

Lilium tigrinum (medication), 235
lipase, 202
listening, to child, 295–296
liver
  defined, 349
  digestion process, 29–30
  disease of, 119
  stool colours, 36
Lockie, Andrew (*Encyclopedia of Homeopathy*), 236
Lomotil (medication), 148–149
loperamide
  constipation causes, 59
  diarrhoea treatment, 59, 154
  faecal incontinence, 268–269
  overview of, 149–150
  travel plans, 259
Lotronex (medication), 152
lower GI series, 349
lower oesophageal sphincter, 26, 50, 349
L-tryptophan, 309
lubricant, 160–161
lubricant enema, 162
lumen, 33
Lycopodium (medication), 235
lymphatic tissue, 29, 48–49

• M •

macrogol, 158
Mag Phos (medication), 235
magnesium, 89–90, 193, 235
magnetic resonance (MR) imaging, 137–138
mail order test, 81
mailing list, 332–333
malabsorption syndrome, 160–161, 349
malnutrition, 30
Manipulation Association of Chartered Physiotherapists, 246
manipulative therapy, 245–246
massage, 244–245, 335
meat, 196, 198
mebeverine, 163, 164
medical expense, 261, 262
medication. *See also specific types*
  abdominal pain, 235, 236
  alcohol interactions, 314
  bloating-reduction tips, 56

medication (continued)
  cause of IBS, 86–87
  constipation remedies, 36, 151–152, 154–162
  cure for IBS, 146, 147
  current drug therapies, 146–147
  depression, 165
  diarrhoea, 59, 148–154, 235, 236
  doctor's attitude toward IBS, 112
  faecal incontinence, 268–269
  gas production, 167
  heartburn, 235
  homeopathic treatment, 234–237
  leaky gut, 48, 49
  liver function, 30
  marketing effects, 300
  morning routine, 279
  muscle spasms, 163–164, 167
  nausea reduction, 52
  online information, 305
  overmedication, 321–322
  overview, 146
  pain management, 163–167
  research, 147–148
meditation, 239, 327, 335
men, as IBS sufferers, 94–97
menstrual period, 97–99, 142, 199
menthol, 60
menu planning, 196–197
Merbentyl (medication), 163
mercury, 87–88
meridian, 237
methylcellulose, 151
metronidazole, 314
micowaving food, 198
microvilli, 68
midgut motility disorder, 55, 61
milk of magnesia, 158–159
Mind/Body Medical Institute, 240
mind-body relationship, 19, 82–83, 248
mineral oil, 160
mineral salt, 159
mint, 52
mistaken identity, 66
mixed bowel habit, 13
monounsaturated fat, 187, 188
morning symptoms
  children's stress, 290–291
  common types, 14–15
  diarrhoea-predominant IBS, 58
  medications, 236

mild cases of IBS, 16–17
  planning tips, 325
  work issues, 277–279
motility, 46, 61
mould, 49
mouth, 24–25, 40
Movicol (medication), 158
moxabustion, 238
MR (magnetic resonance) imaging, 137–138
MSG (flavour enhancer), 24, 87
mucosa, 68, 349
mucous colitis, 350
mucus
  common IBS symptoms, 15
  defined, 350
  digestion process, 25
  good versus bad bacteria, 33
  large intestine function, 31
  leaky gut, 48–49
  stool consistency, 37
multifactorial disease, 46–47
muscle contraction
  large intestine function, 32
  medication, 163–164, 166
  vomiting process, 51
muscle strength, 206, 207, 209

• N •

nails, 119
nap, 181
National Council for Hypnotherapy, 242, 336
National Institute of Diabetes and Digestive
  and Kidney Diseases, 332
Natrum cabonicum (medication), 235
naturopathic medicine, 248–249
nausea
  common IBS symptoms, 15
  low blood sugar, 80
  overview of, 50–52
  remedies, 52
negative thinking, 218, 296–298
nerve growth factor, 208
nervous system
  digestive controls, 38
  faecal incontinence, 61–62
  gut motility, 46
  hypersensitive gut causes, 41–44
  immune system malfunction, 70

incomplete evacuation, 62–63
serotonin research, 307–308
neurotransmitter, 51, 165, 350
New England Journal of Medicine, 332
NHS expense, 262
niacin, 309
nicotine, 88
non-steroidal anti-inflammatory drugs
    (NSAID), 49, 314, 321–322
nutrients
  digestion process, 26
  digestion time, 39
  food record, 185
  gluten intolerance, 139
  good versus bad bacteria, 33
  stool consistency, 37
Nutrition Society, 122
nutritionist, 121–122
nuts, 197
Nux vomica (medication), 236

• *O* •

occult bleeding, 350
odour. *See* smells
odynophagia, 16
oesophageal sphincter, 26, 50, 349
oesophagus
  defined, 350
  digestion process, 26
  heartburn, 50
  less frequent IBS symptoms, 16
oestrogen, 98
oil, 197, 198, 243
older people, 36, 110, 143
olive oil, 98
omega-6 fatty acid, 188
omega-3 fatty acid, 188
one-legged forward bend, 214–215
online support group. *See also* support group
  overview of, 331
  resources, 301–303, 331–333
  social life, 272–273
opiate, 314
opioid analogue, 149
oregano, 201
organisation, IBS. *See specific organisations*
oriental medicine, 237

orthomolecular medicine, 252
osmotic laxative, 158
osteopathy, 245–246
osteoporosis, 143

• *P* •

padded pant, 266
pain. *See* abdominal pain/spasm
pain threshold
  antidepressant effects, 165
  anxiety effects, 83
  culture, 101, 102
  defined, 350
  exercise benefits, 210
  men versus women, 97
  visceral hypersensitivity, 43
pale skin, 119
PALS (Patient Advice and Liaison Service),
    331
pancreas, 28, 30, 350
panic, 218–219, 226, 263
panty liner, 265–266
papaya, 202
paraffin, 160
parasite, 33
passive coping, 288
pathogenic bacteria, 48
Patient Advice and Liaison Service (PALS),
    331
pectin, 152
pelvic examination, 133
pelvic pain, 99
peppermint oil
  aromatherapy, 243
  constipation, 60
  muscle spasms, 163, 164
  overview of, 201
pepsin, 202
peptidase, 202
peristalsis, 350
peritoneum, 350
pharmacy, 233
pharynx, 26
phenolphthalein, 160
phosphate salt, 159
physical examination, 118–120, 130–131
physical stressor, 84

PI-IBS (post-infectious IBS), 67–68
Pilates exercise, 334
piles. *See* haemorrhoid
PIT (Psychodynamic Interpersonal Therapy), 228
placebo, 56, 233–234
plastic pants, 267
pneumonia, 50
Podophyllum (medication), 236
polyp, 131, 134, 350
polyunsaturated fat, 187, 188, 189
portion size, 184
positive thinking, 82, 224
possible cause, 65
post-infectious IBS (PI-IBS), 67–68
posture, yoga, 213–216
prebiotic food, 33
pregnancy, 199–200, 232
preservative, 49
Prince's Foundation for Integrated Health, 250
probiotic bacteria
  versus bad bacteria, 33, 34
  detoxing tips, 193
  diet guidelines, 323
  infection, 68
  overview of, 153–154
  supplements, 202–203
processed food, 45, 49, 188, 317
proctalgia fugax, 16, 63, 346
proctoscopy, 350
productivity, 276
progesterone, 98
prokinetic agent, 159
promotion, 276–277
propantheline bromide, 163
protein
  digestion rate, 28
  food substitutes, 195, 196
  good versus bad bacteria, 33
  menu plan, 196
  overview of, 187
protozoa, 68, 142
prune, 158
psychoanalysis, 227
Psychodynamic Interpersonal Therapy (PIT), 228
psychological disorder, 19
psychological stressor, 84
psychological therapy. *See also specific types*
  bloating-reduction tips, 56
  children's stress, 293

faecal incontinence, 62
incomplete evacuation, 63
overview of, 223
symptom management, 181–182
therapist selection, 229–230
types, 223–229
psyllium, 151–152, 193
Pub Med (Web site), 332
putrescine, 33

• *Q* •

qi, 237
questions, for doctor, 116–118, 123–125

• *R* •

radiation colitis, 351
radioallergeosorbent test (RAST), 81
raffinose, 79
raw food, 197
receptor, 51
rectum
  bleeding, 109–110
  defined, 351
  doctor's exam, 119–120, 131
  faecal incontinence, 62
  IBS symptoms, 16
red stool, 36
reflexology, 239
reflux, 50
registered dietitian, 121–122
relaxation
  general techniques, 239–241
  herbal remedies, 200
  massage, 244–245
  response, 240
  symptom management, 179–181
  therapy, 225
remedy. *See* treatment
research
  antidepressant studies, 166
  causes of IBS, 11–12
  Internet resources, 303–305, 332
  serotonin studies, 306–310
retching, 51
Richard Ebbs Web Site, 335
roasting food, 198